new ...0. 4/2014 Jm

Prentice Hall Health

Q&A review

of Dental Hygiene

Prentice Hall Health

Q&A review

of Dental Hygiene

Fifth Edition

Caren M. Barnes, RDH, MS
Coordinator of Clinical Research
Professor
Department of Surgical Specialties
College of Dentistry
University of Nebraska Medical Center
Lincoln, Nebraska

and

Michelle L. Sensat, RDH, MS
Assistant Professor of Dental Hygiene
Department of Dental Hygiene
College of Dentistry
University of Nebraska Medical Center
Lincoln, Nebraska

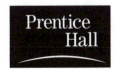

Prentice
Hall

Upper Saddle River, New Jersey 07458

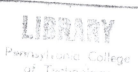
Library of Congress Cataloging-in-Publication Data

Prentice Hall Health's Q & A review of dental hygiene / [edited by] Caren M. Barnes,
Michelle L. Sensat.--5th ed.
      p. ; cm.
   Rev. ed. of: Appleton & Lange's review of dental hygiene. 4th ed. c1995.
   Includes bibliographical references and index.
   ISBN 0-8385-0342-X
      1. Dental hygiene--Examination, questions, etc. I. Title: Q&A review of dental
hygiene. II. Title: Review of dental hygiene. III. Barnes, Caren M. (Caren Marguerite)
IV. Sensat, Michelle L. V. Appleton & Lange's review of dental hygiene.
   [DNLM: 1. Oral Hygiene--Examination Questions. 2. Dental Hygienists--Examination
Questions. WU 18.5 P927 2001]
RK60.5 .A67 2001
617.6'01'076--dc21   2001026705

Notice: The author and publishers of this volume have taken care that the information and technical recommendations contained herein are based on research and expert consultation, and are accurate and compatible with the standards generally accepted at the time of publication. Nevertheless, as new information becomes available, changes in clinical and technical practices become necessary. The reader is advised to carefully consult manufacturers' instructions and information material for all supplies and equipment before use, and to consult with a health care professional as necessary. This advice is especially important when using new supplies or equipment for clinical purposes. The authors and publisher disclaim all responsibility for any liability, loss, or damage incurred as a consequence, directly or indirectly, of the use and application of any of the contents of this volume.

Publisher: Julie Levin Alexander
Acquisitions Editor: Mark Cohen
Managing Development Editor: Marilyn Meserve
Director of Production and Manufacturing: Bruce Johnson
Managing Production Editor: Patrick Walsh
Production Editor: Inkwell Publishing Services
Production Liaison: Danielle Newhouse
Manufacturing Buyer: Pat Brown
Design Director: Cheryl Asherman
Design Coordinator: Maria Guglielmo
Interior and Cover Designer: Janice Bielawa
Electronic Art Creation: Barb Cousins, Hutchison Studios
Marketing Manager: David Hough
Product Information Manager: Rachele Triano
Printer/Binder: Banta Book Group
Composition: Inkwell Publishing Services

Pearson Education LTD.
Pearson Education Australia PTY, Limited
Pearson Education Singapore, Pte. Ltd.
Pearson Education North Asia Ltd.
Pearson Education Canada, Ltd.
Pearson Education Educación de Mexico, S.A. de C.V.
Pearson Education – Japan
Pearson Education Malaysia, Pte. Ltd

10 9 8 7 6 5 4 3 2
ISBN 0-8385-0342-X

To my son, Clay,
with all my love
C.M.B.

In memory of my grandfather and grandmother,
G. Truman Hall and Lucille H. Hall
M.L.S.

Contents

Contributors

We wish to thank the following contributors for their expertise and contributions to the previous editions of this book:

Nancy A. Anderson Kesselring, RDH, MEd
Provision of Dental Hygiene Care

Caren M. Barnes, RDH, MS
Oral Histology and Embryology

J. Stansill Covington, III, BS, MS, DDS
Biomaterials

David F. Greer, DMD, MSD
Radiology

Bereneice M. Madison, BS, MEd, PhD
Microbiology

Judith A. Mills, BS, MS, PhD
Nutrition

Morris L. Robbins, Jr., DDS, FACD
Pharmacology

Brad K. Rodu, DDS
General Pathology, Oral Pathology

David A. Tipton, DDS, PhD
Oral Microbiology

Virginia S. Volker, MS, MPA
Anatomy and Physiology, Head and Neck Anatomy

Margaret B. Waring, RDH, MS, EdD
Research and Statistics

Nancy Johnson Williams, RDH, MS, EdD
Community Dental Health

Kimberly R. Winchester, RDH, BS, MA
Dental Morphology and Occlusion

While all chapters have been revised for the fifth edition, the core content was contributed by these individuals.

Preface

If you are planning to prepare for the National Board Dental Hygiene Examination or for a comprehensive written test in conjunction with a state or regional examination, *Prentice Hall Health Q&A Review of Dental Hygiene* is designed for you. This book is a comprehensive review source with over 1,280 board-type questions with answers and explanations referenced from the most current texts and related sources.

This book is organized to cover basic science and dental science subjects that are encountered on the National Board Dental Hygiene Examination. The following sixteen chapters are included this book: Anatomy and Physiology, Head and Neck Anatomy, Biomaterials, Provision of Dental Hygiene Care, Periodontics, Community Dental Health, Dental Morphology and Occlusion, Radiology, Oral Histology and Embryology, Microbiology, Oral Microbiology, Nutrition, General Pathology, Oral Pathology Pharmacology, Research and Statistics, as well as Case Studies. The content in this book is vast, as every page has vital information.

In each chapter, the question sections are followed by a section containing the answers, explanations, and references, which will give you the answer to the question, an explanation of why the answer is correct, background information on the subject matter, and the source of more in-depth information on the topic. You can use the specific references provided with each explanation to further supplement your exam preparation. The website to accompany this book will further enhance your knowledge on this subject. This book should prove to be a valuable resource to you in your preparation for the National Board Dental Hygiene Examination.

Caren M. Barnes, RDH, MS
Michelle L. Sensat, RDH, MS

Introduction

SUCCESS ACROSS THE BOARDS: THE PRENTICE HALL HEALTH REVIEW SERIES

The Prentice Hall Health Review Series was designed to provide you with a multimedia package to prepare for the National Board Dental Hygiene Examination. By using one or all of the elements in this review system, you can increase your probability of success. The Series presents information in multiple formats and includes vital information about certification, the certification test, and test-taking strategies. For those not studying for a certification exam but rather interested in honing your skills, this series provides a challenge you will enjoy.

Increase your likelihood of success by using these review books and follow the study and test-taking strategies presented later in this chapter.

COMPONENTS OF THE SERIES

The series is made up of a book and Companion Website that supports the book.

Q&A Review of Dental Hygiene by Caren Barnes and Michelle Sensat

About the Book

Content Review: Key topics that may be covered on the National Board Dental Hygiene Examination are included in this book. The book is organized to cover basic science and dental science subjects that are included on the exam.

Extensive case studies are also included.

In each chapter, the question sections are followed by a section containing the answers, explanations, and references, which will give you the answer to the question, an explanation of why the answer is correct, background information on the subject matter, and the source of more in-depth information on the topic. You can use the specific references provided with each explanation to further supplement your exam preparation.

Companion Website for Dental Hygiene Review

Visit the Companion Website at www.prenhall.com/review for additional practice, information about the exam, and links to related resources. Because the site was designed as a supplement to both books in the series, you will want to bookmark it and return frequently for the most current information on your path to success.

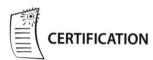

CERTIFICATION

The purpose of the National Board Dental Hygiene Examination is to assist state boards in assessing the cognitive skills essential for the competent practice of dental hygiene. The National Board Dental Hygiene Examination fulfills a written requirement of testing for the licensing process. Currently all 50 states, the District of Columbia, Puerto Rico, and the Virgin Islands recognize National Board results. Some states place limits on acceptance of National Board scores, requiring, for example, that the score be earned in the last 5 or 10 years. The Joint Commission on National Dental Examinations is the agency responsible for the construction and administration of the National Board Dental Hygiene Examination. You may write to them to request a current copy of the *Candidate's Guide.* Applications for the examination and further information on the National Board Dental Hygiene Examination may be obtained by writing:

> Joint Commission on National Dental
> Examinations
> 211 East Chicago Avenue, Suite 1846
> Chicago, Illinois 60611-2678

Qualifications for the Dental Hygienist

To participate in the National Board Dental Hygiene Examination, a candidate must have graduated from a program accredited by the Commission on Dental Accreditation or be within four months of issuance of a degree or certificate from an accredited dental hygiene program. Applications for the exam may be obtained from the Joint Commission, and are due approximately one month before the date of examination. An examination fee is required. A candidate whose application is accepted will receive an admission card approximately two weeks before the testing date. A candidate information booklet will be included with the examination, as well as instructions for completing the application

ABOUT THE EXAM

Each National Board Dental Hygiene Examination is a comprehensive examination consisting of approximately 400 multiple-choice items. Each multiple-choice item consists of a stem, which poses a problem. The candidate then selects the answer from a list of possible answers. Only one answer can ever be correct. The test also contains 14 case studies with corresponding questions, which constitute one-half of the total examination. The National Board Dental Hygiene Examination is a function-oriented examination and includes only functions that a dental hygienist is expected to be able to perform in a majority of states. The examination covers the following major areas:

1. The scientific basis for the practice of dental hygiene (anatomy and physiology, biochemistry and nutrition, microbiology and immunology, pathology and pharmacology).

2. The provision of clinical dental hygiene services (patient assessment, radiographic technique and interpretation, planning and managing dental hygiene care, periodontal procedures, use of preventive agents, and providing supportive treatment).

3. Community health activities (including health promotion and disease prevention within groups, participating in community programs, and analyzing scientific information and application of research findings).

The examination is scored as a single unit, but is divided into two sections: a morning session from 8:30 am to 12:00 PM and an afternoon session from 1:00 PM to 5:00 PM. All candidates are required to attend both sessions. In addition, instructions for the examination are given at 8:15 AM. Candidates should report to the examination site at 8:00 AM.

The candidate's score is determined by (1) the number of correct answers selected by the candidate and (2) by the conversion scale (norm-based) for the examination. There is no penalty for scoring incorrect answers; therefore the candidate should answer each question, even if it is with a guess. The minimum passing score is 75. The examination may be repeated if failed, following guidelines established by the Joint Commission on National Dental Examinations.

Information about examinations may change, so be sure to obtain current information by contacting the Joint Commission on National Dental Examinations.

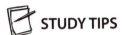 STUDY TIPS

Review Materials

Choose review materials that contain the information you need to study. Save time by making sure that you aren't studying anything you don't need to. For preparation before the exam, the best study resource would be this book. Use the alternate references in this book to easily find related textbooks if additional study is required.

Set a Study Schedule

Use your time-management skills to set a schedule that will help you feel as prepared as you can be. Consider all the relevant factors: the materials you need to study; how many months, weeks, or days until the test date; and how much time you can study each day. If you establish your schedule ahead of time and write it in your date book, you will be much more likely to follow it.

Take Practice Tests

Practice as much as possible, using the questions in this book and on the Companion Website. These questions were designed to follow the format of questions that appear on the exam you will take, so the more you practice with these questions, the better prepared you will be on test day.

The printed practice test in the book will give you a chance to experience the exam before you actually have to take it and will also let you know how you're doing and where you need to do better. For best results, we recommend you take a practice test two to three weeks before you are scheduled to take the actual exam. Spend the next weeks targeting those areas in which you performed poorly by reviewing questions in those areas.

Practice under test-like conditions—in a quiet room, with no books or notes to help you, and with a clock telling you when to quit. Try to come as close as you can to duplicating the actual test situation.

TAKING THE EXAMINATION

Prepare Physically

When taking the exam, you need to work efficiently under time pressure. If your body is tired or under stress, you might not think as clearly or perform as well as you usually do. If you can, avoid staying up all night. Get some sleep so that you can wake up rested and alert.

Eating right is also important. The best advice is to eat a light, well-balanced meal before a test. When time is short, grab a quick-energy snack such as a banana, orange juice, or a granola bar.

The Examination Site

The examination site must be located prior to the required examination time. One suggestion is to find the site and parking facilities the day before the test. Parking fee information should be obtained so that sufficient money can be taken along on the examination day.

Allow plenty of time for travel to the site in case of unexpected mishaps such as traffic snarls. During travel, think positive thoughts (e.g., "My preparation for the exam was thorough, so I'll be able to answer the questions easily"). Maintain a confident attitude to prevent unnecessary stress.

Materials

Be sure to take all required identification materials, registration forms, and any other items required by the testing organization or center. Read information and instructions supplied by the testing organizations thoroughly to be sure you have all necessary materials before the day of the exam.

Read Test Directions

Read the examination directions thoroughly! Because some board examinations have different test sections with different question formats, it is important to be aware of changes in directions. Read each set of directions completely before starting a new section of questions.

Machine-scored tests require that you use a special pencil to fill in a small box on a computerized answer sheet. Use the right pencil (usually a number 2) and mark your answers in the correct space. Neatness counts on these tests, because the computer can misread stray pencil marks or partially erased answers. Periodically, check the answer number against the question number to make sure they match. One question skipped can cause every answer following it to be marked incorrect.

Selecting the Right Answer

Keep in mind that only one answer is correct. First read the stem of the question with *each* possible choice provided and eliminate choices that are obviously incorrect. Be cautious about choosing the first answer that *might* be correct; all possibilities should be considered before the final choice is made; the best answer should be selected.

If a question is complicated, try to break it down into small sections that are easy to understand. Pay special attention to qualifiers such as *only, except,* etc. For example, negative words in a question can confuse your understanding of what the question asks ("Which of the following is *not* ...").

Intelligent Guessing

If you don't know the answer, eliminate those answers that you know or suspect are wrong. Your goal is to narrow down your choices. Here are some questions to ask yourself:

- Is the choice accurate in its own terms? If there's an error in the choice—for example, a term that is incorrectly defined—the answer is wrong.

- Is the choice relevant? An answer may be accurate, but it may not relate to the essence of the question.

- Are there any qualifiers, such as *always, never, all, none, or every?* Qualifiers make it easy to find an exception that makes a choice incorrect.

Mark answers you aren't sure of and go back to them at the end of the test.

Ask yourself whether you would make the same guesses again. Chances are that you will leave your answers alone, but you may notice something that will make you change your mind—a qualifier that affects meaning or a remembered fact that will enable you to answer the question without guessing.

Watch the Clock

Keep track of how much time is left and how you are progressing. Wear a watch or bring a small clock with you to the test room. A wall clock may be broken, or there may be no clock at all.

Some students are so concerned about time, that they rush through the exam and have time left over. In such situations, it's easy to leave early. The best approach, however, is to take your time. Stay until the end so that you can check your answers.

KEYS TO SUCCESS ACROSS THE BOARDS

Study, Review, and Practice

- Keep a positive, confident attitude.
- Follow all directions on the examination.
- Do your best.

Good luck!

You are encouraged to visit http://www.prenhall. com/success for additional tips on studying, test-taking, and other keys to success. At this stage of your education and career you will find these tips helpful.

Some of the study and test-taking tips were adapted from Keys to Effective Learning, *Second Edition, by Carol Carter, Joyce Bishop, and Sarah Lyman Kravits.*

1 Anatomy and Physiology

DIRECTIONS Each of the questions below is followed by several suggested answers. Select the best answer in each case.

---

1. The physiological concept that refers to the maintenance of a constant internal environment is

   A. hemostasis

   B. dynamic equilibrium

   C. homeostasis

   D. interdependence

   E. induction

2. The organelles that contain enzymes capable of digesting and destroying cellular debris, shown in Figure 1-1, are called

   A. endoplasmic reticulum

   B. Golgi apparatus

   C. mitochondria

   D. lysosomes

   E. ribosomes

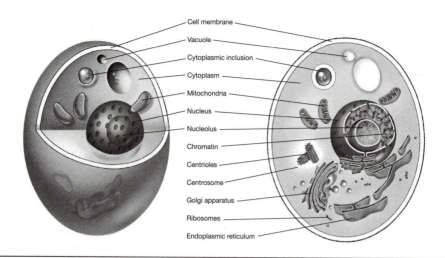

FIGURE 1-1. Two views of a cell, based on what can be seen through the electron microscope. (*From Jacob SW, Francone CA:* Structure and Function in Man, *5th ed. Philadelphia: Saunders, 1982.*)

3. Transport of water across a cell membrane, as illustrated in Figure 1-2, takes place by
   A. osmosis
   B. facilitated diffusion
   C. active transport
   D. diffusion

4. The direction and rate of diffusion of an ion are influenced by the
   A. concentration gradient
   B. hydrostatic pressure gradient
   C. electrical gradient
   D. all of the above

5. Active transport differs from facilitated diffusion in that active transport
   A. moves a substance against a concentration gradient
   B. requires a carrier
   C. requires energy from magnesius adenosine triphosphate (Mg ATP)
   D. is exemplified by the movement of sodium and potassium across cell membranes
   E. all of the above

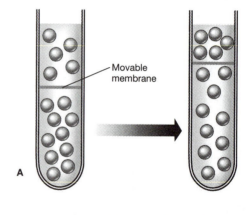

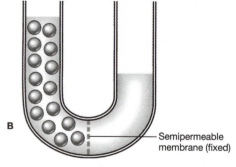

FIGURE 1-2. Diagrammatic representation of osmosis. (A) Osmotic effect on moveable membrane permeable only to water. (B) Osmotic effect of fixed semipermeable membrane. (*From Jacob SW, Francone CA:* Structure and Function in Man, *5th ed. Philadelphia: Saunders, 1982.*)

6. A patient has accidentally been given an intravenous solution that is extremely hypertonic. Which of the following will occur?
   A. Fluid moves from cells to plasma.
   B. The cells shrink.
   C. Crenation is the term to describe the changes that occur.
   D. All of the above are true statements about the events that occur.

7. All of the following are derived from endoderm EXCEPT
   A. epithelial parts of the respiratory system
   B. epithelial parts of the gastrointestinal system
   C. epithelium in the mouth
   D. epithelium of the pharynx

8. Which of the following is derived from mesoderm?
   A. epidermis
   B. nervous system
   C. adrenal medulla
   D. posterior lobe of the pituitary gland
   E. connective tissue

9. The muscles of mastication are derived from which branchial arch?
   A. first
   B. second
   C. third
   D. fourth
   E. fifth

10. The developmental period in which teeth and the palate are MOST susceptible to teratogenic agents is the
    A. third through the fifth week
    B. fourth through the seventh week
    C. fourth through the eighth week
    D. seventh through the eighth week
    E. eighth through the tenth week

11. Gingiva and buccal mucosa, illustrated in Figure 1-3, are
    A. simple squamous epithelium
    B. stratified squamous epithelium
    C. cuboidal epithelium
    D. stratified columnar epithelium
    E. none of the above

12. What type of connective tissue is present in scar tissue?
    A. loose
    B. dense fibrous
    C. lymphatic
    D. reticuloendothelial
    E. adipose

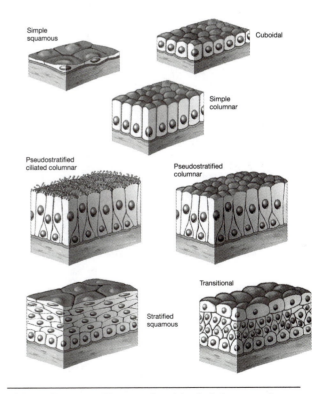

FIGURE 1-3. Types of epithelial tissue, classified according to shape and arrangement of cell layers. (*From Jacob SW, Francone CA: Structure and Function in Man, 5th ed. Philadelphia: Saunders, 1982.*)

13. What kind of cell types line the vascular channels of the body?
    A. stratified squamous epithelium
    B. endothelium
    C. mesothelium
    D. transitional epithelium
    E. pseudostratified columnar epithelium

14. Pleura is a type of
    A. serous membrane
    B. mucous membrane
    C. visceral membrane
    D. parietal membrane
    E. synovial membrane

15. In long bones, the process whereby cartilage cells are replaced by bone cells, organic matrix is laid down, and calcium and phosphate are deposited is known as
    A. intramembranous ossification
    B. endochondral ossification
    C. osteoporosis
    D. erythropoiesis
    E. diaphyseal formation

16. All of the following terms are associated with haversian systems in bone (Fig. 1-4) EXCEPT
    A. canaliculi
    B. lamellae
    C. lacunae
    D. osteocytes
    E. periosteum

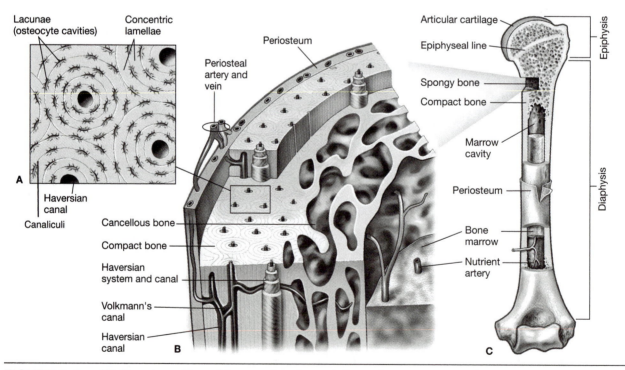

FIGURE 1-4. (A) Cross section of bone, showing relation of osteocytes to haversian system. (B) This section has been magnified out of proportion to show haversian system and lamellae. (Note communication between periosteal vessels and marrow vessels by way of Volkmann's canals.) (C) Diagram of the structure of a long bone (after Lockhart). (*From Jacob SW, Francone CA:* Structure and Function in Man, *5th ed. Philadelphia: Saunders, 1982.*)

17. What kind of joint, as shown in Figure 1-5, is described by the following: joint cavity present; bone ends covered by cartilage; may be separated by a disk; freely movable?
    A. synarthrotic
    B. diarthrotic
    C. cartilagenous
    D. symphysis
    E. synchondroses

18. Which of the following is (are) NOT associated with a skeletal muscle?
    A. sarcolemma
    B. myofibrils
    C. intercalated disc
    D. mitochondria
    E. actin and myosin

19. Actin and myosin are proteins (Fig. 1-6) contained within a
    A. myofibril
    B. myofilament
    C. fiber
    D. sarcoplasmic reticulum

20. A single motor neuron and the muscle cells supplied by its axon branches is termed
    A. an efferent neuron
    B. a motor unit
    C. a motor end plate
    D. a sarcoplasmic reticulum
    E. an annulospiral ending

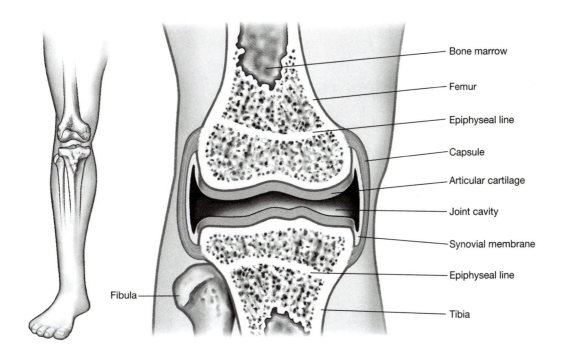

FIGURE 1-5. Frontal section through the right knee joint. (*From Jacob SW, Francone CA:* Structure and Function in Man, *5th ed. Philadelphia: Saunders, 1982.*)

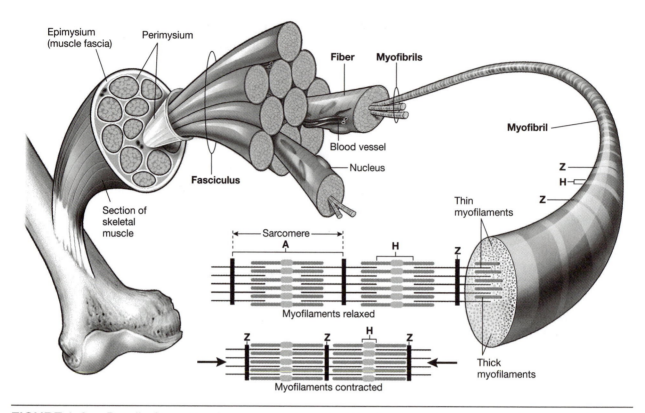

FIGURE 1-6. Detail of muscle showing structure and mechanics of muscular contraction. (*From Jacob SW, Francone CA:* Structure and Function in Man, *5th ed. Philadelphia: Saunders, 1982.*)

21. Which of the following glial cells, shown in Figure 1-7, are responsible for myelin formation in the central nervous system?
    A. ependymal cells
    B. oligodendrocytes
    C. microglia
    D. Schwann cells

22. Depolarization (Fig. 1-8) occurs with
    A. a transfer of sodium ions to the inside of a neuron
    B. a transfer of potassium ions to the outside of a neuron
    C. a reversal of charge across the nerve cell membrane making the outside of the fiber positive with respect to the inside

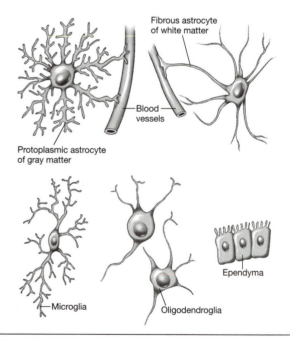

FIGURE 1-7. Neuroglial cells of the central nervous system. (*From Jacob SW, Francone CA:* Structure and Function in Man, *5th ed. Philadelphia: Saunders, 1982.*)

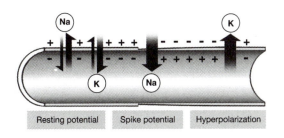

FIGURE 1-8. Conduction of nerve impulse (*From Jacob SW, Francone CA:* Structure and Function in Man, *5th ed. Philadelphia: Saunders, 1982.*)

23. Conduction occurs when a stimulus reduces the membrane potential to a critical level. This level is called
    A. summation
    B. threshold
    C. facilitation
    D. action potential
    E. refractory period

24. Which tract (Fig. 1-9) exerts a facilitative influence on motor neurons in the anterior horn?
    A. lateral corticospinal tract
    B. ventral corticospinal tract

C. lateral reticulospinal tract
D. medial reticulospinal tract
E. ectospinal tract

25. If the ventral root of a spinal nerve were sectioned (Fig. 1-10), what would be the result in the regions supplied by that nerve?
    A. loss of sensation
    B. loss of motor control
    C. loss of sensation and movement
    D. partial loss of sensation and movement
    E. loss of sensation, movement, and control of the degree of constriction of blood vessels

26. Fibers of the corticospinal tract (see Fig. 1-10)
    A. are located in grey columns of the cord
    B. come from neuron cell bodies located in the spinal cord
    C. synapse with neurons in the cerebellar cortex
    D. are descending fibers from the cells in the primary motor cortex of the frontal lobe

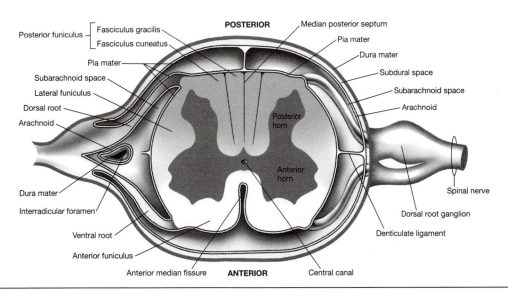

FIGURE 1-9. Cross section of spinal cord illustrating meningeal coverings. (*From Jacob SW, Francone CA:* Structure and Function in Man, *5th ed. Philadelphia: Saunders, 1982.*)

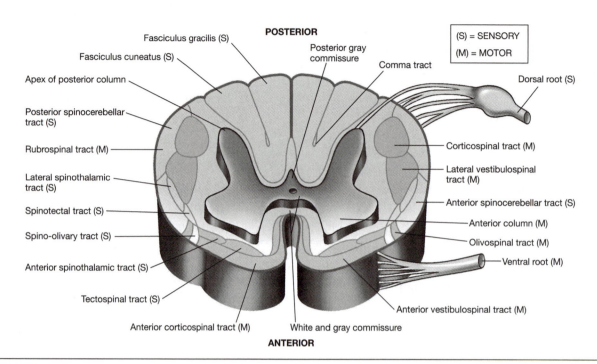

POSTERIOR

Fasciculus gracilis (S)

Fasciculus cuneatus (S)

Apex of posterior column

Posterior spinocerebellar tract (S)

Rubrospinal tract (M)

Lateral spinothalamic tract (S)

Spinotectal tract (S)

Spino-olivary tract (S)

Anterior spinothalamic tract (S)

Tectospinal tract (S)

Anterior corticospinal tract (M)

Posterior gray commissure

Comma tract

(S) = SENSORY

(M) = MOTOR

Dorsal root (S)

Corticospinal tract (M)

Lateral vestibulospinal tract (M)

Anterior spinocerebellar tract (S)

Anterior column (M)

Olivospinal tract (M)

Ventral root (M)

Anterior vestibulospinal tract (M)

White and gray commissure

ANTERIOR

FIGURE 1-10.   Major ascending and descending tracts of the spinal cord. (*From Jacob SW, Francone CA: Structure and Function in Man, 5th ed. Philadelphia: Saunders, 1982.*)

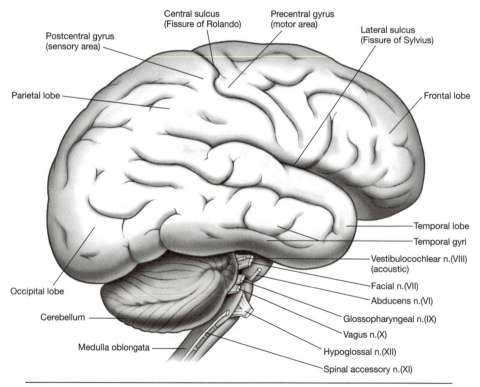

Central sulcus (Fissure of Rolando)

Precentral gyrus (motor area)

Postcentral gyrus (sensory area)

Lateral sulcus (Fissure of Sylvius)

Parietal lobe

Frontal lobe

Temporal lobe

Temporal gyri

Vestibulocochlear n.(VIII) (acoustic)

Facial n.(VII)

Abducens n.(VI)

Glossopharyngeal n.(IX)

Vagus n.(X)

Hypoglossal n.(XII)

Spinal accessory n.(XI)

Occipital lobe

Cerebellum

Medulla oblongata

FIGURE 1-11.   Right side of the brain showing cerebrum, cerebellum, and spinal cord. Several cranial nerves are seen. (*From Jacob SW, Francone CA: Structure and Function in Man, 5th ed. Philadelphia: Saunders, 1982.*)

27. The primary motor area of the brain is the (Fig. 1-11)
   A. precentral gyrus
   B. postcentral gyrus
   C. temporal lobe
   D. occipital lobe
   E. hypothalamus

28. Which of the following functions is (are) conducted in the dorsal columns of the spinal cord (Fig. 1-9), that is, in the fasciculus graciles and cuneatus?
   A. high degree of location
   B. vibratory sense
   C. fine gradations of pressure
   D. kinesthesia
   E. all of the above

29. Damage to the precentral gyrus of the cerebral cortex (Fig. 1-11) can result in
   A. spastic paralysis
   B. sensory loss
   C. intention tremor
   D. tremor at rest
   E. loss of simple reflexes

30. Almost all sensory impulses pass through what structure (Fig. 1-12) on their way to the cerebral cortex?
   A. basal ganglia
   B. corpus striatum
   C. hypothalamus
   D. corpus callosum
   E. thalamus

31. Inability to coordinate muscular activity (Fig. 1-13) can be due to a lesion in the
   A. cerebellum
   B. somesthetic cortex
   C. Broca's area
   D. occipital lobe

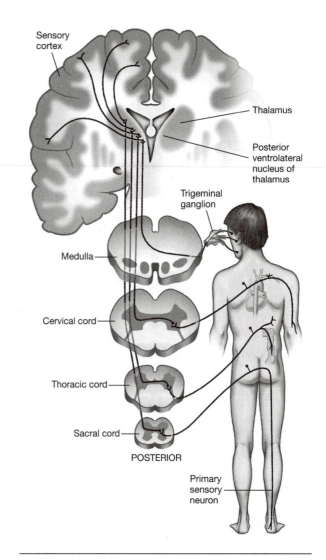

FIGURE 1-12. Lateral spinothalamic tract (pathway for pain and temperature). (*From Jacob SW, Francone CA:* Structure and Function in Man, *5th ed. Philadelphia: Saunders, 1982.*)

32. Which of the following describe(s) the functions of the hypothalamus?
   A. temperature control centers
   B. regulation of visceral activity
   C. synthesis of hormonal releasing factors
   D. influencing basic drives like sex, thirst, hunger
   E. all of the above

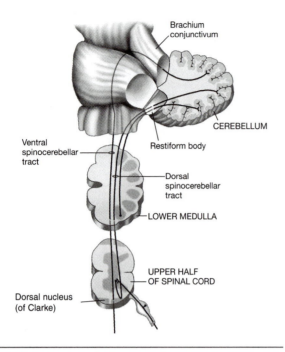

FIGURE 1-13. Proprioceptive cerebellar pathway. (*From Jacob SW, Francone CA: Structure and Function in Man, 5th ed. Philadelphia: Saunders, 1982.*)

33. Important centers for control of respiration and cardiovascular function are located in the
    A. pons
    B. medulla
    C. midbrain
    D. thalamus

34. Which of the following is (are) NOT necessary for any of the responses referred to as reflexes?
    A. autonomic nerves
    B. cerebral cortex
    C. effectors
    D. receptors
    E. synapses

35. A type of receptor that is sensitive to pain is
    A. pacinian corpuscle

B. Meissner's corpuscle
C. free nerve ending
D. end bulb of Krause
E. Ruffin ending

36. Referred pain is
    A. initiated in skin and referred to viscera or muscle
    B. initiated in viscera and referred to the contralateral dermatome
    C. due to converging of pain fibers with other sensory fibers in nuclei of the somesthetic cortex
    D. due to converging of pain fibers with other sensory fibers in the cord and thalamus

37. The autonomic nervous system exerts its influence on
    A. smooth muscle
    B. glandular secretion
    C. cardiac muscle
    D. all of the above

38. The neurotransmitter substance released at the postganglionic terminal of the parasympathetic division of the autonomic nervous system is
    A. norepinephrine
    B. epinephrine
    C. cholinesterase
    D. acetylcholine
    E. gamma-aminobutyric acid

39. Norepinephrine and epinephrine are released from
    A. preganglionic and postganglionic fibers of the sympathetic nervous system
    B. neuromyal junction
    C. postganglionic fibers of the sympathetic nervous system and the adrenal medulla
    D. all of the above

40. All of the following are autonomic effects on the body EXCEPT regulation of
    A. heart rate
    B. digestive secretion
    C. skeletal muscle tone
    D. glandular secretion
    E. blood pressure

41. Extreme excitement in a patient may have which effect(s) on organ systems?
    A. increased blood pressure
    B. decreased heart rate
    C. relaxation of smooth muscles in bronchi
    D. both A and C
    E. both B and C

42. An increase in parasympathetic activity
    A. increases salivation
    B. increases gastrointestinal activity
    C. decreases heart rate
    D. all of the above

43. Hormones
    A. catalyze intracellular biochemical reactions
    B. enter into chemical reactions without being degraded or depleted
    C. are chemical substances that 1) are produced by endocrine glands, 2) travel through the circulatory system, and 3) exert their influence on specific structures
    D. all of the above

44. A tropic hormone
    A. stimulates growth and secretion of a specific glandular tissue
    B. acts by positive feedback control
    C. is produced by the gonads
    D. two of the above

45. Calcium homeostasis is maintained by
    A. mineralocorticoids and adrenocorticotropic hormone (ACTH)
    B. aldosterone and parathyroid hormone
    C. parathyroid hormone and calcitonin
    D. calcitonin and glucagon

46. Calcitonin
    A. potentiates the effect of parathyroid hormone
    B. is secreted by the thyroid gland
    C. is released in response to excess serum calcium
    D. all of the above
    E. B and C only

47. Which hormone promotes glucose transport from blood into cells?
    A. insulin
    B. glucagon
    C. epinephrine
    D. pancreatin

48. Which hormone is LESS involved in a stress reaction?
    A. epinephrine
    B. norepinephrine
    C. cortisone
    D. thyroxin
    E. adrenocorticotropin

49. Cortisol
    A. increases the flux of amino acids in the body
    B. mobilizes stored fat
    C. promotes gluconeogenesis
    D. all of the above
    E. A and C only

50. Insulin has all of the following effects EXCEPT
    A. promotes glucose entry into cells, therefore having a hypoglycemic effect
    B. promotes transport of amino acids into cells, therefore increasing protein synthesis
    C. promotes transport of fatty acids into cells, therefore has a lipogenic effect
    D. promotes liver glycogenolysis, therefore has a hyperglycemic effect
    E. promotes potassium entry into cells, therefore has a hypokalemic effect

51. Antidiuretic hormone is released in direct response to
    A. extracellular potassium levels
    B. extracellular sodium levels
    C. hyperosmolarity of extracellular fluids
    D. hypo-osmolarity of extracellular fluids
    E. degree of hydration

52. Aldosterone
    A. increases reabsorption of water in the distal tubule of the kidney
    B. increases reabsorption of sodium and secretion of potassium
    C. increases reabsorption of sodium and hydrogen ions
    D. decreases reabsorption of sodium in the proximal tubule
    E. increases reabsorption of glucose in the proximal tubule

53. Ovulation
    A. is dependent on a high concentration of LH in the blood
    B. occurs exactly 12 days after the end of menstruation
    C. occurs in one of the uterine tubes
    D. is dependent on high concentrations of estrogen in the blood

54. Which of the following secrete(s) progesterone?
    A. anterior pituitary gland
    B. corpus luteum
    C. corpus albicans
    D. graafian follicles
    E. posterior pituitary gland

55. With inspiration (Fig. 1-14)
    A. volume of the lungs increases, pressure increases
    B. volume of the lungs decreases, pressure increases
    C. volume of the lungs increases, pressure decreases
    D. volume of the lungs decreases, pressure decreases

56. During inspiration (Fig. 1-14),
    A. intrapleural pressure decreases while intra-alveolar pressure increases
    B. both intrapleural and intra-alveolar pressure decrease
    C. intrapleural pressure increases while intra-alveolar pressure decreases
    D. both intrapleural and intra-alveolar pressure increase

57. Respiratory tidal volume is
    A. the amount of air exchanged in the lungs with a normal breath
    B. approximately 1 liter
    C. the maximum amount of air that can be inspired
    D. the volume of air left in the lungs after expiration
    E. the reserve lung volume

58. Which of the following has the highest PCO_2?
    A. atmospheric air
    B. expired air

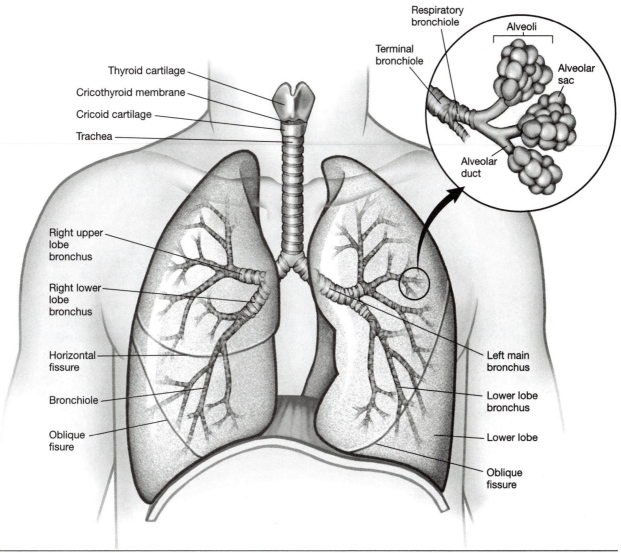

FIGURE 1-14. Distribution of bronchi within the lungs. Enlarged inset shows detail of an alveolus. (*From Jacob SW, Francone CA:* Structure and Function in Man, *5th ed. Philadelphia: Saunders, 1982.*)

C. venous blood

D. interstitial fluid

E. intracellular fluid

59. Oxygen is carried in the blood

    A. as oxyhemoglobin

    B. dissolved in plasma

    C. as carbaminohemoglobin

    D. both A and B

    E. both A and C

60. Carbon dioxide is carried in the blood in all of the following ways EXCEPT

    A. as carbaminohemoglobin

    B. dissolved in plasma

    C. as bicarbonate

    D. as carbonic acid

61. Alveolar ventilation is increased by all of the following EXCEPT
    A. decreased blood pressure
    B. decreased blood pH
    C. increased PCO_2 of arterial blood
    D. decreased PO_2 of arterial blood
    E. metabolic alkalosis

62. Which of the following (Fig. 1-15) is NOT a leukocyte?
    A. neutrophil
    B. thrombocyte
    C. eosinophil
    D. basophil
    E. monocyte

63. A patient with type AB blood can give a transfusion to a patient with type
    A. O
    B. A
    C. B
    D. AB

64. A normal differential blood count shows about 20 to 25 percent of which of the following?
    A. basophils
    B. erythrocytes
    C. lymphocytes
    D. monocytes
    E. neutrophils

65. A patient with hypoproteinemia (low plasma protein levels) may have a tendency to decreased blood volume. The protein fraction that contributes more to colloid osmotic pressure, tending to maintain blood volume by osmotic forces, is
    A. fibrinogen
    B. alpha and beta globulin
    C. gamma globulin
    D. albumin

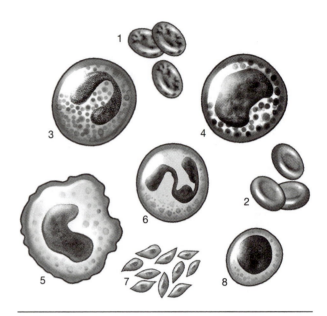

FIGURE 1-15. Blood cells: 1, reticulocyte; 2, erythrocyte; 3, eosinophil; 4, basophil; 5, monocyte; 6, neutrophil; 7, platelets; and 8, lymphocyte. (*From Jacob SW, Francone CA:* Structure and Function in Man, *5th ed. Philadelphia: Saunders, 1982.*)

66. All of the following terms are associated with the ventricles of the heart EXCEPT
    A. chordae tendineae
    B. papillary muscle
    C. sinoatrial node
    D. Purkinje system
    E. endocardium

67. The sinoatrial node (Fig. 1-16) is the normal pacemaker of the heart because
    A. this region has a lower difference between resting membrane potential and threshold than other regions of the heart
    B. this region has more rapid sodium leakage, initiating spontaneous depolarization before other areas

C. this region recovers from the previous refractory period more rapidly than other areas

D. all of the above

E. A and C only

68. Identify the correct sequence of the blood flow through the heart, to the lungs, its return to the heart, and out of the heart to systemic circulation (Fig. 1-16).

A. inferior vena cava, left atrium, bicuspid valves, left ventricle, pulmonary trunk to pulmonary circulation, return via pulmonary veins to right atrium, tricuspid valve, right ventricle, and out through the ascending aorta

B. inferior vena cava, left atrium, tricuspid valves, left ventricle, pulmonary trunk to pulmonary circulation, return via pulmonary veins to right atrium, bicuspid valves, right ventricle, and out through the ascending aorta

C. inferior vena cava, right atrium, triscupid valves, right ventricle, pulmonary trunk to pulmonary circulation, return via pulmonary veins to left atrium, bicuspid valves, left ventricle, and out through the ascending aorta

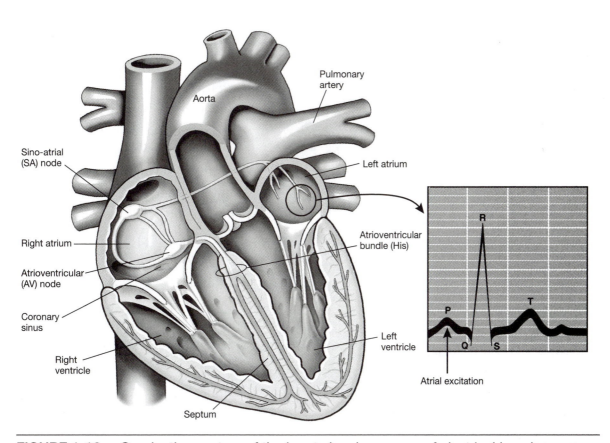

FIGURE 1-16. Conducting system of the heart showing source of electrical impulses produced on electrocardiogram. (*From Jacob SW, Francone CA:* Structure and Function in Man, *5th ed. Philadelphia: Saunders, 1982.*)

69. The pressoreceptor system
    A. responds to an increase in blood pressure at the area of the aortic arch and carotid bodies
    B. operates through the vasomotor center
    C. responds by decreasing the heart rate, strength of contraction, and peripheral resistance
    D. all of the above

70. Mean arterial blood pressure is regulated by
    A. neural mechanisms that control constriction of the arteries
    B. principles of capillary dynamics that regulate blood volume
    C. renal and hormonal mechanisms that regulate blood volume and arteriolar constriction
    D. all of the above
    E. two of the above

71. Diastolic blood pressure is maintained at levels above zero by
    A. peripheral resistance
    B. elasticity of arteries
    C. viscosity of blood
    D. all of the above

72. Which of the following valves (Fig. 1-16) prevent backflow of deoxygenated blood?
    A. pulmonary and aortic valves
    B. pulmonary and right atrioventricular valves
    C. right and left atrioventricular valves
    D. aortic and left atrioventricular valves

73. Cardiac output is the product of the
    A. heart rate and peripheral resistance
    B. heart rate and stroke volume
    C. heart rate and strength of contraction
    D. heart rate and vascular dilatation

74. Blood pressure depends on
    A. heart rate and stroke volume
    B. peripheral resistance
    C. blood volume
    D. blood viscosity
    E. all of the above

75. Oxygenated blood flows through which of the following structures?
    A. pulmonary valve
    B. right atrioventricular valve
    C. pulmonary artery
    D. coronary arteries

76. Digestion means
    A. splitting large chemical compounds in foods into simpler substances that can be absorbed
    B. absorption of small molecular weight end products into body fluids
    C. hydrolysis
    D. A and C only
    E. B and C only

77. All of the following are concerned with protein digestion EXCEPT
    A. pepsin
    B. trypsin
    C. chymotrypsin
    D. carboxypolypeptidase
    E. amylase

78. Rate of gastric emptying is affected by
    A. the quantity of liquid in chyme
    B. neural and hormonal reflexes from the small intestine
    C. the quantity of chyme present in the small intestine
    D. A and C only
    E. all of the above

79. Which of the following is NOT a function of the pancreas?
    A. secretion of digestive enzymes
    B. secretion of insulin
    C. secretion of bile
    D. secretion of glucagon

80. Which gastrointestinal hormone controls secretion of water and bicarbonate by acinar cells of the pancreas?
    A. gastrin
    B. secretin
    C. pancreozymin
    D. cholecystokinin
    E. chymotrypsin

81. An enzyme that hydrolyzes polysaccharides is
    A. lipase
    B. amylase

C. protease
D. trypsin
E. pepsin

82. Functions of the adult liver include all of the following EXCEPT
    A. bile formation
    B. reticuloendothelial activity
    C. glycogenesis, glycogenolysis, and gluconeogenesis
    D. erythropoiesis
    E. detoxication

83. The swallowing mechanism involves which of the following cranial nerves?
    A. trigeminal
    B. facial
    C. glossopharyngeal
    D. vagus and hypoglossal
    E. all of the above

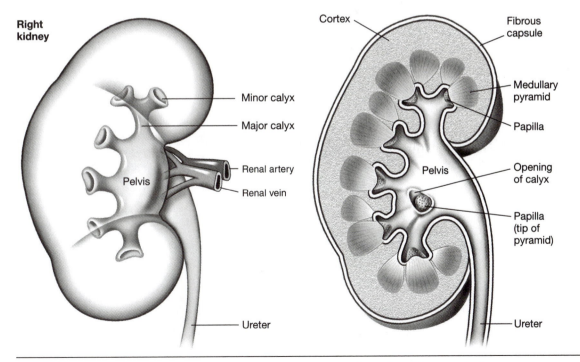

FIGURE 1-17. Entire and sagittal views showing relation of calyces to kidney as a whole. (*From Jacob SW, Francone CA:* Structure and Function in Man, *5th ed. Philadelphia: Saunders, 1982.*)

84. An accumulation of collecting ducts, as seen on gross examination of a kidney (Fig. 1-17), is called
    A. pelvis
    B. calyx
    C. cortex
    D. pyramids

85. Filtration in the kidney (Fig. 1-18) occurs at the
    A. glomerulus
    B. proximal convoluted tubule and loop of Henle
    C. distal convoluted tubule
    D. collecting tubule

86. Reabsorption of water in the distal convoluted tubules and collecting ducts (Fig. 1-19) is regulated by
    A. adrenocorticotropic hormone
    B. antidiuretic hormone
    C. aldosterone
    D. angiotensin

87. Amino acids and glucose are reabsorbed in the proximal tubule (Fig. 1-19) by
    A. diffusion and osmosis
    B. active transport
    C. osmotic forces and pressure gradients
    D. electrochemical gradients

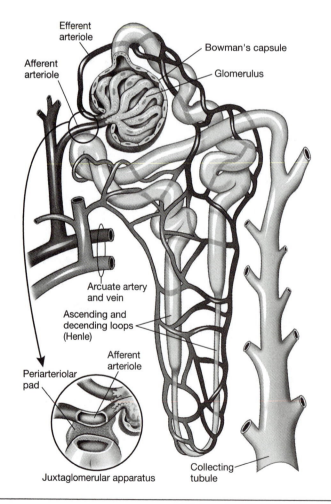

FIGURE 1-18. Detail of nephron showing vascular supply, juxtaglomerular apparatus, and tubule. (*From Jacob SW, Francone CA:* Structure and Function in Man, *5th ed. Philadelphia: Saunders, 1982.*)

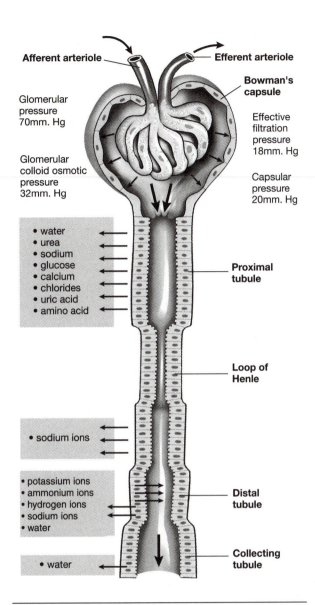

FIGURE 1-19. The normal filtration pressure is about 18 mm Hg. Glomerular hydrostatic pressure (70 mm Hg) minus glomerular colloid osmotic pressure (32 mm Hg) minus capsular pressure (20 mm Hg) equals filtration pressure, 18 mm Hg. The passage of substances in and out of the tubule varies in different portions of the tubule and collecting duct. (*From Jacob SW, Francone CA: Structure and Function in Man, 5th ed. Philadelphia: Saunders, 1982.*)

88. Sodium ions are reabsorbed, and potassium and hydrogen ions are secreted, under the control of
   A. antidiuretic hormone
   B. thyroxin
   C. epinephrine
   D. aldosterone
   E. cortisol

89. Functions of the kidney include all of the following EXCEPT
   A. regulation of hydrogen ion concentration
   B. regulation of body fluid volumes
   C. regulation of serum calcium levels
   D. regulation of serum sodium levels
   E. removal of urea, creatinine, and other metabolic end products

90. Parasympathetic innervation to the lacrimal glands and the secretory glands of the nose and palate is transmitted via the
   A. trigeminal nerve
   B. abducens nerve
   C. facial nerve
   D. glossopharyngeal nerve
   E. vagus nerve

91. The sympathetic innervation to the face and head structures is transmitted via nerves that have cells of origin in the
   A. submandibular ganglion
   B. superior cervical ganglion
   C. oxic ganglion

92. The area of the brain stem that contains cells of origin for the nerves that control motor activity for swallowing is
   A. cerebellum
   B. trigeminal nucleus of the pons
   C. the nucleus ambiguus of the medulla
   D. hypoglossal nucleus of the pons

93. The nerve responsible for constriction of the pupil of the eye is the
    A. optic nerve
    B. oculomotor nerve
    C. abducens nerve
    D. vagus nerve

94. When a person is experiencing much pain, the pupils of the eye will
    A. dilate because it is a parasympathetic response
    B. dilate because it is a sympathetic response
    C. constrict because this is the sympathetic response
    D. not change

95. The human immunodeficiency virus (HIV) can be accurately described by all of the following EXCEPT which?
    A. It damages T4 lymphocytes.
    B. It weakens the immune system in ways that allow opportunistic infections to kill the person that is infected.
    C. HIV is an unstable virus and can be killed by Lysol, Clorox, and proper sterilization methods.
    D. If a person tests HIV-negative, his or her blood and body fluids will contain the virus.
    E. Most scientists think that if a person tests positive for HIV-1 antibodies, the person will eventually develop AIDS.

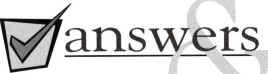

answers & rationales

1.

C. The physiological concept that refers to the maintenance of a constant internal environment is homeostasis. Among the homeostatic control mechanisms now understood are those maintaining normal concentrations of blood constituents, body temperature, volume and pH of the body fluids, blood pressure, and heart rate. While the concept describes a constant state, the constancy is one of dynamic equilibrium in that substances are continually being added to and taken from the internal environment. (1:29–32, 302; 3:5)

2.

D. The organelles that contain enzymes capable of digesting and destroying cellular debris are called lysosomes. Lysosomes are specifically membranous structures containing lytic enzymes capable of breaking down cellular components. Fortunately, they are able to discriminate cellular debris and bacteria from host.(1:20, 24, 302; 3:52–53)

3.

A. Transport of water across a cell membrane takes place by osmosis. In the process of osmosis, water moves from an area of high water concentration into an area of low water concentration. The force with which a solution draws water into it is called osmotic pressure. (1:27–29, 305; 3:56)

4.

D. The direction and rate of diffusion of an ion are influenced by the concentration gradient, hydrostatic gradients, and electrical gradients. Ions diffuse through a semipermeable membrane from an area of high concentration to an area of low concentration. Ions diffuse faster down a pressure gradient and in a direction that tries to equalize electric charges. (1:27–29, 254, 301; 3:56)

5.

E. Active transport moves a substance against a concentration gradient; facilitated diffusion, down a concentration gradient. Active transport requires a carrier and energy. Diffusion and osmosis, on the other hand, are referred to as passive transport because the driving force is the concentration gradient. The continual movement of sodium and potassium across the cell membrane is an example of substances that move by active transport. (1:27–32, 254, 301; 3:56–57)

6.

D. The cells of a patient given an extremely hypertonic solution intravenously will experience crenation and fluid will move from cells to plasma. Water moves from cells by osmosis, into extracellular fluids. As this happens, cells shrink in a process called crenation. (1:27–29, 305; 3:56)

7.

C. Epithelium of the mouth is derived from ectoderm. Specifically, the mouth is lined with stratified squamous epithelium. Epithelial parts of the respiratory system, gastrointestinal system, and pharynx are derived from endoderm. (2:54–55; 3:82)

8.

E. Connective tissue is derived from mesoderm. Mesoderm is also termed mesothelium. The epidermis, nervous system, adrenal medulla, and posterior lobe of the pituitary gland are lined with ectoderm. (2:54–55; 3:82)

9.

A. The branchial arches are condensations of tissue in the neck of the embryo. The human embryo has five branchial arches. The muscles of mastication are derived from the first branchial arch. (2:57–60, 125-128)

10.

D. In general, tissue is more susceptible to developmental derangement at a time when that tissue or system is most rapidly developing. The developmental period in which teeth and the palate are most susceptible to teratogenic agents is during the seventh to eighth weeks in utero. Tetracycline staining is a good example of intrauterine staining of the teeth. (2:112, 268–272)

11.

B. The gingiva and buccal mucosa are composed of stratified squamous epithelium. Stratified squamous epithelium is composed of several layers of flat cells usually located in areas of the body where abrasion and loss of surface cells take place. Human skin is composed of keratinized stratified squamous epithelium. (1:82–83)

12.

B. Dense fibrous connective tissue is present in scar tissue. Dense fibrous connective tissue lends strength to the scar because of its compact arrangement of fibers. Dense fibrous connective tissue is composed of closely arranged tough collagenous and elastic fibers with fewer cells than loose connective tissue. (3:87–88)

13.

B. Endothelial cells line the vascular channels of the body. Endothelium is a type of simple squamous epithelium. It is arranged as a single layer to permit diffusion of substances from one side to the other. (3:82–83, 85)

14.

A. Pleura is a type of serous membrane. Mucous membranes line cavities that open to the exterior. Serous membranes line cavities that do not open to the exterior. (5:94–99)

15.

B. The process by which cartilage trabeculae are invaded by bone cells, organic matrix is laid down, and calcium and phosphate are deposited is known as endochondral ossification. Long bones of the body are formed by endochondral ossification. Flat bones are formed by intramembranous ossification. (1:44; 3:110–111; 5:18–21)

16.

E. Canaliculi, lamellae, lacunae, and osteocytes are associated with haversian systems. The periosteum is the connective tissue covering of bone. The outer layer of periosteum is relatively acellular, dense, and avascular. (1:44; 3:108–109; 5:20–21)

17.

B. Diarthrotic joints have a joint cavity; the bone ends are covered by cartilage. They may be separated by a disk and are freely moveable. A synarthrotic joint, on the other hand, allows little or no movement because fibrous tissue grows between the adjacent bone surfaces. (1:301; 3:150–151)

18.

C. Sarcolemma, myofibrils, mitochondria, actin, and myosin are all associated with skeletal muscle. Skeletal muscle is striated and voluntary. Intercalated discs, representing specialized cell junctions, are present in cardiac muscle only. (1:72; 3:90, 176–177)

19.

A. Actin and myosin are proteins contained within a myofibril. In the process of muscle contraction, actin and myosin interdigitate and shorten in length. Myosin molecules construct thick filaments. (3:168–171)

20.

C. A single motor neuron and the muscle cells supplied by its axon branches are termed a motor end plate. Neurons have two types of processes: axons and dendrites. The axon of the motor nerve divides into several branches, which distribute to different muscle fibers. (1:102–110, 120–123; 3:234–235; 5:38–39)

21.

B. Oligodendrocytes are responsible for myelin formation in the central nervous system. Myelin is a fatty substance that envelops nerve axons. It is segmented periodically by nodes of Ranvier. (2:239)

22.

A. Depolarization is the first stage of conduction. It occurs when the permeability of the cell membrane to sodium increases. In the resting state, the interior of the nerve fiber is negative to the exterior by approximately 70 to 90 millivolts. (1:104–106; 3:239–241)

23.

B. Conduction occurs when a stimulus reduces the membrane potential to a critical level. This level is called threshold. When the transfer of sodium reduces the cell membrane potential to threshold, impulse conduction is initiated. (1:104–106; 3:239–241)

24.

C. The lateral reticulospinal tract exerts a facilitative influence on motor neurons in the anterior horn. Whereas the lateral reticulospinal tract facilitates lower motor neurons, the medial reticulospinal tract exerts an inhibitory influence. Reticulospinal tracts are major pathways to the spinal cord. (1:111; 3:310)

25.

B. Dorsal roots convey predominantly sensory impulses. Ventral roots convey motor impulses. If ventral roots are sectioned, the nerve supply to the skeletal muscle is then disrupted. (1:107, 110, 116, 124–125; 3:267, 270; 5:42–43)

26.

D. Corticospinal tract fibers are descending or motor fibers. The corticospinal tract is the main route for conduction of nerve impulses to skeletal muscles for fine motor control. The corticospinal tracts are known as the pyramidal tracts. The fibers are myelinated and therefore located in the white columns of the spinal cord. (1:101–119; 3:268)

27.

A. Each bulge in the brain is called a gyrus. The motor area of the brain is the precentral gyrus, located in the posterior part of the temporal lobe. The postcentral gyrus is the sensory area of the brain. (1:103–116; 3:249–252; 5:888)

28.

E. The dorsal columns are the fasiculi granicles and cuneatus. The dorsal columns are located in the posterior region of the spinal cord. The dorsal columns contain a high degree of location, vibratory sense, fine gradations of pressure, and kinesthesis. (1:103–116; 3:267–270)

29.

A. Damage to the precentral gyrus of the cerebral cortex can result in spastic paralysis. The precentral gyrus contains cell bodies of motor neurons which innervate skeletal muscle. Damage to this area results in paralysis of a spastic nature because excitatory spinal cord tracts are still intact. (1:135–136; 3:249–252)

30.

E. Almost all sensory impulses pass through the thalamus on their way to the cerebral cortex. The thalamus is a nucleus where secondary ascending sensory neurons synapse with tertiary neurons, which continue conduction to the cerebral cortex. The crude identification of stimuli as pain, temperature, or touch is a result of thalamic integrations. (1:113–115; 3:252, 256–259)

31.

A. Inability to coordinate muscular activity can be due to a lesion in the cerebellum. The cerebellum is located in the posterior cranial fossa, posterior and inferior to the cerebrum. The cerebellum is connected by afferent and efferent pathways with all other parts of the central nervous system. (1:111–113, 300; 3:250–273)

32.

E. The hypothalamus regulates visceral activity and controls temperature centers and synthesis of hormonal releasing factors. It has an important role in maintaining sexual behavior and function. The hypothalamus is located centrally in the brain, lateral and inferior to the third ventricle. (1:111–113, 303; 3:252)

33.

B. The medulla has centers for respiration and cardiovascular activity. The medulla is located posterior and inferior to the pons and is continuous with the spinal cord. All of the afferent and efferent tracts are represented in the medulla. (1:111, 193–194, 236, 304; 3:250–260, 284)

34.

B. The cerebral cortex is not responsible for reflex responses. The cerebral cortex is associated with reception of sensory input, initiation of motor output, and integration of sensory and motor function. More than three-fourths of the cerebral cortex is occupied by association areas. (1:113–115; 3:256)

35.

C. Free nerve endings are receptors sensitive to pain. Free nerve endings are branching fibers. They resemble the appearance of the limbs of a tree in many ways. (1:102–107; 3:233–300)

36.

D. Referred pain is due to converging of pain fibers with other sensory fibers in the cord and thalamus. The brain misinterprets the site of the original stimulus and refers it to another area. Afferent nerves from the viscera terminate in the spinal cord segment that supplies the particular viscus involved. (1:107–113, 124; 3:306)

37.

D. Smooth muscle, glandular secretions, and cardiac muscle are all controlled by the autonomic nervous system (ANS). By acting directly on cardiac muscle, smooth muscle, and glands, the ANS regulates visceral activity. It also helps to control arterial pressure, gastrointestinal mobility, secretion, urinary output, sweating, and body temperature. (1:114–131; 3:293–299; 5:45, 52)

38.

D. Acetylcholine is released from both preganglionic and postganglionic fibers of the parasympathetic division of the ANS. Cholinergic nerves release acetylcholine. Adrenergic nerves release norepinephrine. (1:114–131, 299, 304; 3:294; 5:45)

39.

C. Acetylcholine is released from preganglionic fibers of the sympathetic division. Epinephrine and norepinephrine are released from postganglionic fibers. Norepinephrine and epinephrine are released from the adrenal medulla as hormones. (1:114–131, 299; 3:294; 5:45)

40.

C. Control of heart rate, digestive secretions, glandular secretions, and blood pressure is by the ANS. Skeletal muscle tone is under voluntary control. Visceral activity is under autonomic control. (1:114–131; 3:301)

41.

D. Excitement, fear, and rage increase activity of the sympathetic division of the ANS. In turn, this leads to increased heart rate and stroke volume. This also results in increased blood pressure and relaxation of bronchial smooth muscle to facilitate breathing. (1:119–130, 153–154, 306; 3:243)

42.

D. An increase in parasympathetic activity increases salivation and gastrointestinal activity and decreases heart rate. In general, parasympathetic activity results in visceral function associated with rest and recovery. The cell bodies of preganglionic parasympathetic neurons are located in the second, third, and fourth sacral segments of the spinal cord. (1:119–130; 3:298)

43.

C. Hormones regulate, increase, or decrease activity of particular systems. However, they are utilized or degraded in the process. Enzymes catalyze intracellular biochemical reactions without being degraded or depleted. (1:120, 144–146, 210, 301–302; 3:535–543)

44.

A. A tropic hormone stimulates growth and secretion of a specific glandular tissue. Tropic hormones include adrenocorticotrophic hormone, thyrotrophic hormone, follicle stimulating hormone, and luteinizing hormone. These hormones are released from the anterior lobe of the pituitary gland. (1:44, 111–113, 146–149, 281–292, 302, 305; 3:535–543)

45.

C. Calcium homeostasis is maintained by parathyroid hormone and calcitonin. Parathyroid hormone transfers calcium from bone to blood when blood levels decrease. Calcitonin transfers calcium from blood to bone when blood levels increase. (1:45, 151, 157; 3:113)

46.

E. Calcitonin is secreted by the thyroid gland. It is released in response to excess serum calcium. The effect of calcitonin, or thyrocalcitonin as it is sometimes called, is opposite that of parathyroid hormone. (1:45, 151, 157; 3:556)

47.

A. Insulin, secreted by the beta cells of the pancreas, promotes uptake of glucose by cells. In the liver, insulin increases oxidation of glucose and its conversion to fatty acids. Insulin activity is inadequate in patients with diabetes mellitus. (1:23, 146, 154, 158, 248; 3:556)

48.

D. Thyroxin regulates basal metabolic rate. Thyroxin is a hormone secreted by the thyroid gland. It increases the rate of replacement of cartilage by bone at the growth plate. (1:150–151; 3:549)

49.

D. Cortisol increases the flux of amino acids in the body and mobilizes stored fat. It also promotes gluconeogenesis. Cortisol and other related corticosteriods are produced by the adrenal cortex. (1:146, 153, 157–158, 301; 3:549)

50.

D. Insulin promotes glucose entry into cells, increases protein synthesis, and has a lipogenic effect. It also has a hypokalemic effect. Glycogenolysis, or breaking down of liver and muscle glycogen into glucose, is a function of epinephrine. (1:23, 146, 154, 158, 248, 252; 3:566)

51.

C. Antidiuretic hormone is released in response to hyperosmolarity of extracellular fluids. Antidiuretic hormone, released by the posterior lobe of the pituitary gland, increases renal reabsorption and retention of water to dilute body fluids that are too concentrated. Antidiuretic hormone is also known as vasopressin. (1:146, 148, 156–157, 266–267, 269, 299; 3:547)

52.

B. Aldosterone increases reabsorption of sodium and secretion of potassium. The normal stimuli for increasing aldosterone secretion are hyponatremia, hyperkalemia, or acidosis. Aldosterone is the principal natural mineralocorticoid and is the most active substance known to promote sodium retention. (1:152–153, 157–158, 269–270, 299; 3:558)

53.

A. Ovulation is dependent on a high concentration of luteinizing hormone (LH) in the blood. LH is secreted by the anterior lobe of the pituitary gland. In the male, it controls testicular production of testosterone. (1:147, 291–292, 305; 3:549)

54.

B. The corpus luteum secretes progesterone. After ovulation, the graafian follicle changes its morphology and becomes the corpus luteum. It then functions to secrete progesterone during the last 2 weeks of the menstrual cycle. (1:147, 156, 289–293, 305; 3:612–613)

55.

C. With inspiration, the volume of the lungs increases and pressure decreases. As the size of the thorax and lungs increases, the pressure within the lungs decreases to a level below that of air, according to Boyle's Law. The pressure that is decreased is intrapulmonic pressure. (1:230–231, 236, 303; 3:457–458)

56.

B. Intrapleural pressure is the pressure between the lung surface and the inside of the thoracic cavity. Intra-alveolar pressure is the pressure within the air sacs. Because the lung pleura adheres to the thoracic wall as it expands, the alveoli are stretched to a greater volume. (1:29, 224–239, 268; 3:457–458)

57.

A. Respiratory tidal volume is the amount of air exchanged in the lungs with a normal breath. Tidal volume measured with a spirometer is the volume of air exhaled after a normal inspiration under quiet breathing conditions. The average tidal volume for the adult male is 500 mL. (1:231–234; 3:459–460)

58.

E. Intracellular fluids have the highest PCO_2. CO_2 originates as a by-product of intracellular metabolism. (1:29, 3: 426–442)

59.

D. Each gram of hemoglobin can transport 1.34 mL of oxygen. Normally, 100 mL of blood contains 15 g of hemoglobin. Therefore, 100 mL of blood will contain 15 × 1.34 or 21.1 mL O_2 as oxyhemoglobin. A much lesser amount, approximately 0.3 mL, is dissolved in 100 mL of plasma. (1:23, 165, 234–235, 302; 3:23, 446)

60.

D. Carbon dioxide is carried in the blood as carbaminohemoglobin and bicarbonate and is dissolved in plasma. About one-half of the carbon dioxide in blood is transported as bicarbonate ions. About one-third of CO_2 is transported as carbaminohemoglobin. The remainder of the CO_2 is dissolved in plasma. (1:29; 3:5–6, 462–466)

61.

E. Alveolar ventilation is not increased by metabolic alkalosis. Metabolic alkalosis slows alveolar ventilation in an effort to conserve carbon dioxide. Carbon dioxide combines with water to form carbonic acid, which then dissociates to increase the hydrogen ion concentration. (1:29, 299; 3:587)

62.

B. Thrombocytes are not leukocytes. Granulocytic leukocytes include neutrophils, eosinophils, and basophils. Lymphocytic leukocytes include lymphocytes and monocytes. (1:163–168, 205–206; 3:360–361)

63.

D. A patient can always receive blood from the same type. In addition, type O is in most cases the universal donor. Type AB blood is the universal recipient. (1:170; 3:358–361)

64.

C. A normal differential blood count shows about 70 percent of neutrophils. The normal range of neutrophils is 65 to 75 per 100 white blood cells. For eosinophils, it is 2 to 5 percent; basophils, 0.5 to 1.0%; lymphocytes, 20 to 25 percent; and monocytes, 3 to 8 percent. (1:172; 3:354–356)

65.

D. Because of its large number of small molecules, albumin contributes more to osmotic pressure. Osmotic pressure depends on the total number of particles, either ions or molecules, contained within a given volume, regardless of the size. A patient with hypoproteinemia will therefore lack the normal osmotic pressure necessary to keep the blood volume at normal levels and will have a tendency toward edema and ascites. (1:151–158, 166–172, 224–225; 3:354)

66.

C. The sinoatrial node is not associated with the ventricles of the heart. The sinoatrial node is part of the intrinsic nerve supply to the heart. It is located in the right atria just below the opening from the superior vena cava. (1:181–182; 3:376–377)

67.

D. The sinoatrial node is the normal pacemaker of the heart because 1) this region has a lower difference between resting membrane potential and threshold than other regions of the heart; 2) it has a more rapid sodium leakage; and 3) it recovers from the previous refractory period more rapidly than other areas. These factors result in the sinoatrial node depolarizing more rapidly than other areas. Once depolarization is initiated in any area, it tends to spread over the entire heart; thus the initiating area is the "pacemaker." (1:181–182; 3:376–377)

68.

C. The correct sequence of the blood flow through the heart to the lungs and its return to the heart is as follows: inferior vena cava, right atrium, tricuspid valves, right ventricle, pulmonary trunk to pulmonary circulation and out of the heart to systemic circulation, return via pulmonary veins to left atrium, bicuspid valves, left ventricle, and out through the ascending aorta. (1:178–182; 3:37, 374)

69.

D. The pressoreceptor system responds to an increase in blood pressure at the area of the aortic arch and carotid bodies. It operates through the vasomotor center and responds by decreasing the heart rate, strength of contraction, and peripheral resistance. Conversely, low pressure of blood perfusing the aorta and common carotid arteries reverses the stimulus to effect an increase in sympathetic tone to raise blood pressure. (1:187–190, 198; 3:243)

70.

A. Mean arterial blood pressure is regulated by neural mechanisms that control constriction of the arterioles, principles of capillary dynamics, and renal and hormonal mechanisms. In addition, mean arterial pressure (the approximate average of systolic and diastolic pressures) is affected by the cardiac output. Cardiac output is the volume of blood the heart pumps per minute. (1:187–194, 198; 3:368)

71.

A. Diastolic blood pressure is maintained at levels above zero by peripheral resistance. If diastolic

pressure dropped too low, blood flow would not be continuous and tissue perfusion would be impaired. It is also maintained by the viscosity of blood. (1:187–190, 198, 301; 3:385–392)

72.

B. The pulmonary and right atrioventricular valves prevent backflow of deoxygenated blood. Blood flows through the right atrium, the right atrioventricular valve, the right ventricle, and the pulmonary valve. It then goes to the lungs to be oxygenated. (1:184–185; 3:365–373)

73.

B. The stroke volume is the volume of blood pumped per beat. Multiply volume (approximately 70 mL) by the heart rate (approximately 75 beats/min) to get the cardiac output (the volume of blood pumped per minute). Cardiac output is approximately 5 L/min. (1:177–199; 3:374–376)

74.

E. Blood pressure depends on cardiac output, heart rate, stroke volume, peripheral resistance, blood volume, and blood viscosity. A variation in any of these factors can affect blood pressure, causing it to increase or decrease. Drastic fluctuations are compensated for by adjustments in the remaining factors and by neural and hormonal reflexes. (1:187, 192, 198; 3:386–389)

75.

D. Oxygenated blood flows through the coronary arteries of the heart. The remaining vessels listed contain deoxygenated blood—the pulmonary valve, the right atrioventricular valve, and the pulmonary artery. (1:77–199; 3:371–372)

76.

D. Digestion involves splitting the large chemical compounds in foods into simpler substances that can be absorbed. It also involves hydrolysis. By the process of hydrolysis, or breaking down with the addition of water as H+ and OH-, large molecules are split into particles small enough to be absorbed across the intestinal mucosa. (1:252–259, 301; 3:499–504)

77.

E. Amylase is not concerned with protein digestion. Amylase is an enzyme that hydrolyzes carbohydrates. The remaining four substances split protein into metabolic intermediary products, then into amino acids. (1:254–255, 257, 300; 3:499–504)

78.

E. The rate of gastric emptying is affected by the quantity of liquid in chyme. It is affected by neural and hormonal reflexes from the small intestine and the quantity of chyme in the small intestine. Chyme, in turn, is the term that refers to food products mixed with intestinal secretions in the process of being digested. (1:242, 252–259, 301; 3:499–504)

79.

C. Secretion of bile is not a function of the pancreas. Bile is formed in the liver and stored in the gallbladder. Normally, 500 to 1000 mL of bile is formed in the liver daily. (1:39, 248, 254, 300; 3:16, 478, 491)

80.

B. Secretin controls secretion of water and bicarbonate by acinar cells in the pancreas. Pancreozymin also acts on the pancreas. Pancreozymin controls the quantity of pancreatic enzymes released. (1:145–155, 158, 248–250; 3:503)

81.

B. Amylase hydrolyzes polysaccharides. Lipase hydrolyzes fats. Protease, trypsin, and pepsin are concerned with protein digestion. (1:252–255; 3:512)

82.

D. Erythropoiesis, or red blood cell formation, takes place in the bone marrow, liver, and spleen of the fetus. Liver and spleen are not involved in the adult. The liver forms bile and is involved in reticuloendothelial activity, glucogenesis, glycogenesis, and gluconeogenesis. (1:164–165, 167, 302; 3:512)

83.

E. The trigeminal nerve is the fifth cranial nerve. It innervates the muscles of mastication; the facial nerve innervates muscles of facial expression; the glossopharyngeal muscle innervates the muscles of the pharynx, and the hypoglossal innervates muscle of the tongue. Coordination of all of these muscle groups is necessary for swallowing. (1:118; 3:496; 5:857–859)

84.

D. An accumulation of collecting ducts in the kidney is called pyramids. The collecting ducts form the final segment of the nephron as it transfers glomerular filtrate into the calyces as urine. There are primarily two stages in elaboration of urine by the kidney: the glomerular stage and the tubular stage. (1:148, 152–154, 266–268, 274–275; 3:527)

85.

A. Filtration in the kidney occurs in the glomerulus. The glomerulus is the tuft of capillaries in Bowman's capsule where water, electrolytes, amino acids, glucose, urea, and other small molecular-size constituents are filtered from blood. The capillaries of the glomerulus unite to form the outgoing efferent arteriole. (1:148, 152–154, 266–268, 274–275; 3:523, 544)

86.

B. Reabsorption of water in the distal convoluted tubules and collecting ducts is regulated by the antidiuretic hormone. An increased secretion of antidiuretic hormone by the posterior lobe of the pituitary gland increases the permeability of the distal convoluted tubules and collecting ducts by water so that more is reabsorbed from glomerular filtrate into the blood. (1:148, 152–154, 266–268, 274–275; 3:547)

87.

B. Active transport transfers a substance from an area of low concentration into an area of high concentration with the aid of a carrier and utilization of energy. Diffusion and osmosis are referred to as passive transport because the driving force for transport is the concentration gradient. In passive transport, the net movement of substances is from regions of high concentration to regions of low concentration. (1:27–29, 254, 301; 3:56–57)

88.

D. Sodium ions are reabsorbed and potassium and hydrogen ions are secreted under the control of aldosterone. As each sodium ion is reabsorbed from glomerular filtrate into blood, either a potassium or a hydrogen ion is secreted from blood into glomerular filtrate. The specific ion that is secreted appears to be a matter of numerical chance. (1:148, 152–154, 266–268, 274–275; 3:520–539)

89.

C. Serum calcium levels are regulated principally by increasing or decreasing reabsorption by the intestines. The kidney functions to regulate hydrogen ion concentrations, body fluid volumes, and serum sodium levels. It also helps in the removal of urea, creatinine, and other metabolic end products. (1:43, 46, 61–62, 150–151, 157; 3:520–539)

90.

C. The facial nerve provides parasympathetic fibers to the lacrimal, nasal, palatine, submandibular, and sublingual glands. (1:120; 4:295; 5:862–864)

91.

B. Sympathetic innervation is provided from the superior cervical ganglion via the nerves that course along blood vessels. (1:116, 119, 302; 4:241)

92.

C. The nucleus ambiguus is a collection of neurons in the medulla that sends out branches via cranial nerves IX, X, and XI to control the muscles for swallowing. (1:109, 114–115; 4:282)

93.

B. The oculomotor nerve transmits the impulses to cause constriction of the pupil when a bright light is suddenly focused on the eye. (1:109, 114–115; 4:281; 5:1092)

94.

B. The pupils dilate in response to intense pain because dilation of the pupil is a sympathetic response. (1:23, 130–132; 4:30)

95.

D. If a person tests positive for HIV, the blood and body fluids will contain the virus. All other statements are true. (1:219, 294, 302)

CHAPTER

2 Head and Neck Anatomy

DIRECTIONS Each of the questions below is followed by several suggested answers. Select the best answer in each case.

1. The MOST superior part of the skull (Fig. 2-1) is the
   A. bregma
   B. nasion
   C. lambda
   D. vertex
   E. parietal eminence

2. Which of the following (Fig. 2-2) is located between the greater and lesser wings of the sphenoid bone?
   A. jugular foramen
   B. optic canal
   C. superior orbital fissure
   D. inferior orbital fissure
   E. pterygomaxillary fissure

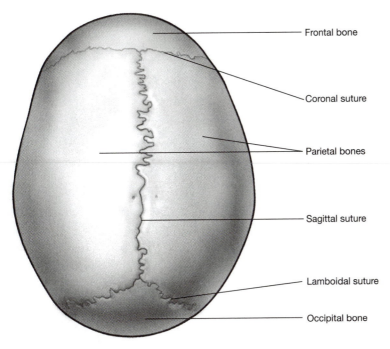

FIGURE 2-1. The skull, viewed from above, showing major features. (*Reed GM, Sheppard VF: Basic Structures of the Head and Neck: A Programmed Instruction in Clinical Anatomy for Dental Professionals. Philadelphia: Saunders, 1976.*)

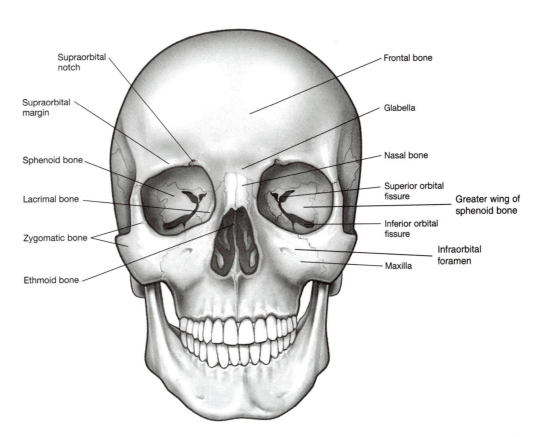

FIGURE 2-2. Openings into the orbit, anterior aspect. (*Reprinted with permission from Wolf-Heidegger G: Atlas of Systematic Human Anatomy, Vol I. Basel: S. Karger AG; reprinted from Reed GM, Sheppard VF: Basic Structures of the Head and Neck. Philadelphia: Saunders, 1976.*)

3. All of the following (Fig. 2-3) are part of the temporal bone EXCEPT
   A. squamous part
   B. mastoid part
   C. tympanic part
   D. mandibular fossa
   E. pterygoid plates

4. The concave area (Fig. 2-4) between the mandibular condyle and coronoid process is the
   A. coronoid notch
   B. maxillary notch
   C. mylohyoid notch
   D. condylar notch
   E. mandibular notch

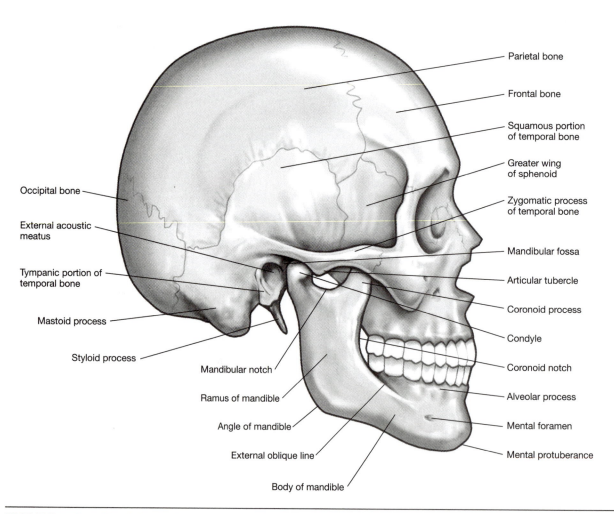

FIGURE 2-3. Skull, lateral aspect, showing the temporal bone. (*Redrawn from Wolf-Heidegger G: Atlas of Systematic Human Anatomy, vol 1. Basel: S. Karger AG; reprinted from Reed GM, Sheppard VF: Basic Structures of the Head and Neck. Philadelphia: Saunders, 1976.*)

5. All the following (Fig. 2-4) are parts of
   the mandible EXCEPT
   A. coronoid process
   B. coronoid notch
   C. mandibular notch
   D. oblique line
   E. coracoid process

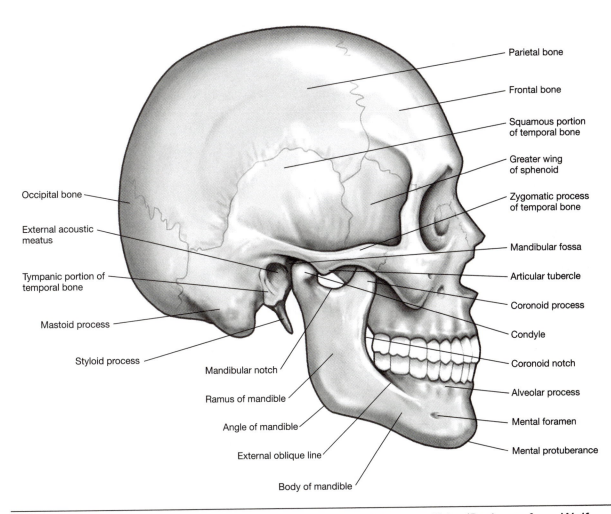

FIGURE 2-4. Skull, lateral aspect, showing the ramus of the mandible. (*Redrawn from Wolf-Heidegger G: Atlas of Systematic Human Anatomy, vol 1. Basel: S. Karger AG; reprinted from Reed GM, Sheppard VF: Basic Structures of the Head and Neck. Philadelphia: Saunders, 1976.*)

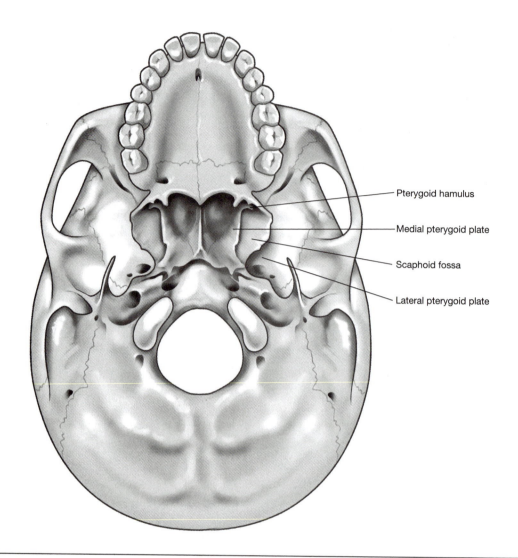

FIGURE 2-5. Pterygoid processes of the sphenoid bone, inferior aspect. (*Redrawn from Wolf-Heidegger G:* Atlas of Systematic Human Anatomy, *vol 1. Basel: S. Karger AG; reprinted from Reed GM, Sheppard VF:* Basic Structures of the Head and Neck. *Philadelphia: Saunders, 1976.*)

6. The pterygoid processes (Fig. 2-5) are part of what bone?
   A. temporal
   B. occipital
   C. sphenoid
   D. ethmoid
   E. maxilla

7. The specialized mechanism that is located in the neck and monitors changes in blood pressure is the
   A. carotid body
   B. carotid sinus
   C. superior cervical ganglion

8. In an interior view of the cranial cavity, extending from front to back, which bones (Fig. 2-6) form the middle part of the base of the skull?

    A. ethmoid, occipital
    B. parietal, frontal, temporal
    C. frontal, sphenoid, occipital, ethmoid
    D. ethmoid, temporal, occipital, frontal
    E. frontal, ethmoid, sphenoid, occipital

9. How is the foramen rotundum, shown in Figure 2-6, oriented in relation to the foramen ovale?

    A. anterolateral
    B. anteromedial
    C. posterolateral
    D. posteromedial
    E. inferior

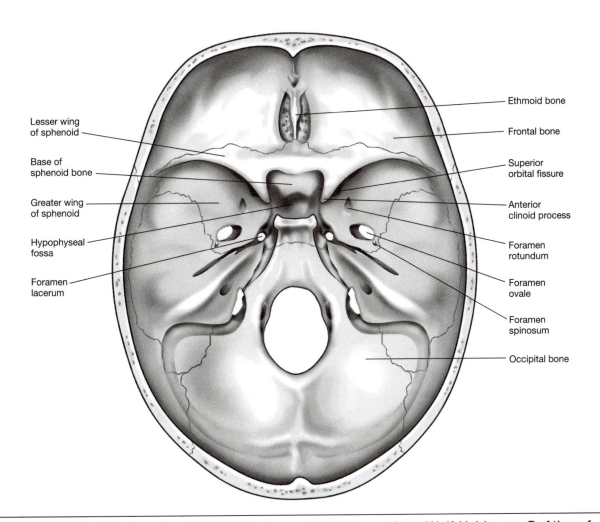

FIGURE 2-6.   Middle cranial fossa, internal aspect. (*Redrawn from Wolf-Heidegger G:* Atlas of Systematic Human Anatomy, *vol 1. Basel: S. Karger AG; reprinted from Reed GM, Sheppard VF:* Basic Structures of the Head and Neck. *Philadelphia: Saunders, 1975.*)

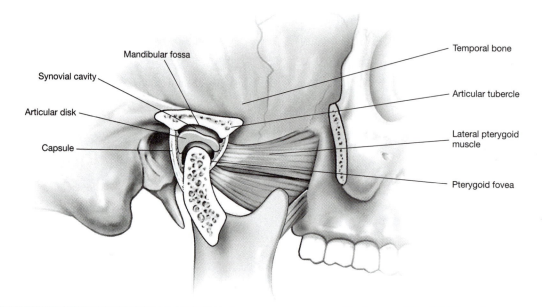

FIGURE 2-7. Right temporomandibular joint, sagittal section. (*Redrawn from Wolf-Heidegger G: Atlas of Systematic Human Anatomy, vol 1. Basel: S. Karger AG; reprinted from Reed GM, Sheppard VF: Basic Structures of the Head and Neck. Philadelphia: Saunders, 1976.*)

10. The mandible (Fig. 2-7) articulates with the
    A. sphenoid bone
    B. maxilla
    C. occipital bone
    D. temporal bone
    E. zygoma

11. The sphenomandibular ligament, shown in Figure 2-8, extends from the spine of the sphenoid to the
    A. external oblique line
    B. pterygoid fovea
    C. lingula
    D. posterior part of the mandibular angle
    E. condyle

FIGURE 2-8. Temporomandibular joint, medial aspect. (*Redrawn from Wolf-Heidegger G: Atlas of Systematic Human Anatomy, vol 1. Basel: S. Karger AG; reprinted from Reed GM, Sheppard VF: Basic Structures of the Head and Neck. Philadelphia: Saunders, 1976.*)

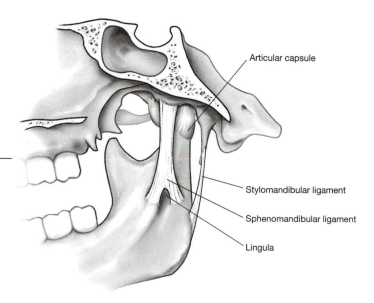

[]

12. All of the following muscles (Fig. 2-9) insert into orbicularis oris EXCEPT
    A. levator labii superioris alaeque nasi
    B. levator labii superioris
    C. zygomaticus muscles
    D. masseter
    E. levator anguli oris

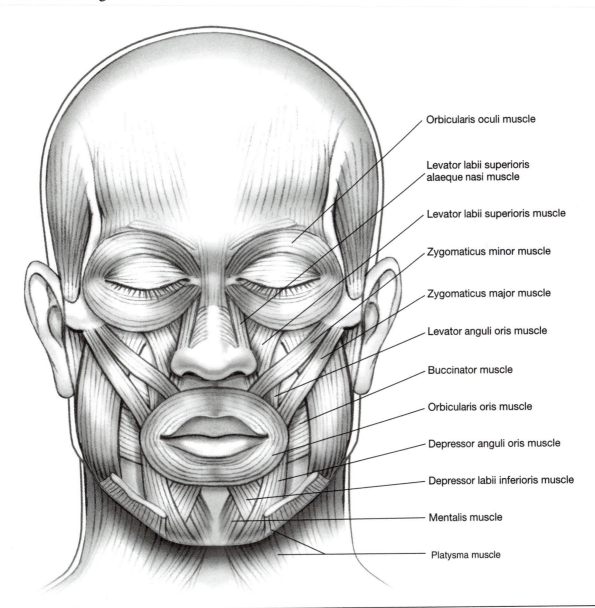

FIGURE 2-9.   Muscles that elevate the upper lip and angle of the mouth. (*Redrawn from Anson (ed.):* Morris' Human Anatomy. *New York: McGraw-Hill, 1966; reprinted from Reed GM, Sheppard VF:* Basic Structures of the Head and Neck. *Philadelphia: Saunders, 1976.*)

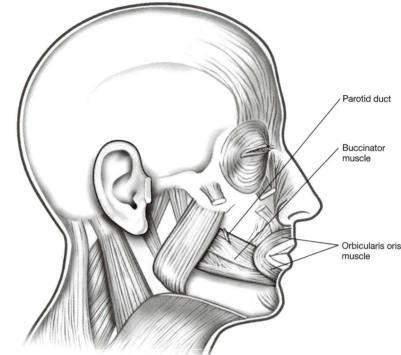

Parotid duct

Buccinator muscle

Orbicularis oris muscle

FIGURE 2-10. Buccinator muscle, lateral aspect. (*Redrawn from Wolf-Heidegger G:* Atlas of Systematic Human Anatomy, *vol 1. Basel: S. Karger AG; reprinted from Reed GM, Sheppard VF:* Basic Structures of the Head and Neck. *Philadelphia: Saunders, 1976.*)

13. The alveolar processes of the maxilla and mandible and the pterygomandibular raphe (Fig. 2-10) are attachments for what muscle?
    A. masseter
    B. medial pterygoid
    C. lateral pterygoid
    D. temporalis
    E. buccinator

14. Which muscle (Fig. 2-11) inserts into the lateral surface of the coronoid process and the anterior border of the ramus of the mandible?
    A. masseter
    B. temporalis
    C. medial pterygoid
    D. buccinator
    E. lateral pterygoid

15. Select the muscle (Fig. 2-12) whose origin is the medial side of the lateral pterygoid plate and whose insertion is the medial surface of the angle and ramus of the mandible.
    A. temporalis
    B. masseter
    C. medial pterygoid
    D. lateral pterygoid
    E. buccinator

16. The lateral pterygoid muscle inserts at the (Fig. 2-12)
    A. pterygoid fovea
    B. pterygoid fovea and articular disc
    C. mandibular condyle
    D. mandibular condyle and articular disc
    E. pterygoid fovea and articular eminence

17. The mandible (Fig. 2-12) is protruded by which muscle?
    A. lateral pterygoid
    B. medial pterygoid
    C. temporalis
    D. buccinator
    E. masseter

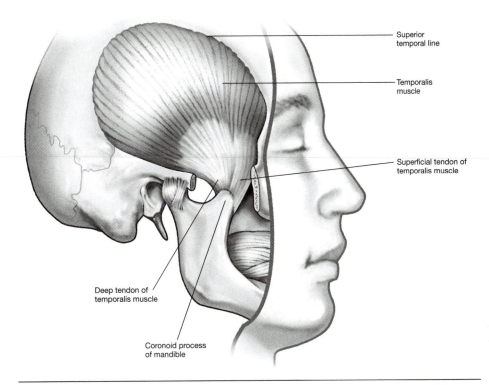

FIGURE 2-11. Temporalis muscle, lateral aspect. (*Redrawn from Wolf-Heidegger G:* Atlas of Systematic Human Anatomy, *vol 1. Basel: S. Karger AG; reprinted from Reed GM, Sheppard VF:* Basic Structures of the Head and Neck. *Philadelphia: Saunders, 1976.*)

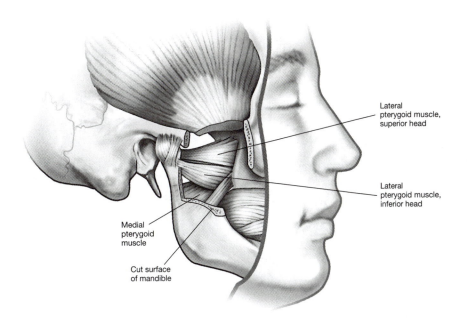

FIGURE 2-12. Pterygoid muscles, lateral aspect (coronoid process and anterior half of ramus of mandible removed). (*Redrawn from Wolf-Heidegger G:* Atlas of Systematic Human Anatomy, *vol 1. Basel: S. Karger AG; reprinted from Reed GM, Sheppard VF:* Basic Structures of the Head and Neck. *Philadelphia: Saunders, 1976.*)

18. Left lateral excursion of the mandible (Fig. 2-12) is accomplished by
    A. contraction of the left lateral pterygoid and relaxation of the right lateral pterygoid
    B. contraction of the right lateral pterygoid and relaxation of the left lateral pterygoid
    C. contraction of the left medial pterygoid and relaxation of the right medial pterygoid
    D. contraction of the right medial pterygoid and relaxation of the left medial pterygoid

19. A patient's jaw deviates markedly to the left when he attempts to protrude the mandible (Fig. 2-12). Which of the following muscles is unable to contract?
    A. right medial pterygoid
    B. left medial pterygoid
    C. right lateral pterygoid
    D. left lateral pterygoid
    E. left temporalis

20. All of the following cranial nerves assist in the movement of the eyeball EXCEPT
    A. optic nerve
    B. oculomotor nerve
    C. trochlear nerve
    D. abducens nerve

21. The mental nerve is responsible for all of the following functions EXCEPT
    A. sensory impulses from the skin of the lower lip
    B. sensory impulses from the chin
    C. sensory impulses from the mucous membranes of the lower lip
    D. sensory impulses from the upper lip, skin, and mucous membrane

22. Which cranial nerve is tested by reading an eye chart?
    A. optic
    B. oculomotor
    C. trochlear
    D. abducens
    E. all of the above

23. Failure to feel pain from an abscessed tooth might be due to an injury of which cranial nerve?
    A. III
    B. IV
    C. V
    D. VII
    E. IX

24. Which of the following cranial nerves does NOT supply sensory or motor fibers to the tongue?
    A. trigeminal
    B. facial
    C. glossopharyngeal
    D. accessory

25. The sense of taste from the posterior third of the tongue is carried by fibers of the
    A. trigeminal nerve
    B. hypoglossal nerve
    C. facial nerve
    D. glossopharyngeal nerve

26. Muscles of mastication are innervated by
    A. efferent fibers of the trigeminal nerve
    B. efferent fibers of the facial nerve
    C. the glossopharyngeal motor nerves
    D. afferent fibers of the facial nerve

27. Pain and temperature sensations from mucous membranes of the cheek, tongue, gingiva, and teeth of the mandible (Fig. 2-13) are innervated by the
    A. mandibular division of the trigeminal nerve
    B. maxillary division of the trigeminal nerve
    C. ophthalmic division of the trigeminal nerve

28. The foramen ovale transmits the
    A. middle meningeal artery
    B. facial nerve
    C. ophthalmic division of the trigeminal nerve
    D. maxillary division of the trigeminal nerve
    E. mandibular division of the trigeminal nerve

29. The mandibular division of the trigeminal nerve innervates the
    A. muscles of mastication
    B. temporomandibular joint
    C. skin around the lower lips
    D. A and B only
    E. A, B, and C

30. Which foramen transmits the nerve that supplies the muscles of mastication?
    A. ovale
    B. rotundum
    C. spinosum
    D. jugular
    E. mental

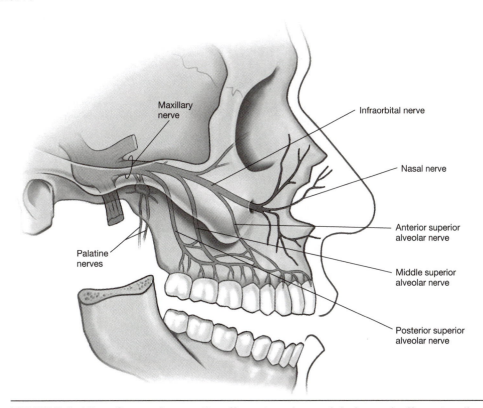

FIGURE 2-13. General somatic afferent and special visceral afferent cell columns in the brainstem viewed from median sagittal surface. (*Redrawn from Truex and Carpenter:* Human Neuroanatomy, *6th ed. Baltimore: Williams and Wilkins; reprinted from Reed GM, Sheppard VF:* Basic Structures of the Head and Neck. *Philadelphia: Saunders, 1975.*)

31. Which of the following nerves innervates the hard palate and the soft palate (Fig. 2-14)?

    A. greater palatine nerve

    B. nasopalatine nerve

    C. posterior superior alveolar nerve

    D. middle superior alveolar nerve

    E. buccal nerve

32. The nerve that innervates the mucous membranes of the pharynx and is the sensory component of the gag reflex is the

    A. facial nerve

    B. glossopharyngeal nerve

    C. hypoglossal nerve

    D. trigeminal nerve

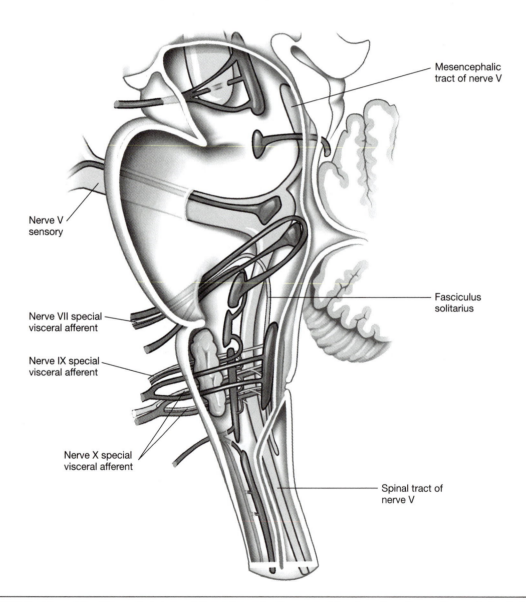

FIGURE 2-14. Maxillary division of the trigeminal nerve (V), showing branches of the infraorbital nerve. (*Redrawn and modified from Woodburne RT:* Essentials of Human Anatomy, *4th ed. New York: Oxford University Press; reprinted from Reed GM, Sheppard VF:* Basic Structures of the Head and Neck. *Philadelphia: Saunders, 1976.*)

33. What type of fiber (Fig. 2-15) is carried in the chorda tympani nerve?

    A. pain and temperature
    B. touch
    C. pressure
    D. parasympathetic and taste
    E. sympathetic

34. Submandibular and sublingual salivary glands (Fig. 2-15) are supplied by what nerve?

    A. trigeminal
    B. facial
    C. glossopharyngeal
    D. vagus
    E. trigeminal and facial

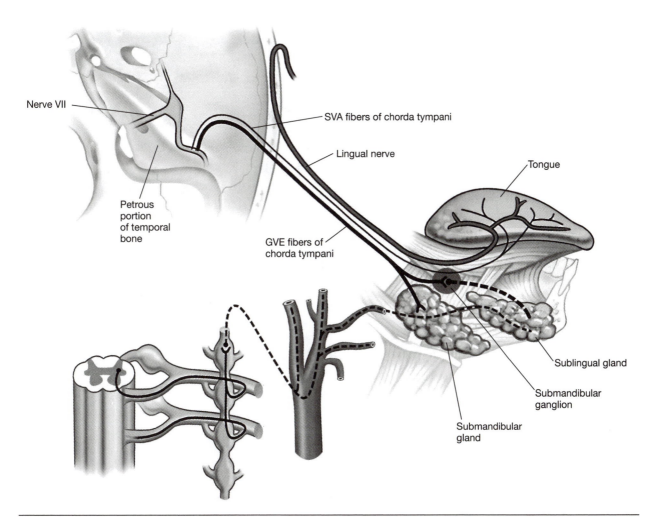

FIGURE 2-15. Distribution of the chorda tympani. (*Redrawn and modified from Woodburne RT: Essentials of Human Anatomy, 4th ed. New York: Oxford University Press; reprinted from Reed GM, Sheppard VF: Basic Structures of the Head and Neck. Philadelphia: Saunders, 1976.*)

35. The parotid gland (Fig. 2-16) is supplied by what fibers of what nerve?

    A. somatic visceral efferent (SVE); trigeminal

    B. general visceral efferent (GVE); facial

    C. general visceral efferent (GVE); glossopharyngeal

    D. general visceral afferent (GVA); vagus

    E. somatic visceral afferent (SVA); facial

36. Sympathetic fibers to the head supply the

    A. lacrimal glands

    B. smooth muscle in walls of blood vessels

    C. smooth muscle in the lower larynx

    D. parotid gland

    E. intrinsic muscles of the tongue

37. Increased intracranial pressure compressing the oculomotor nerve and causing diminished function of the parasympathetic fibers results in

    A. dilated pupils

    B. constricted pupils

    C. inability to move the eye laterally

    D. inability to look downward and laterally

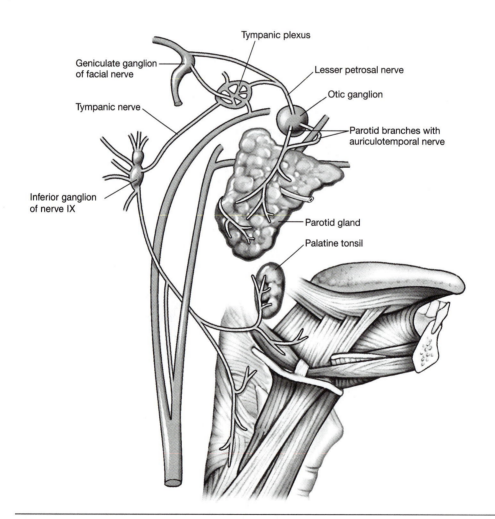

FIGURE 2-16.   General visceral efferent supply of the glossopharyngeal nerve (IX). (*Modified from Woodburne RT: Essentials of Human Anatomy, 4th ed. New York: Oxford University Press; reprinted from Reed GM, Sheppard VF: Basic Structures of the Head and Neck. Philadelphia: Saunders, 1976.*)

38. Postganglionic parasympathetic cell bodies are located in all of the following ganglia EXCEPT
    A. ciliary
    B. pterygopalatine
    C. trigeminal
    D. otic
    E. submandibular

39. All of the following (Fig. 2-17) are parts of the venous dural sinuses EXCEPT
    A. cavernous sinus
    B. ethmoid sinus
    C. transverse sinus
    D. straight sinus
    E. confluence of sinuses

40. The cerebrospinal fluid is produced by the
    A. choroid plexus
    B. subarachnoid granulations
    C. pia mater
    D. falx cerebri

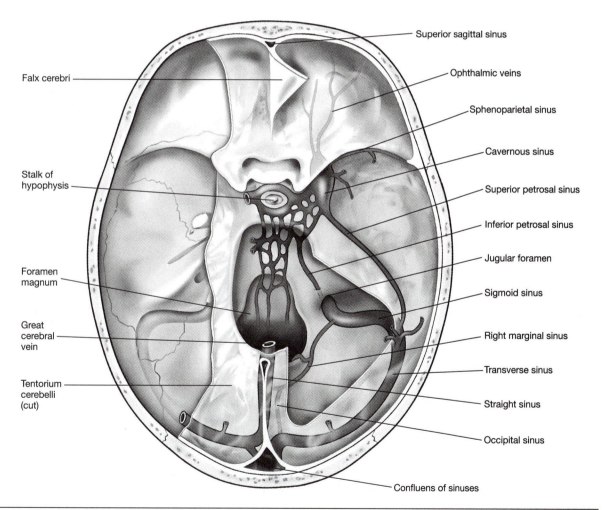

FIGURE 2-17.   Horizontal section showing transverse, sigmoid, and petrosal sinuses. (*Redrawn from Wolf-Heidegger G:* Atlas of Systematic Human Anatomy, *vol. 3. Basel: S. Karger AG; reprinted from Reed GM, Sheppard VF:* Basic Structures of the Head and Neck. *Philadelphia: Saunders, 1976.*)

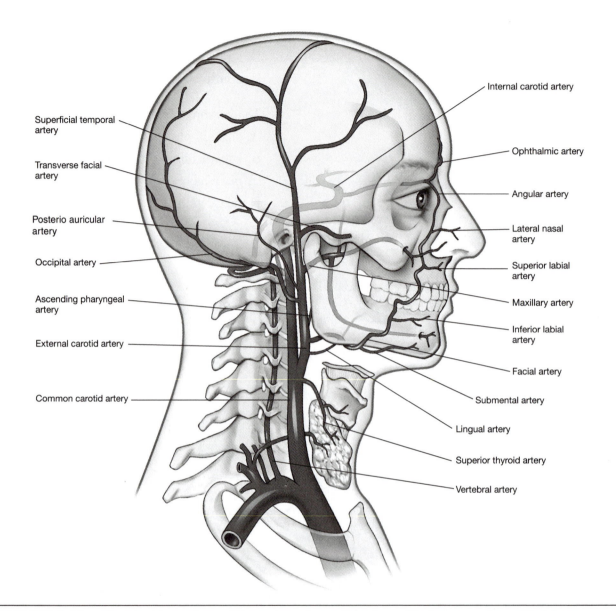

FIGURE 2-18. Terminal branches of the external carotid artery. (*Redrawn and modifed from Jacob and Francone:* Structure and Function in Man, *3rd ed. Philadelphia: Saunders; reprinted from Reed GM, Sheppard VF:* Basic Structures of the Head and Neck. *Philadelphia: Saunders, 1976.*)

41. Terminal branches of the external carotid artery, as shown in Figure 2-18, are the
   A. vertebral and basilar arteries
   B. facial and angular arteries
   C. maxillary and superficial temporal arteries
   D. lingual and inferior alveolar arteries
   E. occipital and posterior auricular arteries

42. The maxillary artery (Fig. 2-18) is a branch of the
   A. internal carotid artery
   B. external carotid artery
   C. common carotid artery
   D. vertebral artery

43. All of the following (Fig. 2-19) are
branches of the facial artery EXCEPT
A. inferior labial artery
B. superior labial artery
C. lateral nasal artery
D. angular artery
E. supraorbital artery

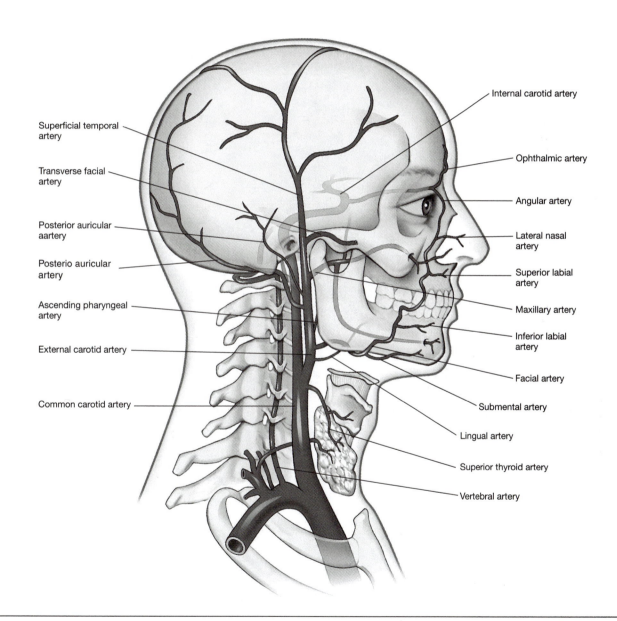

FIGURE 2-19. Course and main branches of the facial artery. (*Redrawn and modifed from Jacob and Francone*: Structure and Function in Man, *3rd ed. Philadelphia: Saunders; reprinted from Reed GM, Sheppard VF*: Basic Structures of the Head and Neck. *Philadelphia: Saunders, 1976.*)

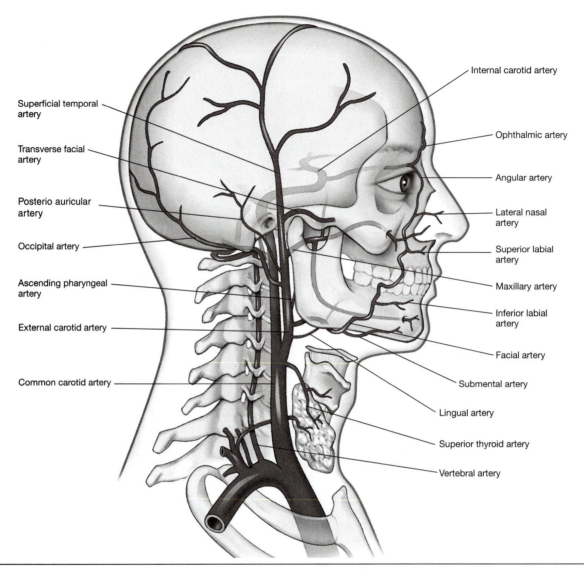

FIGURE 2-20. Main branches of the external carotid artery. (*Redrawn and modifed from Jacob and Francone:* Structure and Function in Man, *3rd ed. Philadelphia: Saunders; reprinted from Reed GM, Sheppard VF:* Basic Structures of the Head and Neck. *Philadelphia: Saunders, 1975.*)

44. Which of the following (Fig. 2-20) is NOT a branch of the external carotid artery?
    A. facial artery
    B. maxillary artery
    C. vertebral artery
    D. occipital artery
    E. superficial temporal artery

45. The lingual artery, shown in Figure 2-21, arises from what artery?
    A. external carotid
    B. submental

C. inferior alveolar
D. hypoglossal
E. ascending pharyngeal

46. Which of the following supplies blood to the temporomandibular joint?
    A. facial artery
    B. pterygoid arteries from the maxillary artery
    C. lingual artery
    D. superficial temporal and maxillary branches
    E. masseteric artery

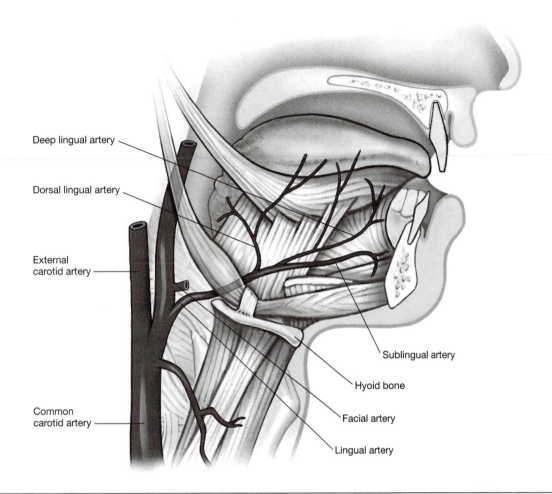

Deep lingual artery

Dorsal lingual artery

External carotid artery

Common carotid artery

Sublingual artery

Hyoid bone

Facial artery

Lingual artery

FIGURE 2-21. Branches of the lingual artery. (*Redrawn and modified from Woodburne RT: Essentials of Human Anatomy, 4th ed. New York: Oxford University Press; reprinted from Reed GM, Sheppard VF: Basic Structures of the Head and Neck. Philadelphia: Saunders, 1976.*)

47. Blood supply to the maxillary molar teeth (Fig. 2-22) is through what artery?
    A. posterior superior alveolar
    B. pterygoid portion of the maxillary
    C. facial
    D. angular
    E. internal carotid

48. Extensive bleeding from a fractured neck of the mandible with medial displacement would most likely be due to rupture of which branch (Fig. 2-23) of the maxillary artery?
    A. sphenopalatine
    B. posterior superior alveolar
    C. descending palatine
    D. inferior alveolar
    E. pharyngeal

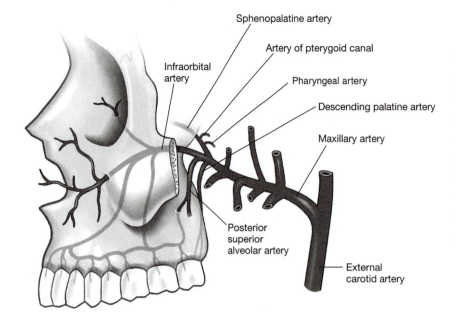

FIGURE 2-22. Main branches of the pterygopalatine region of the maxillary artery seen from the left side. Intraosseous portions are indicated by dotted lines. (*From Reed GM, Sheppard VF:* Basic Structures of the Head and Neck. *Philadelphia: Saunders, 1976.*)

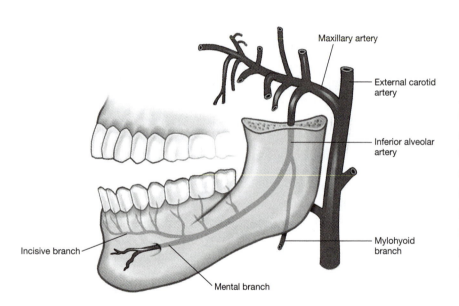

FIGURE 2-23. Branches of the inferior alveolar artery. Intraosseous portions are indicated by dotted lines. (*From Reed GM, Sheppard VF:* Basic Structures of the Head and Neck. *Philadelphia: Saunders, 1976.*)

49. The major artery that extends through the pterygopalatine fossa is the
    A. facial artery
    B. maxillary artery
    C. superficial temporal artery
    D. internal carotid artery

50. The artery that courses through the optic foramen and supplies the orbit and its contents, including the eyeball, is the
    A. anterior optic artery
    B. ophthalmic artery
    C. infraorbital artery of the maxillary artery
    D. supraorbital artery
    E. supratrochlear artery

51. The basilar artery (Fig. 2-24) is anterior and inferior to the

    A. medulla
    B. pons
    C. midbrain
    D. diencephalon
    E. cerebellum

52. The general location of the cerebral arterial circle (Fig. 2-24) is

    A. at the base of the occipital bone
    B. anterior to the clinoid process
    C. encircling the sella turcica
    D. across the petrous bone
    E. inferior to the zygoma

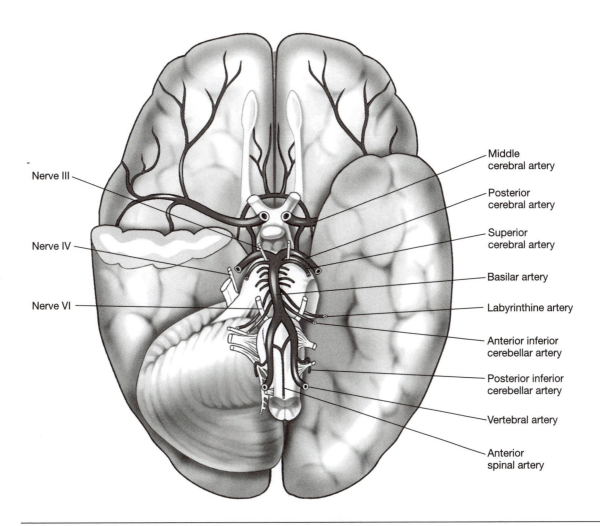

FIGURE 2-24. Blood supply to the brain, ventral aspect showing vertebral artery and branches of the basilar artery. (*Redrawn from Wolf-Heidegger G:* Atlas of Systematic Human Anatomy, *vol. 3. Basel: S. Karger AG; reprinted from Reed GM, Sheppard VF:* Basic Structures of the Head and Neck. *Philadelphia: Saunders, 1976.*)

53. Infectious toxins from maxillary teeth and gingiva drain principally into which lymph nodes (Fig. 2-25)?

    A. retroauricular nodes
    B. orbital lymph nodes
    C. submandibular and facial nodes
    D. facial nodes only
    E. submental and occipital nodes

54. The submandibular lymph nodes, shown in Figure 2-25, receive lymphatic drainage from all of the following regions EXCEPT

    A. chin and cheeks
    B. mandibular teeth
    C. parotid gland
    D. mandibular gingiva
    E. submental and submandibular salivary glands

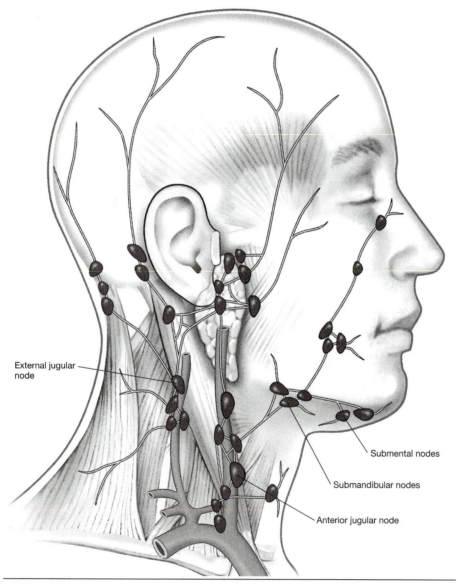

FIGURE 2-25.   Superficial lymph nodes of the neck. *(Redrawn from Woodburne RT: Essentials of Human Anatomy, 4th ed. New York: Oxford University Press; reprinted from Reed GM, Sheppard VF: Basic Structures of the Head and Neck. Philadelphia: Saunders, 1976.)*

55. The infratemporal fossa is important in dentistry because it contains the
    A. origin of the mandibular nerve
    B. facial artery
    C. buccinator muscle
    D. salivary glands
    E. muscles of mastication and many of the nerves and vessels supplying the mouth

56. The slit-like opening between the lateral pterygoid plate and the infratemporal surface of the maxilla (Fig. 2-26) is the
    A. nasopalatine foramen
    B. pterygoid fissure
    C. pterygopalatine fissure
    D. scaphoid fossa
    E. pterygoid canal

57. The communication link between the pterygopalatine fossa and the nasal cavity is the
    A. pterygopalatine fissure
    B. sphenopalatine foramen
    C. pterygomaxillary fissure
    D. nasopalatine foramen
    E. sphenopalatine fissure

58. All of the following are openings from the pterygopalatine fossa EXCEPT
    A. pterygomaxillary fissure
    B. foramen rotundum
    C. foramen lacerum
    D. palatine canal
    E. sphenopalatine foramen

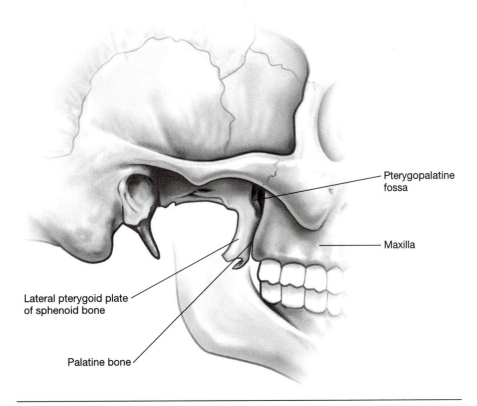

FIGURE 2-26. The pterygopalatine fossa, lateral aspect. (*From Reed GM, Sheppard VF: Basic Structures of the Head and Neck. Philadelphia: Saunders, 1976.*)

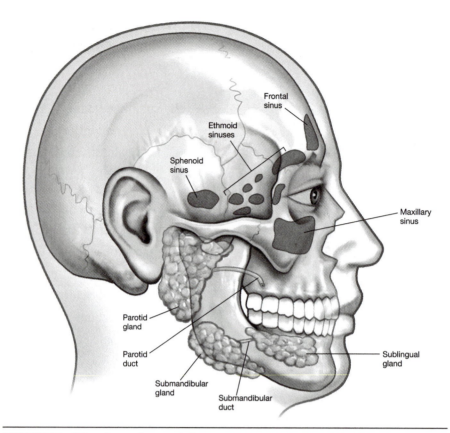

FIGURE 2-27. Locations of the paranasal sinuses. (*Modified from Jacob and Francone:* Structure and Function in Man, *3rd ed. Philadelphia: Saunders; reprinted from Reed GM, Sheppard VF:* Basic Structures of the Head and Neck. *Philadelphia: Saunders, 1976.*)

59. Which of the following bones (Fig. 2-27) does NOT contain a paranasal sinus?
    A. frontal
    B. ethmoid
    C. sphenoid
    D. maxilla
    E. zygomatic

60. The maxillary sinuses develop
    A. during the third month of fetal life
    B. at birth
    C. after the permanent teeth have erupted
    D. during the sixth to eighth years
    E. at about 12 years

61. The maxillary sinus opens into the
    A. frontonasal duct
    B. sphenoethmoidal recess
    C. hiatus semilunaris
    D. bulla ethmoidalis
    E. nasolacrimal duct

62. The maxillary sinus is innervated by the
    A. anterior and posterior superior alveolar nerve
    B. middle superior alveolar nerve
    C. posterior superior alveolar nerve
    D. infraorbital nerve
    E. all of the above

63. The line of demarcation between the loose alveolar mucosa and the more dense alveolar mucosa adjacent to teeth is the
    A. retromolar papilla
    B. palatoglossal fold
    C. mucogingival junction
    D. sulcus terminalis
    E. pterygopalatine junction

64. What muscle (Fig. 2-28) forms a mucosal fold anterior to the palatine tonsil?
    A. stylopharyngeus
    B. levator veli palatini
    C. tensor veli palatini
    D. palatoglossal
    E. palatopharyngeal

65. A fold of mucous membrane that helps anchor the tongue to the mouth floor in the midline is the
    A. fauces
    B. philtrum
    C. frenulum
    D. nasolabial fold
    E. anterior median fold

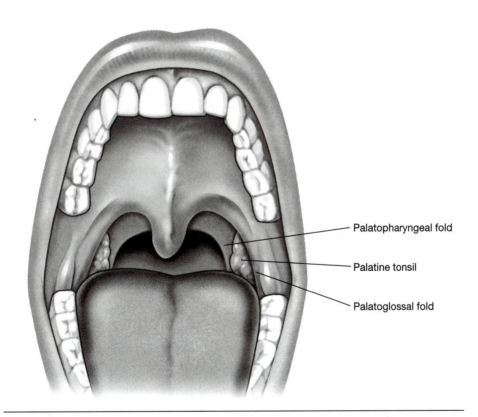

FIGURE 2-28. Interior of mouth, tongue extended, showing palatoglossal and palatopharyngeal folds. (*Redrawn from Wolf-Heidegger G:* Atlas of Systematic Human Anatomy, *vol. 2. Basel: S. Karger AG; reprinted from Reed GM, Sheppard VF:* Basic Structures of the Head and Neck. *Philadelphia: Saunders, 1975.*)

66. All of the following form the floor of the mouth EXCEPT (Fig. 2-29)
    A. mylohyoid muscle
    B. geniohyoid muscle
    C. hyoglossus muscle
    D. styloglossus muscle
    E. sublingual gland

67. Branches of the facial nerve to muscles of the face are enmeshed in which salivary gland?
    A. sublingual
    B. submandibular
    C. parotid
    D. incisive
    E. palatine

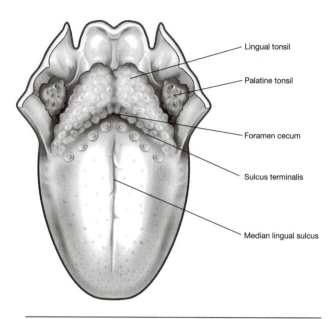

FIGURE 2-30. Dorsum of tongue, showing sulci and lingual tonsil. (*Redrawn from Woodburne RT: Essentials of Human Anatomy, 4th ed. New York: Oxford University Press; reprinted from Reed GM, Sheppard VF: Basic Structures of the Head and Neck. Philadelphia: Saunders, 1976.*)

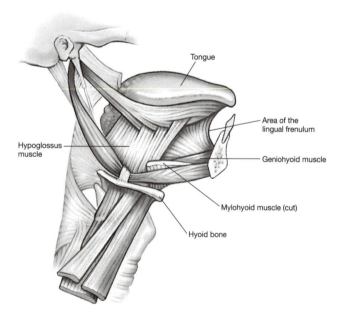

FIGURE 2-29. Muscles supporting the floor of the mouth, lateral aspect. (*Redrawn from Romanes GJ (ed.): Cunningham's Textbook of Anatomy, 10th ed. New York: Oxford University Press; reprinted from Reed GM, Sheppard VF: Basic Structures of the Head and Neck. Philadelphia: Saunders, 1976.*)

68. The V-shaped demarcation that separates the anterior two-thirds of the tongue (Fig. 2-30) from the posterior one-third is the
    A. foramen cecum
    B. medial lingual sulcus
    C. frenulum
    D. sulcus terminalis
    E. lingual groove

69. All of the following nerves supply gingiva EXCEPT
    A. greater and lesser palatine nerves
    B. superior alveolar nerves
    C. infraorbital nerve
    D. nasopalatine nerve
    E. lingual nerve

70. Buccal gingiva of the mandibular molars (Fig. 2-31) is innervated by which of the following nerve(s)?
    A. posterior superior alveolar
    B. buccal
    C. chorda tympani
    D. auriculotemporal bone
    E. all of the above

71. Ventral rami of spinal nerves C5 through T1 form the
    A. cervical plexus
    B. branchial plexus
    C. lumbar plexus
    D. sacral plexus

72. All of the following tracts are located within the spinal cord EXCEPT
    A. lateral spinothalamic
    B. dorsal columns
    C. thalamocortical
    D. lateral corticospinal
    E. reticulospinal

73. The brain structures that lie lateral to the third ventricle are
    A. thalami
    B. hypothalamus
    C. pons
    D. A and B only
    E. A and C only

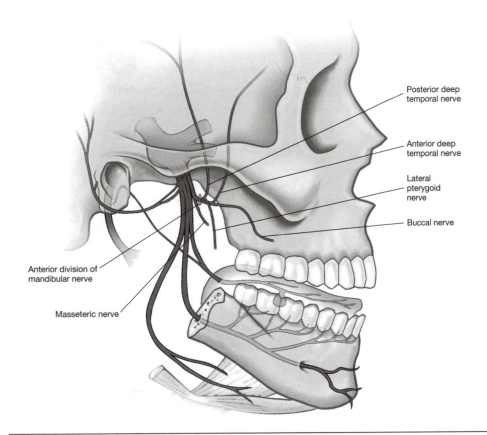

FIGURE 2-31. Branches of the anterior division of the mandibular nerve. (*Redrawn and modified from Woodburne RT:* Essentials of Human Anatomy, *4th ed. New York: Oxford University Press; reprinted from Reed GM, Sheppard VF:* Basic Structures of the Head and Neck. *Philadelphia: Saunders, 1976.*)

74. The superior and inferior ganglia are associated with which cranial nerve?

    A. trigeminal

    B. facial

    C. glossopharyngeal

    D. vagus

    E. hypoglossal

75. Which of the following cranial nerves (Fig. 2-32) contain fibers of the parasympathetic division of the autonomic nervous system?

    A. oculomotor

    B. trigeminal

    C. glossopharyngeal

    D. vagus

    E. all of the above

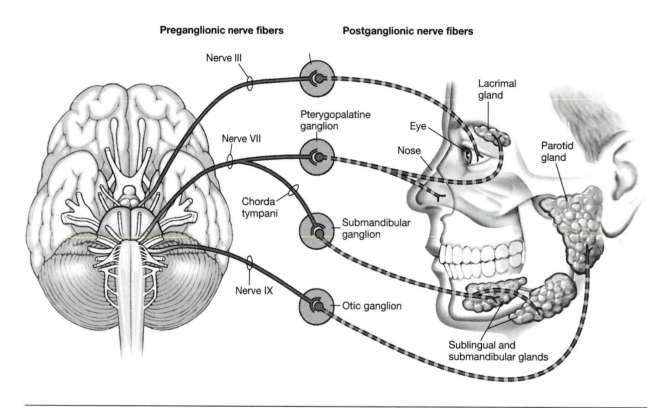

FIGURE 2-32. Parasympathetic nerve supply to the head. (*Modified from Woodburne RT: Essentials of Human Anatomy, 4th ed. New York: Oxford University Press; reprinted from Reed GM, Sheppard VF: Basic Structures of the Head and Neck. Philadelphia: Saunders, 1976.*)

76. Arrange the following in order of blood flow.
    1. vena cava
    2. left atrium
    3. left ventricle
    4. lungs
    5. right atrium
    6. right ventricle
    7. tricuspid valve
    8. mitral valve
    9. pulmonary valve
    10. aortic valve
    11. aorta
        A. 1, 2, 7, 3, 4, 9, 5, 8, 6, 10, 11
        B. 1, 2, 8, 3, 9, 4, 5, 7, 6, 11, 10
        C. 5, 7, 6, 9, 4, 2, 8, 3, 10, 11, 1
        D. 1, 5, 7, 6, 9, 4, 2, 8, 3, 10, 11
        E. 1, 5, 7, 6, 4, 9, 2, 8, 3, 11, 10

77. All of the following are associated with the ventricles of the heart EXCEPT
    A. papillary muscle
    B. chordae tendinae
    C. foramen ovale
    D. septum
    E. myocardium

78. All of the following are direct branches off the aorta EXCEPT
    A. innominate (brachiocephalic) artery
    B. right common carotid artery
    C. coronary arteries
    D. left common carotid artery
    E. celiac trunk

79. Arrange in order the route of blood supply to the right side of the face.
    1. aorta
    2. brachiocephalic trunk
    3. left ventricle
    4. external carotid artery
    5. common carotid artery
    6. internal carotid artery
    7. facial artery
    8. maxillary artery
        A. 1, 3, 2, 5, 6
        B. 1, 3, 5, 4, 6, 7
        C. 3, 2, 1, 5, 6, 7
        D. 3, 1, 5, 4, 7
        E. 3, 1, 2, 5, 4, 7

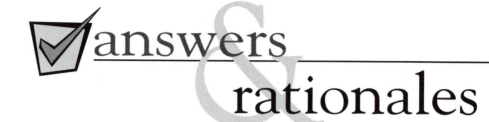
answers & rationales

1.

D. The most superior part of the skull is the vertex. The vertex in most individuals is located about one-half to two-thirds of the distance from the coronal junction to the lambdoidal junction. The vertex is located on the parietal bone. (2:839, 842; 4:97)

2.

C. The superior orbital fissure is located between the wings of the sphenoid bone. The superior orbital fissure transmits nerves to the muscles of the eye and the ophthalmic vein. Specifically, the supraorbital fissure transmits the third, fourth, and part of the fifth cranial nerves. (1:226; 2:845; 3:123; 4:102)

3.

E. The pterygoid plates are part of the sphenoid bone. The pterygoid plates are part of the pterygoid processes. The pterygoid fossa is also part of the pterygoid plates. (2:841; 3:124, 126; 4:98)

4.

E. The concave area between the mandibular condyle and coronoid process is the mandibular notch. The mandibular notch transmits arteries and nerves to the masseter muscle. The mandibular notch is also known as the coronoid notch. (3:130; 4:105)

5.

E. The coracoid process is not a part of the mandible. The coracoid process is part of the scapula. Landmarks of the mandible include the coronoid process, the coronoid notch (mandibular notch), and the external oblique line. (1:46, 51–56; 2:669; 3:130–133; 4:105; 5:206–208)

6.

C. The pterygoid processes are part of the sphenoid bone. The pterygoid processes provide attachment for the medial and lateral pterygoid muscles, which are the muscles of mastication. The pterygoid processes include the medial and lateral pterygoid plates and the pterygoid fossa. (1:226; 2:841; 3:124–126; 4:98; 5:203)

7.

B. The specialized mechanism that is located in the neck and monitors changes in blood pressure is the carotid sinus. The carotid sinus contains receptors that are sensitive to the stretch in the walls of the common carotid arteries. (1:194)

8.

E. The frontal, ethmoid, sphenoid, and occipital bones extending from front to back form the medial part of the base of the skull. These bones, located in the midline, are at the three levels forming the anterior, middle, and superior cranial fossae. The frontal, ethmoid, sphenoid, and occipital bones are not paired. (1:51–57; 2:834, 842–843; 4:82–99)

9.

B. The foramen rotundum is anteromedial to the foramen ovale. The foramen rotundum transmits the maxillary division of the trigeminal nerve. The foramen ovale transmits the mandibular division of the trigeminal nerve. (1:51–57; 2:845–846; 3:124–126; 4:94, 102, 226; 5:203)

10.

D. The mandible articulates with the temporal bone. The articulation is termed the temporomandibular joint. The temporomandibular joint is a hinge joint. The temporomandibular joint is also classified as a synovial joint. (1:65; 2:923–925; 3:152–157; 4:103–105; 5:283–288)

11.

C. The sphenomandibular ligament extends from the spine of the sphenoid bone to the lingula. The lingula is a small extension of bone located inferomedial to the mandibular foramen. It partially covers the opening of the mandibular foramen. (2:923–924; 3:133; 4:203, 221)

12.

D. Levator lavii superioris alaeque nasi, levator labii superioris, zygomaticus muscles, and the levator anguli oris all insert into the oblicularis oris. The masseter muscle is in another category. It is a muscle of mastication, whereas the other muscles are muscles of facial expression that insert into the oblicularis oris. (1:76; 2:852–855; 3:161; 4:156–160; 5:226–227)

13.

E. The alveolar processes of the maxilla and mandible and the pterygomandibular raphe are attachments for the buccinator muscle. The buccinator muscle forms the muscular substance of the cheek just lateral to the teeth. The buccinator muscle is a muscle of mastication. (1:77; 2:852–854; 3:133; 163, 167, 180; 4:156–160; 5:228)

14.

B. The temporalis muscle inserts into the lateral surface of the coronoid process and the anterior border of the ramus of the mandible. The temporalis muscle originates in the infratemporal fossa. If the entire temporalis muscle contracts, the overall action is to pull upward on the coronoid process and elevate the mandible. (1:77; 2:920; 3:142; 4:204–205, 223)

15.

C. The medial pterygoid muscle has its origin in the medial side of the lateral pterygoid plate. Its inser-

tion is in the medial surface of the angle and ramus of the mandible. The medial pterygoid muscle assists in closing the mandible. (1:179, 190–191; 2:920; 4:204, 207, 223; 5:217)

16.

B. The lateral pterygoid muscle inserts at the pterygoid fovea and articular disc. Its superior origin arises from the infratemporal crest of the greater wing of the sphenoid bone and the inferior origin arises from the lateral side of the pterygoid plate. The lateral pterygoid muscle assists in protrusion and depression of the mandible. (1:78; 2:920; 3:138; 4:204, 207, 223; 5:217)

17.

A. The mandible is protruded by the lateral pterygoid muscle. Because the insertion of the lateral pterygoid muscles on the neck of the mandible is posterior to the origin at the pterygoid plates, contraction of this muscle pulls the mandible forward. The lateral pterygoid muscle also assists in the depression of the mandible. (1:78; 2:920; 3:142–143; 4:204, 207, 223; 5:217)

18.

B. Left lateral excursion of the mandible is accomplished by contraction of the right lateral pterygoid and relaxation of the left lateral pterygoid. Lateral excursion of the mandible follows contraction of the opposite lateral pterygoid muscle, with relaxation of the lateral pterygoid on the side of the shift. The superior head of the lateral pterygoid functions only in the action of biting. (1:78; 2:926; 3:143–144; 4:204, 207, 223; 5:217)

19.

D. If a patient's mandible deviates markedly to the left when he attempts to protrude the mandible, the left lateral pterygoid muscle is unable to contract. Protrusion of the mandible is accomplished by bilateral contraction of the lateral pterygoid muscles. When only one lateral pterygoid muscle is contracted, there will be lateral excursion to the opposite side of the contracted muscle. (1:78; 2:926; 3:143–144; 4:204–207, 223; 5:217)

20.

A. The optic nerve serves a sensory function to the eye and functions in vision. The oculomotor nerve, trochlear nerve, and abducens nerve all have a motor function and assist in the movement of the eyeball. (4:182–185, 280–285)

21.

D. The mental nerve provides sensory innervation to the skin of the lower lip, chin, and mucous membranes of the lower lip. The upper lip is innervated by the superior labial branches of the infraorbital nerve. (4:161–162, 215, 291, 294)

22.

A. The optic nerve is tested when reading an eye chart. The optic nerve is sensory for vision. The oculomotor, trochlear, and abducens nerves are motor nerves to the eyeball. (1:119; 2:1083–1084; 3:187; 4:173, 182, 280–281)

23.

C. Failure to feel pain from an abscessed tooth might be due to an injury of the fifth cranial nerve. The trigeminal nerve is the general somatic nerve to the mouth. It provides sensory and motor functions to the oral cavity. (1:118; 2:1083–1084; 3:187–197; 4:174, 184, 213, 241, 279, 281, 285)

24.

D. The trigeminal, facial, glossopharyngeal, and hypoglossal cranial nerves supply sensory and motor functions to the tongue. The anterior two-thirds of the tongue are supplied by fibers for general sensation that are part of the trigeminal nerve; taste fibers from the posterior one-third of the tongue are carried by the glossopharyngeal nerve. The hypoglossal nerve is motor to muscles that move the tongue. (2:1083–1084; 3:97–102; 4:239; 5:242–253)

25.

D. The sense of taste from the posterior third of the tongue is carried by the glossopharyngeal nerve. The facial nerve carries taste sensation from the anterior two-thirds on the tongue; the glossopharyngeal nerve is motor to muscles that move the tongue. (2:1083–1085; 4:239)

26.

A. Muscles of mastication are classified as muscles of branchiomeric origin; this means that they are derived from embryonic branchial arches. For this reason, they are placed in the "special" category of functional components. Efferent implies motor nerves. Muscles of mastication are supplied by fibers from the trigeminal nerve. (1:77; 2:1096; 4:202–204, 215)

27.

A. The mandibular division of the trigeminal nerve contains sensory and motor components. It provides sensory innervation to the mucous membranes of the cheek, tongue, gingiva, and teeth of the mandible. (4:291–292)

28.

E. The foramen ovale transmits the mandibular division of the trigeminal nerve. The mandibular division of the trigeminal nerve, like the ophthalmic and maxillary divisions, contains a large number of general somatic afferent fibers conveying general sensation. The mandibular division, however, differs from the other divisions in that the mandibular nerve is joined just after it leaves the foramen ovale by the motor root of the trigeminal nerve. (1:119; 2:845–846; 4:77, 99, 102, 174, 213, 241, 291; 5:242–250)

29.

E. The mandibular division of the trigeminal nerve innervates the muscles of mastication and the skin of the lower face, cheek, lower lip, ear, external acoustic meatus, temporomandibular joint, and skin of the temporal region. It also supplies the mucous membranes of the cheek, tongue, mandibular teeth, gingiva, mastoid air cells, mandible, and portions of the dura mater. (4:161–162, 213–215, 291–292)

30.

A. The foramen ovale transmits the nerve that innervates the muscles of mastication. The muscles of mastication are innervated by the mandibular division of the trigeminal nerve. The mandibular division of the trigeminal nerve exits the skull through the foramen ovale. (1:119; 2:845–846; 3:124–125; 4:106)

31.

A. The greater palatine nerve innervates the soft palate, hard palate, gingiva, and mucous membranes as far anteriorly as the incisive teeth. (4:290)

32.

B. The mucous membranes of the pharynx and the associated gag reflex receive sensory innervation from the glossopharyngeal nerve. (4:298–299)

33.

D. Parasympathetic fibers and taste fibers are carried in the chorda tympani nerve. The chorda tympani nerve conveys general visceral efferent fibers of the parasympathetic division of the autonomic nerve. It carries special visceral afferent fibers for taste. (2:923, 944; 4:188, 214, 241, 293, 297)

34.

B. Submandibular and sublingual salivary glands are supplied by the facial nerve. The parotid salivary gland is supplied by the glossopharyngeal nerve. The facial nerve is sensory and motor in function, as is the glossopharyngeal nerve. (3:195–198; 4:162, 174, 188, 193, 197, 281, 294)

35.

C. The parotid gland is supplied by the general visceral efferent fibers of the glossopharyngeal nerve. General visceral efferent fibers are motor fibers of the parasympathetic division of the autonomic nervous system. The glossopharyngeal nerve also supplies a motor function to the pharynx. (2:1083–1085; 3:195–198; 4:174, 188, 195, 282, 298; 5:275–276)

36.

B. Sympathetic fibers to the head supply the smooth muscle in walls of blood vessels. A normal sympathetic tone transmitted to smooth muscle in the blood vessels maintains the lumen in a partly constricted state. A decreased sympathetic tone allows vessels to dilate; an increased sympathetic tone causes the vessels to constrict. (2:32; 4:25–28, 326)

37.

A. Increased intracranial pressure compressing the oculomotor nerve and causing diminished function of the parasympathetic fibers results in dilated pupils. General visceral efferent fibers (parasympathetic) of the oculomotor nerve supply muscles that constrict the pupil. When these are inoperable, the pupil dilates. (2:905; 4:173, 179, 182, 282–285, 325, 327)

38.

C. Postganglionic parasympathetic cell bodies are not located in the trigeminal nerve. The parasympathetic nerve supply to the head includes preganglionic and postganglionic fibers of the oculomotor, facial, glossopharyngeal, and vagus nerves. Preganglionic fibers of the oculomotor nerve synapse with postganglionic neurons in the ciliary ganglion; fibers of the facial nerve synapse with the pterygopalatine and submandibular ganglia; those of the glossopharyngeal nerve synapse with the optic ganglion. (2:1083–1085; 4:30, 327)

39.

B. The ethmoid sinus is not a part of the venous dural sinuses. The ethmoid sinus is an air sinus, considered part of the paranasal sinus. The venous dural sinuses drain deoxygenated blood from the brain. (2:959–960; 4:231)

40.

A. Cerebrospinal fluid is produced by the choroid plexus. The choroid plexus is a membranous partition extending into the cavity of each of the ventricles. It forms a semipermeable partition that filters cerebrospinal fluid from blood. (2:891; 4:266, 275, 319)

41.

C. Terminal branches of the external carotid artery are the maxillary and superficial temporal arteries. The maxillary artery supplies maxillary teeth, muscles of mastication, the palate, dura mater, and part of the nasal cavity. The superficial temporal artery supplies the external ear, the scalp above the ear, and the temporomandibular joint. (2:948, 1018; 4:141, 144, 155, 163, 192–193, 195–196, 211, 225, 232, 235, 254, 320)

42.

B. The maxillary artery is a branch of the external carotid artery. The maxillary artery, like all extracranial arteries except the superior orbital, is a branch of the external carotid artery. The internal carotid artery is not a branch of the external carotid artery. (1:552, 557; 2:920, 922; 3:171–177; 4:141, 192, 193–195, 254, 320)

43.

E. The supraorbital artery is not a branch of the facial artery. The supraorbital artery originates within the skull and extends forward through the orbit. The facial artery is a branch of the external carotid artery and it supplies the skin and muscles of facial expression. (1:185; 2:873–874, 913, 1018; 3:171; 4:155, 164, 328)

44.

C. The vertebral artery is not a branch of the external carotid artery. The vertebral artery is a branch of the subclavian artery. The main branches of the external carotid artery are the facial, lingual, and maxillary arteries. (2:894, 1027; 3:171; 4:137, 276, 330)

45.

A. The lingual artery arises from the external carotid artery. The lingual artery supplies structures of the floor of the mouth and the posterior and inferior surface of the tongue. The lingual artery branches off the external carotid artery below the facial artery. (2:1018; 3:171; 4:143, 212, 239, 242, 321)

46.

D. The superficial temporal and deep auricles supply arterial blood to the temporomandibular joint. The deep auricular artery is a branch of the maxillary artery. Both the superficial temporal artery and the maxillary artery are terminal branches of the external carotid artery. (2:920, 1018; 3:152–157; 4:144, 155, 163, 192–193, 196, 325)

47.

A. The posterior superior alveolar artery supplies blood to the maxillary molar teeth. The superior alveolar artery is a branch of the maxillary artery. The posterior superior alveolar artery comes out of the pterygopalatine fossa through the pterygomaxillary fissure and descends onto the maxillary tuberosity, entering the bone behind the third molar. (2:922; 3:175; 4:211–212, 225)

48.

D. Extensive bleeding from a fractured neck of the mandible with medial displacement would most likely be due to the rupture of the inferior alveolar artery. The inferior alveolar branch of the maxillary artery descends from a position medial to the neck of the mandible to enter the mandibular foramen inferiorly. The inferior alveolar artery sends off branches into each of the mandibular teeth and into bone. (2:920; 3:171–177; 4:212, 235)

49.

B. The major vessel that extends through the pterygopalatine fossa is the maxillary artery. The maxillary artery extends from a point anterior to the ear through the infratemporal fossa. It also extends into the pterygopalatine fossa where it divides its terminal branches. (2:950, 952; 4:144, 163, 192, 196, 211, 232, 235, 325)

50.

B. The ophthalmic artery exits from the skull through the optic foramen and supplies the orbit and the eyeball. (4:185)

51.

B. The basilar artery is anterior and inferior to the pons of the brain. Vertebral arteries ascend in the transverse process of cervical vertebrae, lie anterior to the medulla, and join to form the basilary artery. The basilary artery is anterior and inferior to the pons. (2:894-895; 4:276)

52.

C. The general location of the cerebral arterial circle is encircling the sella turcica. When the cerebral arterial circle is viewed on the inferior surface of the brain, it encircles the pituitary stalk and optic chiasma. The stalk leads to the pituitary gland in the sella turcica or hypophyseal fossa. (2:895–896; 4:276)

53.

C. Infectious toxins from maxillary teeth and gingiva drain principally into the submandibular and facial lymph nodes. The submandibular lymph nodes are located medial to the angle of the mandible. The facial lymph nodes are located in the area of the zygomatic muscles. (2:1012; 3:198–199; 4:312, 315)

54.

C. The submandibular lymph nodes do not receive lymphatic drainage from the parotid gland. Lymphatic drainage from the parotid gland enters the deep parotid lymph nodes. Parotid lymph nodes are also known as auricular nodes. (2:869–870, 964; 3:201–203; 4:311, 314)

55.

E. The infratemporal fossa is important in dentistry because it contains the muscles of mastication and many of the nerves and vessels supplying the mouth. The infratemporal fossa is the area extending inferiorly below the zygomatic arch. It extends medially, deep to the ramus of the mandible. (4:77, 202–203, 323)

56.

B. The slit-like opening between the lateral pterygoid plate and the infratemporal surface of the maxilla is the pterygoid fissure. The pterygoid fissure is continuous with the pterygopalatine fossa. The pterygopalatine fossa contains the terminal branches of the maxillary artery. (2:950; 4:94)

57.

B. The communication link between the pterygopalatine fossa and the nasal cavity is the sphenopalatine foramen. The sphenopalatine artery and the nasopalatine nerve extend through the sphenopalatine foramen. The sphenopalatine artery supplies most parts of the nasal cavity. (2:956, 958; 3:175–176; 4:94)

58.

C. The foramen lacerum is not an opening from the pterygopalatine fossa. The foramen lacerum is on the base of the skull. The pterygopalatine fossa is the origin of the muscles of mastication. (2:845–846, 893; 4:98, 102)

59.

E. The zygoma does not contain a paranasal sinus. Paranasal sinuses are air sinuses. Venous dural sinuses contain deoxygenated blood. (2:834, 957–959; 3:127–140; 4:229–234, 326)

60.

C. The maxillary sinuses develop after the permanent teeth have erupted. The growth of the maxillary air sinus continues through adulthood. The maxillary air sinus sometimes infringes on the maxillary alveolar bone. (2:959; 3:127-140; 4:76, 231)

61.

C. The maxillary sinus opens into the hiatus semiluminaris. The hiatus semiluminaris is a groove in the middle meatus of the lateral nasal cavity. It also contains the openings of the frontonasal duct and the anterior ethmoid air cells. (2:956; 4:76, 230–231)

62.

E. The maxillary sinus is innervated by the anterior superior alveolar nerve, middle superior alveolar nerve, posterior superior alveolar nerve, and infraorbital nerve. General visceral afferent nerve fibers to the maxillary sinus convey pain, temperature, touch, and pressure. (1:227; 2:959; 4:76, 231, 291)

63.

C. The line of demarcation between the loose alveolar mucosa and the denser alveolar mucosa adjacent to the teeth is the mucogingival junction. The mucogingival junction is visible as the demarcation between the reddish loose mucosa and the pink alveolar mucosa adjacent to the teeth. The attached gingiva extends from the base of the gingival sulcus to the mucogingival junction. (2:929–930; 3:2, 295; 4:36, 325)

64.

D. The palatoglossal muscle forms a mucosal fold anterior to the palatine tonsils. The palatoglossal fold is medial to the palatine tonsils. The palatopharyngeal fold is lateral to the palatine tonsils. (2:936–938; 3:9, 164; 4:245)

answers & rationales

65.

C. A fold of mucous membrane that helps anchor the tongue to the floor of the mouth is the frenulum. Sometimes the lingual frenulum is excessively tight, limiting movement of the tongue. The terms *frenum* and *frenulum* are used interchangeably. (2:941; 3:9–11; 4:37)

66.

D. The styloglossus muscle does not form a part of the floor of the mouth. The styloglossus muscle extends from the styloid process on the skull to the posterior tongue. The styloglossus muscle pulls the tongue backward and upward. (3:98; 4:198, 239; 5:224)

67.

C. Branches of the facial nerve to muscles of the face are enmeshed in the parotid gland. The parotid gland is medial, posterior, and lateral to the neck of the mandible. The facial nerve extends from the stylomastoid foramen laterally around the neck of the mandible through the gland. (1:250, 283–284; 2: 870, 1084–1085; 4:162, 174, 188, 193, 197, 281; 5:250-251)

68.

D. The V-shaped demarcation that separates the anterior two-thirds of the tongue from the posterior one-third is the sulculus terminalis. Along this V-shaped demarcation, the circumvallate papillae are found. The anterior two-thirds and the posterior one-third of the tongue are derived from two different embryological origins. (2:940; 4:37, 238)

69.

C. The infraorbital nerve does not supply the gingiva. The infraorbital nerve supplies the anterior cheek. It also supplies the skin of the nose, lower eyelid, skin, mucosa of the upper lip, and maxillary labial gingiva. (3:194; 4:161, 291)

70.

B. Buccal gingiva of the mandibular molars is innervated by the buccal nerve. The buccal nerve is a branch of the mandibular division of the trigeminal nerve. The trigeminal nerve is the fifth cranial nerve. (2:860–861; 3:192–195; 4:161, 213, 293)

71.

B. Spinal nerves C5 through T1 form the branchial plexus. The branchial plexus is a network of fibers originating from C5 to T1 spinal cord levels. The plexus redivides into nerves that supply the arm and part of the neck. (1:116, 126–128; 4:116, 134–135)

72.

C. The thalamocortical tract is not located within the spinal cord. The thalamocortical tract extends from the thalamus to the cerebral cortex. (1:111–113)

73.

A. The bilateral deep cerebral nuclei located just lateral to the third ventricle are the thalami. The thalami are sites of synapse of ascending sensory neurons with cell bodies of the other nuclei whose processes extend to the postcentral gyri of the cerebral cortex. (1:111–113)

74.

D. The superior and inferior ganglia are associated with the vagus nerve. The superior and inferior ganglia are located within the jugular foramen. The vagus nerve is the tenth cranial nerve. (2:1083–1085; 3:188, 199–200; 4:148–149, 323)

75.

E. The oculomotor, trigeminal, glossopharyngeal, and vagus nerves contain fibers of the parasympathetic division of the autonomic nervous system. Parasympathetic nerves are general visceral efferent fibers. (4:326)

76.

D. The order of blood flow is as follows: the vena cava to the right atrium to the tricuspid valve to the right ventricle to the pulmonary valve to the lungs to the left atrium to the mitral valve to the left ventricle to the aortic valve to the aorta. The one-way flow of blood through the heart is ensured by the pattern of contraction of the atria and ventricles and by the placement of the valves. (1:178)

77.

C. The foramen ovale is not associated with the ventricles of the heart. The foramen ovale is an opening in the septum between the atria in fetal life. It closes at birth and forms a solid partition between these chambers. (1:177)

78.

B. The right common carotid artery does not branch off the aorta. The right common carotid artery is a branch of the brachiocephalic trunk. The left common carotid artery branches directly off the aorta. (1:177–182; 3:171; 4:141, 195, 319)

79.

E. The route of the blood supply to the right side of the face is the left ventricle to the aorta, brachiocephalic trunk, common carotid artery, external carotid artery, and the facial artery. The brachiocephalic trunk branches off the aorta side only to divide into the subclavian and common carotid arteries. (1:177–182)

3 Biomaterials

DIRECTIONS
Each of the questions below is followed by several suggested answers. Select the best answer in each case.

1. Diagnostic casts made from alginate impressions are used routinely for all of the following reasons EXCEPT
    A. to determine occlusion
    B. as the cast used to fabricate a fixed partial denture
    C. to present a treatment plan to the patient
    D. to compare with subsequent models

2. The two principal methods of forming metallic objects used in dentistry are
    A. cast and wrought
    B. stamped and forged
    C. distilled and cast
    D. wrought and synthetic

3. The three methods of inducing a polymerization reaction in dentistry include all of the following EXCEPT
    A. light curing
    B. radioactive curing

C. heat curing

D. self-curing

4. Pit and fissure sealants represent a trade-off with composite resins in terms of physical and mechanical properties. In order to get the viscosity low enough to flow into the pits and fissures of teeth, what characteristic must be sacrificed?

A. color stability

B. strength

C. the ability to use a light gun to cure it

D. the ability to use it on primary teeth

5. The resistance to flowing demonstrated by a fluid is known as

A. thickness ratio

B. viscosity

C. polymerization

D. liquid density

6. What do pit and fissure sealants, composite resins, acrylic appliances, and elastomeric impression materials have in common?

A. They are all polymers.

B. They all have to be heated before using.

C. They can all be used as anterior filling materials.

D. They are all products of secondary reactions.

7. Placing a base in the "bottom" of a cavity preparation serves what purpose?

A. It helps hold the restoration in place.

B. It helps insulate the pulpal tissue from the external environment.

C. It kills any residual bacteria.

D. It serves to add bulk to the cavity preparation.

8. Which of the following acts as an electrolyte in conjunction with a metal restoration to make up an electric cell and cause galvanism?

A. bone

B. enamel

C. dentin

D. saliva

9. The brief but sharp electrical sensation one can receive when two dissimilar metals come into contact in the mouth is called

A. galvanic shock

B. alternating current corrosion

C. electrolyte explosion

D. electromagnetic pulse

10. Which of the following dental materials is a poor thermal conductor?

A. gold crowns

B. amalgam

C. composite resins

D. gold foil restorations

11. All of the following are primary factors when considering the ideal restorative material EXCEPT

A. sustaining biting forces

B. resistance to abrasion

C. adaptability to the walls of the cavity

D. indestructibility in the fluids of the mouth

E. color

12. One should approach the subject of dental materials from the standpoint of

A. what the material is chemically

B. what happens to the material physically

C. how the material is manipulated technically

D. all of the above

13. The preferred method for altering the gelation period of an alginate impression material is to change the
    A. water–powder ratio
    B. temperature of the water
    C. spatulation time of a mix
    D. quantity of the reactor in the powder
    E. quantity of the retarder in the powder

14. A complex set of chemical reactions that can weaken and eventually destroy a metal is called
    A. tarnish
    B. rust
    C. hydrogen depletion
    D. corrosion

15. The delayed expansion or secondary expansion that some zinc-containing amalgams exhibit for many months after their placement is thought to result from
    A. poor quality control at the factory
    B. moisture contamination during placement
    C. overtrituration
    D. mercury allergy in the patient

16. An increase in the temperature of the water used in mixing irreversible hydrocolloids will
    A. prevent setting
    B. shorten time to set
    C. lengthen time to set
    D. not affect time to set

17. What component of many cements has a definite soothing property on pulpal tissue?
    A. zinc oxide
    B. methyl methacrylate
    C. bis-GMA
    D. eugenol

18. The chief difference between model plaster powder and dental stone powder is
    A. shelf life
    B. chemical formula
    C. solubility in water
    D. particle size and shape

19. On a percentage basis, the main ingredient of a reversible hydrocolloid is
    A. water
    B. agar-agar
    C. calcium alginate
    D. potassium sulfate

20. The safety of the interaction of dental materials and tissue in the oral cavity (as well as the rest of the body) is assessed in studies grouped under the heading of
    A. radioactivity studies
    B. biocompatibility
    C. carcinogenic potential
    D. antigenic potential

21. There are several disadvantages associated with use of base metal dental casting alloys. Which of the following is an advantage that base metal alloys have over the noble metal alloys?
    A. Base metal is easier to cast and finish.
    B. Base metal has a stronger porcelain bond.
    C. Base metal is much heavier (denser) than noble metal alloys.
    D. Base metal is stronger and thus more suited to long-span fixed bridges.

22. Which of the following would NOT be a likely test used to assay a material's biocompatibility?
    A. toxicity test using bacterial cultures
    B. pulp response using extracted human teeth

C. carcinogenic potential using mice

D. antigenic potential using rabbits

23. What purpose does acid etching serve in the application of pit and fissure sealants and composite resins?

A. It kills bacteria.

B. It puts a glaze over the tooth.

C. It increases the surface area available for sealant/composite bonding.

D. It provides activation molecules to start the chemical reaction.

24. What appearance does a properly acid-etched surface have?

A. slightly pink with a definite shine

B. dull white and chalky

C. somewhat gray in color

D. identical to natural dentition

25. Which of the following is NOT true concerning dental porcelain?

A. Dental porcelains are ground glass with small amounts of tooth-colored paints added.

B. Many porcelains rust at a temperature of over 2000°F.

C. The glaze firing is the last firing and it produces a smooth, translucent surface.

D. Dental porcelain has good biocompatibility, but is very brittle.

26. If an acid-etched surface is contaminated with saliva, you can correct it by blowing a high volume of dry air over it for 15 seconds.

A. true

B. true if the air is completely dry

C. true, but this air may upset the setting of the following restorative material

D. false

27. If an alginate impression cannot be poured immediately, what must be done?

A. The impression must be heated to body temperature for 15 minutes.

B. The impression must be placed in a bowl of very cold water.

C. The impression must be immersed in a solution of 15% calcium sulfate for 10 minutes.

D. The impression must be kept in an environment of 100% relative humidity, such as in damp paper towels or a humidor.

28. If the dental amalgam alloy particles and mercury are undertriturated, the resulting amalgam restoration may

A. contract

B. dissolve

C. fracture

D. liberate heat

29. Of the factors that influence the physical properties of a silver amalgam restoration, which is the MOST likely to cause delayed expansion?

A. moisture contamination

B. overtrituration of amalgam

C. too much mercury in the mix

D. inadequate condensing pressures

30. Which of the following is the MOST accurate definition for the term amalgam?

A. the metallic substance, supplied in the form of fillings, which is mixed with mercury

B. a metallic substance composed of two or more metals that are mutually soluble in a molten state

C. an alloy of two or more metals, one of which is mercury

D. a metallic substance composed of silver, copper, zinc, and tin

31. Which of the following does NOT contribute to the expansion of an amalgam restoration?
    A. overtrituration
    B. smaller percentage of tin in the alloy
    C. excess mercury present in the alloy
    D. greater percentage of silver in the alloy

32. Which of the following is the BEST definition of an alloy?
    A. a metal at room temperature
    B. a mixture of two or more metals
    C. a pure compound that is metallic
    D. a metal containing mercury

33. The process of mixing an amalgam is known as
    A. amalgamation
    B. condensation
    C. trituration
    D. carving

34. The forcing of the plastic mass into the prepared cavity is known as
    A. condensation
    B. trituration
    C. amalgamation
    D. homogenization

35. Which of the following sequences is proper when considering the placement of an amalgam alloy?
    A. condensation, carving, trituration
    B. carving, trituration, condensation
    C. carving, condensation, trituration
    D. trituration, condensation, carving

36. Excessive mercury in the amalgam
    A. causes increased expansion
    B. causes decreased expansion
    C. has no effect on expansion

37. Glass ionomer restorative materials have been developed by combining the technology of two other dental materials. These are
    A. silicates and bis-GMA resins
    B. zinc phosphate cements and bis-GMA resins
    C. silicates and zinc polyacrylates (polycarboxylates)
    D. silicones and polyethers

38. Amalgam for tooth restoration was introduced into this country during the early
    A. 20th century
    B. 19th century
    C. 18th century
    D. 16th century

39. Which of the following groups of metallic elements would be called precious or noble for their ability to resist corrosion?
    A. gold, silver, and platinum
    B. silver, copper, and mercury
    C. silver, gold, and annealed copper-ruthenium
    D. copper, palladium, and silver

40. Direct placement resins for anterior teeth are available in filled and unfilled versions. To what does filled refer?
    A. The material expands slightly on setting and fills the cavity completely.
    B. An inert filler is present in the resin.
    C. The dispensing containers were filled at the factory.
    D. Filled is a term used by the manufacturer to imply the resin is not synthetic.

41. The principal purpose of trituration is to
    A. coat the alloy particles with mercury
    B. dissolve all the alloy particles in the mercury
    C. reduce the size of the crystals as rapidly as they form
    D. reduce the size of the original alloy particles as much as possible

42. All elastomeric impression materials
    A. contract slightly during curing
    B. expand slightly during curing
    C. contract initially and then expand during curing
    D. expand initially and then contract during curing

43. Several polymer systems are used in dentistry. Which of the following systems is used MOST frequently?
    A. methyl methacrylate
    B. bis-GMA
    C. polyether
    D. polyvinyl

44. A disadvantage of acrylic resin as a dental restorative material is
    A. poor initial esthetics
    B. high insolubility in saliva
    C. high modulus in elasticity
    D. high thermal coefficient of expansion

45. Some impression materials are most accurate when at least 3 mm of space is present between the impression tray and the oral tissue. Which of the following impression material types shows this characteristic?
    A. irreversible hydrocolloids
    B. polyethers
    C. polymethacrylates
    D. polysulfides

46. Which of the following terms describes one aspect of the polymerization reaction of methyl methacrylate?
    A. isotopic
    B. ionic
    C. covalent ion exchange
    D. exothermic

47. The powder used in mixing acrylic resin is referred to as the
    A. monomer
    B. dimer
    C. polymer
    D. initiator

48. One failing of many dental restorative materials is their inability to completely seal out the external environment. The process by which fluids, microorganisms, and debris from the oral cavity penetrate between the tooth and the restoration is known as
    A. syneresis
    B. microleakage
    C. imbibition
    D. trans-ionic transfer

49. Direct placement resins harden by two methods. What are these?
    A. autopolymerization and self-curing
    B. cold-curing and self-curing
    C. autopolymerization and light-initiated polymerization
    D. heat cure and cold cure

50. The characteristic exhibited by gold of being able to be pulled into a long thin wire is an example of
    A. casting
    B. case hardening
    C. reverse ionic transfer
    D. ductility

51. The main purpose of adding copper to an amalgam alloy is to
    A. increase the silver-tin phase
    B. increase the silver-mercury phase
    C. increase the tin-mercury phase
    D. decrease the tin-mercury phase

52. The primary property that causes the composites in a Class II restoration to fail is
    A. low abrasive resistance
    B. high flow
    C. low compressive strength
    D. marginal percolation

53. Zinc phosphate cement powder is composed chiefly of
    A. zirconium
    B. zinc oxide
    C. zinc stearate
    D. zinc carbonate

54. A glass slab should be cooled when mixing zinc phosphate cement to
    A. maintain free zinc oxide in the set cement
    B. maintain the proper acid–water ratio
    C. accelerate the setting time
    D. increase the powder–liquid ratio

55. The frozen-slab method of mixing zinc phosphate cement has which of the following advantages?
    A. It significantly increases the ultimate compressive strength and increases the setting time.
    B. It increases the working time but decreases the setting time once placed in the mouth.
    C. It decreases the working time but increases the setting time once placed in the mouth.
    D. It significantly improves the film thickness and ultimate compressive strength.

56. Zinc phosphate cement liquid that has lost some of its water content will affect the mix in that the
    A. setting time will be lengthened
    B. setting time will be accelerated
    C. film thickness will be increased
    D. viscosity of the mix will be increased

57. The setting time of a zinc oxide-eugenol impression paste may BEST be accelerated by
    A. increasing the amount of eugenol
    B. adding a drop of water to the mix
    C. chilling the mixing slab and spatula
    D. adding a drop of oleic acid to the mix

58. Color can be described in terms of three standard components. Which of the following is NOT a standard component used to describe a color?
    A. hue
    B. intensity
    C. chroma
    D. value

59. Which of the following is NOT a characteristic of polysulfide rubber impression materials?
    A. They have a strong odor.
    B. They have a short setting time.
    C. They deform readily when removed from undercut areas.
    D. They have a good tear resistance.

60. One beneficial feature of the zinc polyacrylate (polycarboxylate) cements over zinc phosphate cements is that
    A. The zinc polyacrylates provide some true adhesion by a chelation between calcium and carboxylate groups.
    B. The zinc polyacrylates have a much lower film thickness.
    C. The zinc polyacrylates have a significantly greater compressive strength.
    D. The zinc polyacrylates stimulate the formation of secondary dentin.

61. Mixing zinc phosphate cement very rapidly will
    A. have no effect on the final compressive strength of the cement
    B. decrease the final compressive strength of the cement
    C. increase the final compressive strength of the cement
    D. produce an endothermic reaction

62. Zinc phosphate cement, upon setting, will
    A. shrink slightly
    B. expand slightly
    C. neither shrink nor expand

63. The MOST effective dental cement in stimulating the growth of reparative dentin is
    A. zinc phosphate cement
    B. calcium hydroxide cement
    C. zinc silicophosphate cement
    D. carboxylate cement

64. In a technical sense, which of the following materials is the MOST recyclable?
    A. polymethyl methacrylate
    B. dental stone
    C. polysulfide impression materials
    D. polyether impression materials

65. There are four types of gypsum products approved for use in dentistry. Which of the following types is NOT used today?
    A. Type I impression plaster
    B. Type II model plaster
    C. Type III dental stone
    D. Type IV die stone

66. Why is dental stone vibrated after mixing?
    A. The mixing is not uniform and vibration completes the mixing.
    B. The vibration shakes up any remaining particles.
    C. The vibration makes the mixture more dense by removing any trapped air pockets.
    D. The vibration halts the reaction and allows extended pouring times.

67. Modern high-copper dental amalgam alloys generally demonstrate improved physical properties when the
    A. gamma II phase is increased
    B. gamma II phase is decreased
    C. gamma phase is decreased
    D. gamma III phase is increased
    E. gamma III phase is decreased

68. Which of the following metals contributes to the corrosion resistance of a dental casting gold alloy?
    A. zinc
    B. gold
    C. nickel
    D. copper

69. Which of the following alloys is MOST likely to make appliances of the same dimension most rigid?
    A. wrought gold
    B. cobalt–chromium
    C. palladium (white gold)
    D. partial denture cast gold

70. If a topical fluoride is to be used in conjunction with a pit and fissure sealant, which sequence is used?
    A. Fluoride before sealant.
    B. Fluoride should not be used.
    C. Fluoride after sealant.
    D. It doesn't make any difference.

71. Which of the following is NOT a criterion for electing to use a pit and fissure sealant on a patient?

    A. caries susceptibility

    B. caries activity

    C. length of time tooth has remained caries-free

    D. knowing that orthodontics will be started soon

72. Which of the following types of compounds are MOST commonly used as a pit and fissure sealant?

    A. cyanoacrylate resins

    B. polyurethane resins

    C. bis-GMA resins

    D. poly(methyl methacrylate) resins

73. Inhibitors are added to the monomer of the denture base resins to

    A. activate the monomer

    B. increase shelf life

    C. speed up the reaction

    D. produce a softer polymer

74. In mixing dental stone, why should the powder be sprinkled onto the water in the bowl?

    A. This process results in better powder mixing and reduced chance for air bubbles.

    B. The powder is added to the water to avoid using more than one bowl.

    C. The addition of powder last prevents the mix from becoming exothermic.

    D. This is not recommended; the water should be added to the powder.

75. Plasticizers are sometimes added to denture base resin to

    A. produce a softer final polymer

    B. cause an opaque material

    C. eliminate oxidative decomposition

    D. speed up the peroxide decomposition

76. Dental acrylic resin is a

    A. natural thermoset resin

    B. synthetic thermoset resin

    C. natural thermoplastic resin

    D. synthetic thermoplastic resin

77. Which of the following properties contributes greatly to the strength of a polymer?

    A. covalent addition

    B. biochemical adhesion

    C. cross-linking

78. A cause of localized porosity positioned sporadically (not just in the thickest parts) on the surface of or within the structure of a cured acrylic denture results from

    A. the monomer not being diffused homogeneously throughout the resin dough before curing

    B. use of acrylic resin of sticky consistency for packing the denture mold

    C. insufficient pressure on the acrylic resin in the denture mold

    D. use of only a boiling water bath for curing purposes

79. The use of composite resins in posterior teeth should be approached with caution. Which of the following reasons BEST explains why this is true?

    A. Posterior composites can cause corrosive breakdown of crowns and bridges.

    B. Posterior composites, when next to amalgams, can accelerate mercury release.

    C. Posterior composites do not have suitable physical and mechanical properties for use in posterior teeth.

    D. All of the above.

80. The single MOST important development in the reduction of atmospheric mercury found in dental offices is
    A. the development of the gamma II phase
    B. high copper amalgams
    C. the introduction of pre-encapsulated amalgam alloys
    D. the high speed triturator

81. The cast chromium–cobalt alloy used for removable partial dentures has many advantages. Which of the following properties is NOT an advantage of this alloy system?
    A. low specific gravity
    B. high flexibility
    C. corrosion resistance
    D. high strength

82. The denture base resins should have which of the following physical properties?
    A. adequate strength
    B. satisfactory thermal properties
    C. low specific gravity
    D. all of the above

83. In general, what is the difference between precious metals and nonprecious metals that makes precious metals so desirable for intraoral use?
    A. their cost
    B. the inherent corrosion resistance
    C. the low specific gravity
    D. the high melting point

84. Proper monitoring of oral hygiene around implants is absolutely imperative. Which of the following reasons BEST explains why?
    A. Plaque around the implant could cause corrosion, leading to failure of the implant from metal fatigue.
    B. Improper brushing techniques could lead to calculus buildup on the implant.
    C. Because there is no direct connective tissue attachment, the potential for infection is high.
    D. There are no special precautions used to clean implants because they are not real teeth.

85. In casting a restoration for a patient, the proper sequence of events is
    A. cast, wax, polish, invest, burn out
    B. polish, wax, invest, burn out, cast
    C. wax, invest, burn out, cast, polish
    D. invest, wax, cast, burn out, polish

86. After an alloy is cast for a dental restoration, a surface oxide must often be removed prior to polishing the restoration. This process is known as
    A. investing
    B. pickling
    C. flux addition
    D. passivation

87. One disadvantage of dental porcelain restorations is
    A. brittleness
    B. matching tooth color
    C. expansion
    D. radioactivity

88. Which of the following is true concerning the first application of dental porcelain to a restoration?
    A. The first layer is called body and is very translucent.
    B. The first layer is called incisal and provides a stable substrate for additional layers.
    C. The first layer is called glaze and provides reduction of surface oxides on the metal casting.
    D. The first layer is called opaque and effectively covers the metallic sheen of the underlying casting.

89. Which of the following agents is used as both a cement and a restorative agent?
    A. zinc oxide–eugenol
    B. zinc phosphate
    C. silicates
    D. glass ionomer

90. When a material has stresses and resulting strains that are in proportion to each other, it is obeying
    A. Hooke's Law
    B. covalent-ionic equations
    C. stress-induced fatigue
    D. elongation ductility

91. Which of the following does NOT involve a polymerization reaction?
    A. the setting of amalgam
    B. the curing of a denture
    C. making an impression using rubber-base material
    D. cementing a crown

92. Considering the different stages in a polymerization reaction, most of the reaction takes place during the
    A. initiation stage
    B. propagation stage
    C. cross-link stage
    D. termination stage

93. The constituent that contributes the tarnish resistance to a chrome–cobalt alloy is
    A. carbon
    B. cobalt
    C. chromium
    D. nickel

94. Most polymerization reactions are one of two types. They are
    A. free-radical and heat cure
    B. cross-link and condensation
    C. cross-link and chain-lengthening
    D. addition and condensation

95. The chemical resistance of the stainless steels is due largely to the presence of
    A. chromium
    B. cobalt
    C. nickel
    D. carbon

96. The 18-8 stainless steel indicates that the composition includes
    A. 18% cobalt and 8% nickel
    B. 18 parts chromium and 8 parts nickel, in 56 total parts
    C. 18% chromium and 8% nickel
    D. 18% chromium and 8% cobalt

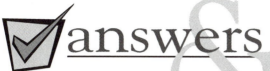
answers
& rationales

1.

B. Diagnostic casts can be made of the patient's mouth to study the dentition and to educate the patient. At the time the casts are made, the patient will be interested in seeing the arrangement of the teeth. Tooth form and arrangement of the dentition can be observed. These casts are not of sufficient precision to allow fabrication of fixed dental prostheses. (1:52–54, 67–73)

2.

A. Casting involves heating a metal until molten and pouring or forcing it into a mold for it to harden. Some metals that are not brittle can be formed into useful shapes by the use of mechanical forces, such as rolling or wire drawing. Inlays, crowns, bridges, and partial denture frameworks are usually cast, while wires and most orthodontic appliances are wrought. (1:151–157)

3.

B. No polymers in dentistry use radioactive materials to effect the polymerization reaction. Heat curing is most commonly used for denture base resins, while light-cured and self-curing resins have many dental applications. (1:108, 120)

4.

B. The strength of a sealant is sacrificed in order to make it flow into the pits and fissures. Sealants are completely unfilled, making them weak as compared to composites. This is the primary reason that sealants that are left high in occlusion usually come out quickly. (1:136–137)

5.

B. Viscosity is a term describing how well a liquid flows under pressure. With water being given a value of 1.0, most dental liquids have a viscosity reading in the tens of thousands. The manufacturers of cements and cavity liners strive for low viscosity in their products, as long as they maintain their other physical properties. (3:77–79)

6.

A. All of the items listed are polymers. They all have long chains of identical repeating units known as "mers." (1:102–103)

7.

B. A base is used to provide thermal insulation to protect the pulp. This is especially important in metallic restorations on the posterior teeth, as they conduct temperature well. (1:12)

8.

D. A cause for sensitivity is the small currents created whenever two metals are present in the oral cavity. Because both restorations are wet with saliva, a small battery exists between the two metallic restorations. When the two restorations touch during mastication, the current produced by the battery may irritate the pulp and produce a sharp pain. These currents are referred to as galvanic currents. (3:46–47)

9.

A. Galvanic shock is a type of electrical short circuit that can occur in the mouth. It usually involves two different metallic restorations that are not normally in contact. The amount of electricity involved in galvanic shock can range up to 1.0 microamperes and 500 millivolts. (3:46–47)

10.

C. Composite resins, as a group, are poor thermal conductors. Metals, as a group, are excellent thermal conductors. (1:32)

11.

E. The properties of restorative materials that are of primary importance are: 1) indestructibility in the fluids of the mouth, 2) adaptability to the walls of the cavity, 3) freedom from shrinkage or expansion following placement in the cavity form, 4) resistance to attrition, and 5) sustaining power against the force of mastication. Properties of restorative materials of secondary importance are: 1) color or appearance, 2) low thermal conductivity, 3) convenience of manipulation, and 4) resistance to tarnish and corrosion. (1:14–39)

12.

D. One should approach the subject of dental materials from the point of view of determining what the material is chemically, why it behaves as it does physically and mechanically, and how it is manipulated technically to develop the most satisfactory properties. (1:4–5)

13.

B. The setting time of alginate impression material can be altered by changing the water–powder ratio or the mixing time. Neither of these methods is recommended, however, because slight deviations in proportions or mixing time can diminish certain properties of the gel. If gelation time is to be altered, the best method is to vary the temperature of the water used in making the mix. The higher the water temperature, the shorter the gelation time. (2:146-152)

14.

D. Tarnish is a very mild form of corrosion that usually involves a loss of luster on the surface of a metal and is often associated with some surface deposit. Rust is a type of corrosion most often involving the oxidation of iron. Corrosion is a very complex phenomenon involving not only the metal structure, but also the environment in which the metal is placed. (3:49)

15.

B. Moisture contamination is to be avoided in all amalgam placements, but zinc-containing amalgams are especially sensitive to moisture. The actual chemical reaction is not fully understood, but apparently, the offending element is zinc. This delayed expansion takes place over several months and can result in expansion of up to 4%. (3:234)

16.

B. If gelation time of the alginate is to be altered, the best method is to vary the temperature of the water used in making the mix. The higher the water temperature, the shorter the gelation time. (2:146–152)

17.

D. Eugenol, a natural plant oil, is an important component of the zinc oxide–eugenol cements that are used to cement the temporary restorations on teeth during the period between tooth preparation and final restoration seating. (2:123–125)

18.

D. Plaster, stone, and improved stone are made up of hemihydrate particles whose size, shape, and porosity differ for each material. These physical differences in the hemihydrate particles are the basic factors that determine the manipulative conditions for mixing the particles and the properties and usage of the hardened gypsum product. (1:40–56)

19.

A. While the basic constituent of reversible hydrocolloid impression materials is agar-agar, present in a concentration of 8 to 15%, the principal ingredient by weight (approximately 80 to 85%) is water. (1:67–73)

20.

B. Biocompatibility is a broad term used to describe how safe a material is. The potential for cancer or allergy are just two types of tests performed. The American Dental Association and the U.S. Food and Drug Administration have responsibility for assessing a material's safety. (3:141–177)

21.

D. While base metal dental casting alloys are very sensitive in terms of the techniques used to cast, finish, and apply porcelain, they are quite strong. Many noble metal alloys are not suited for a long-span fixed bridge (from a mechanical standpoint) due to a tendency to flex under loading, which could pop the porcelain off. Base metal alloy advantages are principally found only in their strength and low density. (1:191–202; 2:222–223, 230)

22.

B. While pulpal response is an important aspect of the biocompatibility of dental materials, the testing must be on intact teeth in a living subject. If the safety of the product has been established, human subjects are often used; if not, monkeys are appropriate. Because it uses living teeth, pulpal response is usually one of the last tests performed; all toxicity tests must have been performed prior to this. (3:141–177)

23.

C. Acid etching preferentially dissolves part of the enamel matrix of the tooth, making for a surface that is very rough microscopically. This produces a greatly increased surface area over which the sealant or composite can bind, which improves the strength of the attachment. (1:130–131)

24.

B. A properly acid-etched surface has a distinctive appearance of dull white and chalky. Any other appearance is an indication that the acid etching has been contaminated and must be reapplied. (1:130–131)

25.

A. Dental porcelain is a mixture of feldspar and quartz. These two materials have extremely high (over 2000°F) fusing temperatures—much higher than that of glass. Metallic oxides are used to impart the proper shade to the porcelain. Paints would decompose at such temperatures. (1:227–229)

26.

D. The only remedy for a contaminated acid-etched surface is to completely re-etch. (1:131)

27.

D. Alginate impressions are very susceptible to loss of water, which has a drastic effect on the accuracy of the resulting cast. While it is best to pour an alginate impression immediately, it may be held for approximately 30 minutes in a humid atmosphere such as damp paper towels or a humidor. (1:72)

28.

C. The undermixed (undertriturated) mass is crumbly and not convenient to manipulate during insertion. It is dull in appearance and shows a slight increase in expansion. Of greater importance is the reduction in strength observed in undermixed amalgams. (1:180–183)

29.

A. Moisture contamination of the amalgam mass from any source will result in an excessive delayed expansion after the restoration has been placed for several hours or days. (3:234)

30.

C. Any alloy containing mercury is called an amalgam. (1:165)

31.

A. The overmixed mass exhibits reduced expansion. The overmixed mass may be considered synonymous with an overworked mass. (1:180–183)

32.

B. An alloy is defined as a mixture of two or more metals. A related definition is that an alloy containing mercury is an amalgam. (1:141)

33.

C. An alloy, known as the amalgam alloy, is made by the manufacturer and generally is cut into small particles or filings. The mixing of these particles with mercury is known as trituration. (1:165, 180–183)

34.

A. The dentist forces the plastic mass into the cavity preparation by condensation, using specially designed instruments. (1:183–184)

35.

D. The amalgam is mixed (trituration), then placed in the cavity (condensation), and then is formed to duplicate the anatomy lost (carving). (1:165)

36.

A. Excess mercury retained in the amalgam restoration leads to additional reaction expansion and a loss of strength in the restoration. (1:178–180)

37.

C. The favorable properties of both silicates and polyacrylates are demonstrated by the glass ionomer restoratives. Dissolution of the material liberates fluoride ions, which impart a degree of caries resistance to the tooth, and the presence of polyacrylic acid provides for a chelation reaction between the ionomer mix and the calcium on the surface of the tooth structure, producing adhesion. (1:239–245)

38.

B. Amalgam for the restoration of tooth tissue is reported to have been first used in 1826 in France in the form of a silver–mercury paste. Soon afterward, in 1833, it was introduced into the United States. (1:164)

39.

A. There are five elements generally regarded as members of the precious metal group: gold, silver, palladium, platinum, and ruthenium. Of these, the first four have significant dental uses. (1:195)

40.

B. An inert filler is present in the matrix of the resin to modify the mechanical properties of the resin. The presence of filler makes the resin a composite resin, meaning that the resin is a blend of filler and resin. Composite resins have been so successful that unfilled resins are rarely used. (1:119)

41.

A. The object of trituration is to bring about an amalgamation of the mercury and alloy. Each individual alloy particle is coated with a slight film of oxide that prevents penetration by the mercury. During trituration, this film is rubbed off and the clean metal is then readily attacked by the mercury. (1:180–183)

42.

A. Setting contraction of all rubber impression materials is a consistent dimensional change. These changes have been measured both directly and indirectly. (3:283–285)

43.

A. The methyl methacrylate system is the one used most frequently in dentistry. It is used in denture bases, denture teeth, custom impression trays, temporary restorations, and mouth splints. The bis-GMA system, while used for composite resin restorations and sealants, is a distant second. (1:106, 107, 119, 128)

44.

D. Ideal dental restorative materials should have a coefficient of thermal expansion similar to enamel (very low). Those with high coefficients often leak at the margins. (3:43)

45.

A. Irreversible hydrocolloid (alginate) is most accurate when at least 3 mm of space exists between the impression tray and the tissue. The other impression material types are most accurate when a small but definite space exists between the impression tray and the tissue. (1:68–73)

46.

D. The polymerization of methyl methacrylate is exothermic, meaning that heat is given off by the reaction. Neither ionic nor covalent is appropriate, as the reaction proceeds by the free radical (not charges) mechanism. (1:108)

47.

C. The methyl methacrylate system often comes as a powder and liquid. The powder is composed primarily of beads of prepolymerized methacrylate. (1:107–108)

48.

B. Currently, no dental material completely and permanently seals out the oral environment. (1:8–9)

49.

C. Autopolymerizing resins begin to set shortly after the two components are mixed together. Light-cured resins are already mixed together but will not begin to set until a bright light is placed close to the resin to initiate the polymerization reaction. Auto-cure, cold-cure, and self-cure are synonyms. (2:61)

50.

D. The ability to form a wire from a metal is ductility. A related term is malleability, which describes a metal being able to be hammered into a thin sheet without rupture. (1:27)

51.

D. Copper combines with the tin, preventing the formation of the tin–mercury phase (gamma II), which is the most corrosive and weakest phase. (1:170–172)

52.

A. The lack of resistance to wear appears to be the greatest deterrent to the use of composite resins in stress-bearing restorations, even though their superior aesthetics and low thermal conductivity are advantages when compared to amalgam. (2:59-60, 62)

53.

B. Zinc phosphate cement powders consist primarily of calcined zinc oxide and magnesium oxide in the approximate ratio of 9 to 1. (1:258–259)

54.

D. A cool mixing slab should be employed. The temperature of the slab should not be below the dew point of the room; however, the cool slab delays the setting and allows the operator to incorporate the maximal amount of powder before the crystallization proceeds to a point at which the mixture stiffens. (3:182)

55.

B. The advantages of the frozen-slab method are a substantial increase in the working time of the mix on the slab and a shorter setting time of the mix after placement in the mouth. Compressive and tensile strengths of cements prepared by the frozen-slab method are not significantly different from those prepared from normal mixes. Film thickness is not altered. (3:182)

56.

A. The addition of water to the liquid shortens the setting time and a concentration of the liquid prolongs it. (2:122–123)

57.

B. The addition of a drop of water or alcohol when mixing will speed the set. The setting can be slowed by the addition of inert oils, such as olive oil, mineral oil, or petroleum, during mixing. (2:125)

58.

B. The three standard descriptions of color are hue, chroma, and value. Intensity is not used, but instead is included in the term *value*. (1:34–36)

59.

B. The setting time of polysulfide rubber impression materials is long (from 20 minutes) after placement in the mouth. The odor and ability to stain clothing require caution when using these materials. The presence of undercuts in the patient should be cause to use another material. (2:163–165)

60.

A. One advantage of the zinc polyacrylate cements is the adhesion to enamel and dentin, which is attributed to the ability of the carboxylate groups in the polymer molecule to chelate to calcium. (1:266–268)

61.

B. A proper mixing technique assures a greater powder–liquid ratio for the consistency of cement desired, and this increases the compressive strength of the cement mass. Ninety seconds of mixing appears to be an adequate length of time to accomplish a proper zinc phosphate cementing mass. (1:264–265)

62.

A. Zinc phosphate cements shrink slightly during setting. The cement shrinks much more when it is in contact with air than when it is under water. Thus, the cement should not be allowed to dry out. (1:266–267)

63.

B. A cement material used for capping the pulp of a tooth unavoidably exposed during a dental operation is calcium hydroxide. It is generally believed that the calcium hydroxide tends to accelerate the formation of secondary reparative dentin over the exposed pulp. Secondary dentin is an effective barrier to further irritants. Usually, the thicker the reparative dentin between the floor of the cavity and the pulp, the better is the protection from chemical and physical trauma. (1:236–237)

64.

B. Dental stone is the most recyclable material as its setting is a hydration reaction, which means to reuse it you could grind it up and place it in an oven to drive off the water. The other materials are set in such a way that reuse is not feasible. (1:43–44)

65.

A. Type I dental impression plaster is not used at all today due to the tremendous improvement in other impression-making systems. (1:40–43)

66.

C. As the stone is mixed, air bubbles are incorporated into the mix. Vibration forces the air bubbles (which are less dense) to the surface of the mixture, making the entire mix more dense. (1:49)

67.

B. The gamma II phase (tin–mercury) is decreased in most high-copper modern amalgam restorations. The copper reacts with the tin and prevents formation of the gamma II phase (which demonstrates the most creep and is the weakest and most corrosive phase). (1:170–172)

68.

B. The chief contribution of gold is to increase the tarnish resistance of the alloy. The tarnish resistance is in almost direct proportion to the gold content where the gold is combined with base metals. It has been estimated that the gold content of a successful dental gold alloy should be at least 75% by weight in order to resist tarnish in the mouth. (1:194–195)

69.

B. The modulus of elasticity of the cobalt–chromium alloys is approximately twice that of the Type IV (partial denture) casting gold alloys. Consequently, it can be expected that cobalt–chromium dental appliances may be stiffer than those made from gold alloys. (2:22–23)

70.

C. Sealants should be applied first. If fluoride is applied first, the efficiency of the acid etching is diminished. (3:270–274)

71.

D. A patient's beginning orthodontic treatment should not have an effect on the decision of whether or not to use pit and fissure sealants. (3:270–274)

72.

C. While all four systems have been used, virtually all systems today use the bis-GMA system. (3:270, 274)

73.

B. The liquid is methyl methacrylate. A small amount of an inhibitor such as hydroquinone is usually present to aid in preventing polymerization of the monomer during storage. (3:135)

74.

A. The physical and mechanical properties of dental stones are greatly reduced when the water–powder ratio is inaccurate or when air bubbles are trapped in the mix; thus, all avenues to produce a consistent mix are employed. (1:44–47)

75.

A. Plasticizers are sometimes added to the monomer of a denture base resin to produce a softer, more resilient final polymer. They are generally relatively low-molecular-weight esters. (2:142, 260, 263)

76.

D. Synthetic resins are usually molded under heat and pressure. If the resin is molded without a chemical change occurring, as by softening it under heat and pressure and then by cooling it to form a solid, it is classified as thermoplastic. (1:101–102)

77.

C. Cross-linking, the chemical attachment of one polymer strand to another, greatly increases the physical and mechanical properties of a polymer. (1:105–106)

78.

A. A cause of porosity in an acrylic denture base is a lack of homogeneity in the dough or gel at the time of polymerization. It is probable that some regions will contain more monomer than others; these regions will shrink more during polymerization than the adjacent regions, and such a localized shrink will tend to produce voids. Porosity in the thickest portions is due to too rapid a heating rate early in the curing process, boiling the monomer. (2:258–259)

79.

C. Although research is very active in this area, composites are still too weak for widespread use in posterior teeth. Also, they are very difficult to place and contour properly. Class II cavity preparations are especially difficult to place due to inability to maintain dryness in the proximal box. (2:1–2, 60)

80.

C. The pre-encapsulated amalgam alloy capsules greatly reduce exposure to elemental mercury. A spill of bulk mercury in an office is a serious problem requiring specialized equipment to properly contain it. (1:187–190)

81.

B. Chromium–cobalt alloys are quite inflexible. They have essentially no ductility or malleability after they are cast. All of the other properties seen in the question are advantages of chromium–cobalt alloys. (1:199)

82.

D. A number of authors have listed the optimum properties of a denture base resin. The following desirable qualities indicate the wide variety of requirements; the order in which these properties are listed does not represent their relative importance: 1) adequate strength characteristics; 2) satisfactory thermal properties; 3) dimensional stability in or out of oral fluids; 4) low specific gravity; 5) good chemical stability; 6) insolubility in and low sorption of fluids present; 7) absence of taste, odor, and oral tissues; 8) natural appearance; 9) stability of color and translucency; 10) reasonable adhesion to other plastics; 11) ease and accuracy in fabrication and repair; and 12) moderate cost. (2:263–265)

83.

B. Precious metals as a group exhibit excellent corrosion resistance. Base metal alloys depend on a thin layer of corrosion products on the surface (called a passivation layer) for corrosion resistance. (1:194–195)

84.

C. Any infection resulting from improper cleaning in this area could migrate down the implant toward the bone. This infection could have results ranging from simple implant failure to a life-threatening infection for the patient. Assurance that the patient can and will keep the implant clean is one of the most important criteria in patient selection. (4:419)

85.

C. The wax pattern is encased in a special gypsum product (invest), which is placed in a hot oven (burn out), and molten metal is forced into the space provided by the burning out process (casting). The restoration is then polished. (1:216–221)

86.

B. The flux is used while the alloy is on the molten stage. With pickling, the casting is placed in an acidic solution which reduces the surface oxides. (1:222)

87.

A. The compressive strength of ceramic bodies is greater than either their tensile or their shear strength. The tensile strength is low because of the unavoidable surface defects. The shear strength is low because of the lack of ductility or ability to shear, caused by the complex structure of the glass ceramic materials. The shear and tensile strengths of the fired porcelain are so low that the slightest imperfection in the preparation of the cavity in the tooth may cause the jacket crown to fracture in service. (2:23–24)

88.

D. The sequence of porcelain application is opaque, body, incisal, and glaze. (3:477)

89.

D. Only glass ionomer serves dual purposes of a cement and a restorative material. (1:231, 240–242, 268–269)

90.

A. Up to the proportional limit, when a material has stresses and resulting strains in proportion to each other, it is obeying Hooke's Law. Past the proportional limit, permanent deformation occurs. (1:23)

91.

A. The setting of amalgam involves a reaction of mercury and silver in which a plastic mixture forms and hardens. Most cements, impression materials, and resins involve polymerization reactions. In denture curing, the addition of heat begins the reaction, while most reactions involving impression materials and cements begin when the components are mixed together. (1:170–172)

92.

B. The propagation stage constitutes the bulk of the reaction (over 90%). It is during this stage that the polymer grows in length. Cross-linking reactions, while minor in number, often greatly add to the strength of the resulting polymer. (1:104–105)

93.

C. The chromium content is responsible for the tarnish resistance and stainless properties of the cobalt–chromium alloys. It is thought that for dental chromium alloys to have good tarnish-resistant properties, they should also contain a minimum of 20% chromium. (1:195)

94.

D. Addition polymerization involves the adding of the units on each side of the carbon–carbon double bond. No ionic forms are involved, as a rule, with the entire reaction sequence being carried out by free-radical chemical species. Condensation polymerization often involves ionic species and produces a small molecule (usually the water of an alcohol) as a by-product of each step of the reaction. (1:83, 102)

95.

A. The chemical resistance of stainless steel is due largely to the presence of chromium in the alloy. No other element added to iron has been so effective in producing resistance to corrosion. (1:195)

96.

C. The austenitic (18-8) group represents the alloy used most extensively for dental appliances in the mouth. The popular 18-8 alloys are of this type and contain approximately 18 percent chromium and 8 percent nickel. (1:282)

4 Provision of Dental Hygiene Care

DIRECTIONS Each of the questions below is followed by several suggested answers. Select the best answer in each case.

1. Before the patient is seated for an appointment, the dental chair should be in which of the following positions?

   A. chair at patient's waist level; back down

   B. chair at low level; back lowered

   C. chair up as far as it will go, so the operator can adjust the chair according to the patient's height

   D. chair at low level; back upright

   E. chair lowered with back parallel to floor

2. Which of the following is NOT a type of mirror surface?

   A. plane

   B. concave

   C. flat

   D. convex

   E. front surface

3. The reflection of light from the lingual aspect through the teeth as they are examined from the facial aspect is called
   A. indirect vision
   B. direct vision
   C. illumination
   D. transillumination

4. The reason(s) for using a modified pen grasp for periodontal instrumentation is (are) because this grasp
   A. allows the clinician to rotate the instrument with the fingers
   B. ensures control of the working end
   C. allows for controlled strokes for deposit removal
   D. all of the above

5. Which of the following parts of an instrument should be considered when determining accessibility of working end to a deep periodontal pocket?
   A. the handle
   B. the shank
   C. the nib
   D. the blade
   E. the cutting edge

6. The operating distance from the patient's mouth to the eyes of the operator should be approximately
   A. 8 inches
   B. 12 inches
   C. 16 inches
   D. 24 inches

7. Normal adult body temperature range is
   A. 97.0–99.6°F
   B. 94.0–99.0°F
   C. 95.0–100.5°F
   D. 97.0–101.0°F

8. Which of the following factors influence body temperature?
   A. time of day, hemorrhage, pathology, application of external heat
   B. heart rate, pathology, hemorrhage
   C. respiration, time of day, application of external heat
   D. hemorrhage, respiration, heart rate, time of day

9. When taking a patient's oral temperature, the thermometer should be in place for how long?
   A. 30 seconds
   B. 1 minute
   C. 2 minutes
   D. 2 1/2 minutes
   E. 3 minutes

10. Normal respiration rate for an adult is which of the following?
    A. 14–20 per minute
    B. 25–40 per minute
    C. 30–40 per minute
    D. 60–80 per minute

11. If a radial pulse cannot be found or taken, which of the following alternative areas can be used?
    A. femoral artery or jugular artery
    B. brachial artery or facial artery
    C. facial artery or temporal artery
    D. jugular artery or temporal artery

12. Which of the following ingredients serves to retain moisture in a commercial toothpaste?
    A. detergent
    B. humectant
    C. surfactant
    D. binder
    E. surface agent

13. Which of the following types of dentifrices has a drug or chemical agent added for a specific preventive or treatment action?
    A. therapeutic
    B. caustic
    C. detersive
    D. prophylactic

14. Which of the following permanent teeth are utilized to classify occlusion?
    A. second molars
    B. second premolars
    C. first premolars
    D. first molars

15. Which of the following types of mouth-washes are prepared to relieve pain?
    A. astringents
    B. anodynes
    C. buffering agents
    D. oxygenating agents

16. A hypertonic sodium chloride solution contains
    A. 1/2 teaspoon salt added to 8 ounces of water
    B. 1 teaspoon salt added to 8 ounces of water
    C. 11/2 teaspoons salt added to 8 ounces of water
    D. 2 teaspoons salt added to 4 ounces of water
    E. 1/4 teaspoon salt added to 8 ounces of water

17. A hypochlorite solution for cleaning dentures contains which of the following ingredients?
    A. Calgon™, chlorine bleach, and water
    B. acetic acid, water, and chlorine bleach
    C. chlorine bleach, water, and vinegar
    D. water, Calgon™, and sodium chloride

18. A line where two surfaces meet on an instrument is termed a
    A. nib
    B. shank
    C. blade
    D. cutting edge

19. Which of the following factors is responsible for the effectiveness of chlorhexidine against bacterial plaque?
    A. limited absorption
    B. substantivity
    C. high alcohol content
    D. oxygenating properties
    E. low pH

20. An exploratory stroke utilizes which of the following?
    A. heavy pressure
    B. light pressure
    C. moderate pressure
    D. intermittent pressure

21. The facial surface of a curette is
    A. a convex curve
    B. between the lateral surfaces
    C. the cutting edge

22. In scaling the line angles of a tooth, which of these factors is (are) important to remember?
    A. The tip must be kept against the tooth surface to avoid laceration.
    B. Often a deposit is left if the blade is not extended to the gingival attachment.
    C. One must be aware of the contour of the teeth and the relationship of the tip of the instrument to the interdental papillae.
    D. A fulcrum must be established to help ensure control of the instrument.
    E. All of the above.

23. Two opposite curette blades of area-specific curettes must be used to scale facial or lingual surfaces of any given anterior tooth because
    A. one blade will not adapt to both the mesial and distal of any given tooth surface
    B. one side of the blade must be used from midline to mesial, and the other side of the blade from midline to distal
    C. both A and B

24. In order for a curette blade to be properly activated against the tooth surface, the _____ surface must be placed at an angle of at least _____ and not more than _____ to the tooth surface. Select the correct completions from the following.
    A. cutting; 90°; 45°
    B. facial; 60°; 30°
    C. cutting; 60°; 30°
    D. cutting; 90°; 30°
    E. facial; 45°; 90°

25. A sickle scaler with a curved blade is referred to as
    A. a contra-angled sickle scaler
    B. a straight sickle scaler
    C. a curved sickle scaler
    D. a posterior scaler
    E. an anterior scaler

26. The following description is of which instrument? The instrument has multiple cutting edges lined up as a series of miniature hoes on a round, oval, or rectangular base. Multiple blades are at 90° or 105° angles with the shank.
    A. file
    B. chisel
    C. hoe
    D. carver

27. Which of the following is NOT a major part of a scaler?
    A. working end
    B. handle
    C. shank
    D. nib
    E. cutting edge

28. Ultrasonic scaling is based on the principle of
    A. rapid electrical impulses
    B. a jet stream of water
    C. pressure
    D. high-frequency sound waves

29. Which of the following is (are) contraindicated when polishing, due to the production of increased frictional heat?
    A. rapid abrasion
    B. coarse abrasive polish
    C. dry agents
    D. heavy pressure
    E. all of the above

30. A material composed of particles of sufficient hardness and sharpness to cut or scratch a softer material when drawn across its surface is called
    A. an abrasive
    B. a cleanser
    C. a polish
    D. a dentifrice

31. When taking an oral cytology smear, how should the scraped cells be put on the slide?
    A. Wipe the tongue blade across the slide once.
    B. Wipe the tongue blade back and forth across the slide several times.
    C. Scrape them off of the tongue blade with a sharp object.
    D. Scrape the tongue blade against the slide several times.

32. Some loss of tooth structure occurs during polishing; therefore, which of the following must be applied in an attempt to replace the lost protection?
    A. sealants
    B. fluoride
    C. an amalgam
    D. a varnish

33. Which of the following is considered the MOST effective treatment for hypersensitive teeth?
    A. acidulated phosphate fluoride
    B. sodium fluoride
    C. stannous fluoride
    D. A and B only
    E. B and C only

34. Diastolic pressure represents which of the following?
    A. aortic pressure
    B. ventricular relaxation
    C. heart rate
    D. ventricular contraction

35. Which of the following blood pressures is considered normal?
    A. 100/80 mm Hg
    B. 120/80 mm Hg
    C. 130/120 mm Hg
    D. 140/60 mm Hg
    E. 150/100 mm Hg

36. The process by which all forms of life, including bacterial spores and viruses, are destroyed describes the process of
    A. sterilization
    B. cleaning
    C. disinfecting
    D. decontamination

37. The following description is of which instrument? Single, straight cutting edge; blade at 99° to 100° angle to the shank; cutting edge beveled at 45° angle to the end of the blade; used for removing large, tenacious, accessible supragingival calculus.
    A. chisel
    B. hoe
    C. file
    D. sickle scaler

38. When is a tooth MOST susceptible to a dental caries attack?
    A. a year after eruption
    B. soon after eruption
    C. the tooth is consistently susceptible

39. Prolonged use of hydrogen peroxide is most likely to produce which of the following conditions?
    A. black hairy tongue
    B. gingival hypersensitivity
    C. decalcification
    D. geographic tongue
    E. candidiasis

40. A retrognathic profile is usually associated with which of the following classifications of malocclusion?
    A. Class I
    B. Class II
    C. Class III

41. A prognathic profile is usually associated with which of the following classifications of malocclusion?
    A. Class I
    B. Class II
    C. Class III

42. Instruments receive the MOST wear from
    A. autoclaving
    B. scaling
    C. gas sterilization
    D. sharpening
    E. ultrasonic cleaning

43. A mesial cavity in a mandibular right second premolar is classified as a
    A. Class I
    B. Class II
    C. Class III
    D. Class IV
    E. Class V

44. Subgingival calculus differs from supragingival calculus in
    A. location
    B. density
    C. color
    D. A and C only
    E. A, B, and C

45. Which of the following types of dental stains can become embedded in decalcified surface enamel?
    A. orange stain
    B. black line stain
    C. brown stain
    D. green stain

46. A patient taking diphenylhydantoin sodium probably has
    A. rheumatic fever
    B. tuberculosis
    C. rheumatism
    D. diabetes
    E. epilepsy

47. The MOST frequent error in the use of alginates for impressions is
    A. having too much water in the mix
    B. delaying the pouring of the cast
    C. having too much powder in the mix
    D. water added to the powder is too hot
    E. wax is not added to the tray

48. Which of the following is (are) the BEST reason(s) for using compressed air during an oral prophylaxis?

    A. to dry calculus, making it more visible
    B. to dry the gingival sulcus
    C. to expose dental caries that are sensitive to air
    D. to dry calculus, making it easier to remove
    E. all of the above

49. Repeated application of a topical fluoride will NOT cause enamel mottling because
    A. topical fluoride is too weak to produce mottling
    B. the tooth is already calcified and cannot be altered
    C. the glycerin base of the polishing agent will protect the tooth from mottling
    D. both A and C

50. Oral irrigators (water irrigation devices) are NOT useful for
    A. removing bacterial plaque
    B. stimulating the gingiva
    C. dislodging debris from orthodontic appliances
    D. all of the above

51. Match each of the following Gracey curettes with its intended area of use. (Letters may be used more than once.)

    1. Gracey 1/2   ____   A. anterior teeth
    2. Gracey 3/4   ____   B. anterior and bicuspid teeth
    3. Gracey 5/6   ____   C. anterior teeth, proximal surfaces
    4. Gracey 7/8   ____   D. posterior teeth, mesial surfaces
    5. Gracey 9/10   ____   E. posterior teeth, distal surfaces
    6. Gracey 11/12 ____   F. posterior teeth, palatal surfaces
    7. Gracey 13/14 ____   G. posterior teeth, buccal surfaces

52. The effectiveness of topical anesthetic agents is increased by
    A. drying the tissue before application
    B. placing the topical agent interproximally
    C. isolating the area to prevent dilution
    D. both A and C
    E. A, B, and C

53. Which of the following will decrease the retention and effectiveness of a pit and fissure sealant?
    A. improper technique
    B. abrasive dentifrice
    C. water contamination of the etched enamel
    D. consistent use of a hard-bristle toothbrush
    E. all of the above

54. A chisel is best designed for removing supragingival calculus deposits from
    A. interproximal surfaces of anterior teeth
    B. interproximal surfaces of posterior teeth
    C. lingual surfaces of posterior teeth
    D. buccal surfaces of posterior teeth

55. Which of the following working strokes is BEST used with the hoe for removal of calculus?
    A. push-pull
    B. wrist
    C. rotary wrist
    D. push
    E. pull

56. During mouth-to-mouth resuscitation or rescue breathing, the emergency operator should breathe into the victim's mouth and release at a rate of
    A. 6–7 times per minute
    B. 10 times per minute
    C. 12–20 times per minute
    D. 30 times per minute
    E. 60 times per minute

57. When performing cardiopulmonary resuscitation, the ratio of compressions to breaths is
    A. 10 compressions, then 1 breath
    B. 15 compressions, then 2 breaths
    C. 12 compressions, then 2 breaths
    D. 8 compressions, then 1 breath

58. When performing the Heimlich maneuver or abdominal thrusts, where do you place your fist and how are the thrusts given?
    A. at the lower tip of the breastbone and with an upward thrust
    B. on the navel and with a straight back thrust
    C. just above the navel and well below the lower tip of the breastbone with a quick upward thrust

59. A toxic reaction to a local anesthetic (due to intravascular injection) is treated with
    A. oxygen and supportive therapy
    B. mouth-to-mouth resuscitation
    C. barbiturates for convulsions and supportive therapy
    D. administration of an antihistamine and supportive therapy

60. Nitroglycerine (glyceryl trinitrate) is used for the treatment of
    A. diabetes
    B. epilepsy
    C. convulsions
    D. angina pectoris
    E. hypertension

61. Which of the following is the MOST effective chemotherapeutic agent against bacterial plaque?

A. Listerine™

B. zinc chloride

C. chlorhexidine

D. hydrogen peroxide

E. sodium perborate

62. Which of the following vitamins requires sunlight in order to be synthesized?

A. vitamin A

B. vitamin B12

C. vitamin C

D. vitamin D

E. vitamin K

63. Which of the following instruments is designed primarily for a push-type working stroke?

A. scaler

B. hoe

C. Gracey curette

D. file

E. A push-type stroke is not recommended for any of the instruments listed.

64. If a patient has recently suffered a myocardial infarction, elective dental and dental hygiene appointments should be postponed for

A. six weeks

B. one month

C. three months or longer

D. more than one year

65. Which of the following stains of the teeth will show up brilliant yellow under ultraviolet light?

A. chromogenic stain

B. erythroblastosis fetalis

C. fluorosis

D. tetracycline

66. A disturbance of the shape of the permanent teeth (and sometimes primary teeth) is referred to as

A. taurodontism

B. hypophosphatasia

C. dentinal dysplasia

D. enamel hypoplasia

67. Which of the following tooth-numbering systems assigns the numbers 1 through 32 to the permanent teeth?

A. Universal Numbering System

B. Two-Digit System

C. Fédération Dentaire Internationale System

D. Palmer System

68. A tooth in supraversion is

A. in a position labial to normal

B. in a position lingual to normal

C. elongated above the line of occlusion

D. in a position buccal to normal

69. The source of minerals for subgingival calculus is

A. saliva

B. blood

C. gingival sulcular fluid

D. food

70. Mucoceles are usually the result of

A. mechanical trauma

B. coagulation of serum

C. bacterial invasion

D. the etiology is unknown

71. Which of the following surface disinfectants has residual biocidal action?

A. chlorines

B. iodophors

C. quaternary ammonium compounds

D. phenols

72. Chemical agents that are EPA registered for surface disinfection include
    A. quaternary ammonia compounds, iodophors, alcohol
    B. alcohol, sodium hypochlorite, glutaraldehydes
    C. sodium hypochlorite, iodophors, synthetic phenols
    D. glutaraldehydes, quaternary ammonia compounds, sodium hypochlorite

73. Which of the following terms is used to describe a flat, nonraised lesion?
    A. vesicle
    B. macule
    C. bulla
    D. ulcer

74. A small, circumscribed, fluid-filled lesion with a thin surface covering is called a
    A. macule
    B. papule
    C. plaque
    D. vesicle

75. The incubation period for hepatitis B virus is
    A. 2–6 days
    B. 2–6 weeks
    C. 2–6 months

76. The first step in the prevention of disease transmission is
    A. washing of the operator's hands
    B. placing gloves on the operator's hands
    C. taking the patient's medical history
    D. being sure the dental operatory is disinfected and instruments are sterilized

77. Which of the following will contribute to the prevention of disease transmission and lessen the chance of cross-contamination?
    A. utilization of barriers
    B. high-volume aspiration
    C. antiretraction valves
    D. flushing water lines
    E. all of the above

78. To adapt any of the Gracey curettes to tooth surfaces, which of the following must be parallel to the surface to be scaled?
    A. handle
    B. terminal shank
    C. cutting edge
    D. face of the curette

79. Which of the following methods of sterilization kills bacterial spores in the shortest time?
    A. dry heat oven
    B. chemical vapor
    C. steam autoclave
    D. ethylene oxide

80. When performing gingival curettage, the face of the curette blade forms which angle with the soft-tissue pocket wall?
    A. 45°
    B. 60°
    C. 70°
    D. 90°

81. When sharpening instruments with a flat stone, the angle between the instrument and the stone should be between
    A. 70° and 80°
    B. 80° and 90°
    C. 90° and 100°
    D. 100° and 110°

82. A scientifically effective face mask will
    A. prevent passage of microorganisms
    B. have minimal marginal leakage
    C. filter particles
    D. all of the above

83. The goal(s) of instrument sharpening is (are)
    A. to remove the metal uniformly and preserve the original shape
    B. to restore and maintain a knifelike cutting edge
    C. to increase the working efficiency of the instrument
    D. all of the above

84. The most widely used local anesthetics are
    A. amides
    B. esters
    C. ethyls
    D. amines

85. Of all the topical anesthetics, which of the following types is the LEAST desirable?
    A. ointment
    B. gel
    C. liquid
    D. spray

86. The most widely used method of conscious sedation is
    A. hypnosis
    B. nitrous oxide–oxygen
    C. tranquilizers
    D. intravenous administration of sedatives

87. When using topical anesthetics to alleviate tissue discomfort and to relieve patient anxiety, it is important to limit
    A. the amount applied
    B. the concentration used
    C. the area of application
    D. A and B only
    E. A, B, and C

88. Which of the following is added to local anesthetics to decrease absorption into the blood, thus increasing duration of the anesthetic and decreasing toxicity of the anesthetic?
    A. epinephrine
    B. paraben
    C. sodium metabisulfite
    D. sodium chloride

89. Which of the following design characteristics is NOT useful in a curette used to reach heavy, tenacious calculus in a deep pocket on a molar?
    A. a long shank
    B. a multiangled shank
    C. a fine, flexible shank

90. Acquired pellicle is initially derived from
    A. saliva
    B. tooth structure
    C. bacterial products
    D. dietary components

91. A patient experiencing tachycardia has a pulse rate
    A. less than 140 bpm
    B. greater than 70 bpm
    C. less than 50 bpm
    D. greater than 150 bpm

92. Fluoride-induced enamel hypoplasia or hypocalcification is
    A. more caries-prone
    B. caries-resistant
    C. hypersensitive to temperature changes

93. In order to open the angulation of a curette blade in relation to the tooth surface, the shank must be moved
    A. toward the tooth
    B. away from the tooth
    C. parallel to the tooth
    D. perpendicular to the tooth

94. Airabrasive polishing is contraindicated in patients with
    A. respiratory conditions
    B. exposed cementum or dentin
    C. soft, spongy gingiva
    D. composite restorations
    E. a sodium-restricted diet
    F. A and D only
    G. A, B, C, D, and E

95. The standard regimen for antibiotic pre-medication is
    A. 2 grams of clindamycin 1 hour before the appointment
    B. 2 grams of amoxicillin 1 hour before the appointment
    C. 2 grams of amoxicillin 1 hour before the appointment and 1 gram 6 hours later
    D. 2 grams of clindamycin 1 hour before the appointment and 1 gram 6 hours later

96. Overheating during amalgam polishing may cause injury to
    A. osteoclasts
    B. ameloblasts
    C. osteoblasts
    D. odontoblasts

97. Which of the following is the MOST important factor to remember?
    A. changing gloves between patients
    B. using protective attire and barrier techniques
    C. treating all patients as though they are infectious
    D. minimizing the formation of droplets, splatters, and aerosols

98. Instruments should be sharpened
    A. at the first sign of dullness
    B. after every use
    C. before every use

99. Ending instrument sharpening strokes on a downward strike will assist in
    A. rounding of the edge
    B. preserving the contour of the blade
    C. preventing dullness of the blade
    D. preventing formation of a wire edge

100. When using an ultrasonic scaler, the patient may experience sensitivity. Which of the following alterations in technique can be made to lessen sensitivity?
    A. Lighten the pressure of the instrument against the tooth or deposit.
    B. Lower the power setting.
    C. Increase the water flow.
    D. Maintain constant motion.
    E. All of the above.

101. The initial instruction in patient education is best given at the beginning of the appointment because
    A. the patient will see the importance of home care because the hygienist has placed emphasis on its importance
    B. at the end of the appointment, time may be limited, the patient may be tired, and the gingiva may be sensitive
    C. after the plaque and calculus are removed, the opportunity to show the patient what is to be accomplished is lost
    D. A and B only
    E. B and C only
    F. A, B, and C

102. MOST fluoride is excreted through the
    A. small intestine
    B. kidneys
    C. liver
    D. feces
    E. sweat glands

103. MOST fluoride is absorbed in the
    A. liver
    B. small intestine
    C. sweat glands
    D. urine
    E. kidneys

104. The pH of acidulated fluoride gels is in the range of
    A. 1–3
    B. 3–5
    C. 5–7
    D. 7–9
    E. 9–11

105. Fluorosis may result from excessive fluoride consumed during
    A. the mineralization stage of tooth development
    B. the maturation stage of tooth development
    C. either the mineralization or the maturation stage of tooth development

106. Which of the following is an advantage of a school-based fluoride program?
    A. It is the most effective method of reducing dental caries.
    B. It can be implemented by nondental personnel.
    C. It can achieve maximum effectiveness with monthly application.
    D. It is the least expensive method of administering fluoride.

107. In communities without fluoridated water supplies, the most cost-effective method of delivering fluoride to 6- to 12-year-old children is through
    A. fluoride tablets
    B. school water fluoridation
    C. brushing with a fluoride gel

D. a fluoride mouthrinse program

108. Which of the following factors need NOT be considered in deciding whether pediatric fluoride supplements should be prescribed?
    A. age of the patient
    B. amount of fluoride in the drinking water
    C. conscientiousness of the patient or parents
    D. type of topical fluoride applied professionally

109. A three-year-old child who lives in a non-fluoridated area has rampant decay. Which of the following home-care regimens, with parental supervision, is suitable for this child?
    A. fluoride tablets
    B. fluoride dentifrice
    C. fluoride mouthrinse
    D. brush-on gel
    E. fluoride drops

110. Which of the following have been demonstrated to be the MOST effective in inhibiting microbial plaque?
    A. fluoride
    B. antibiotics
    C. chlorhexidine
    D. water irrigation devices

111. Toothbrush selection for a patient should be primarily and most importantly based on which of the following?
    A. whether the toothbrush is ADA-approved
    B. type of bristles
    C. state of health of the periodontium
    D. anatomic configuration of the teeth and gingiva
    E. individual patient's needs

112. In order to clean properly and most efficiently, in general, patients should be advised to floss
   A. before bedtime
   B. as often as possible
   C. before brushing
   D. after brushing

113. Fluoride uptake in teeth depends on which of the following factors?
   A. amount of fluoride delivered
   B. type of fluoride delivered
   C. form of fluoride delivered
   D. length of time of exposure to fluoride delivered

114. Ideally, the optimum concentration of fluoride in community drinking water is in the range of
   A. 0.2–1.0 parts per million (ppm)
   B. 0.6–1.2 ppm
   C. 1.0–2.0 ppm
   D. 1.2–2.5 ppm

115. Which of the following types and concentrations of fluoride should be recommended to a head and neck cancer patient for home-care custom tray use?
   A. 0.4% stannous fluoride
   B. 1% neutral sodium fluoride
   C. 1.23% acidulated phosphate fluoride
   D. A and C only
   E. A and B only
   F. A, B, and C

116. Which of the following types of fluoride is reported to cause staining of demineralized enamel and porcelain?
   A. stannous fluoride
   B. acidulated phosphate fluoride
   C. neutral sodium fluoride

117. A symptom is referred to as any departure from the normal that may be indicative of disease. Which of the following are symptoms observed by the patient?
   A. objective symptoms
   B. subjective symptoms
   C. cardinal symptoms
   D. signal symptoms

118. Which of the following fluorides is recommended for a patient with bulimia nervosa?
   A. stannous fluoride
   B. neutral sodium fluoride
   C. acidulated phosphate fluoride

119. Which of the following is an advantage of ethylene oxide sterilization?
   A. Sterilization is achieved at a low temperature.
   B. A short cycle is required.
   C. It is nonirritating.
   D. It is nonexplosive.

120. Bruxism can cause
   A. acute pulpitis
   B. wear facets
   C. occlusal trauma
   D. muscle fatigue and limited opening
   E. B, C, and D only
   F. A, B, C, and D

121. The length of time of retention of sealants depends almost entirely on
   A. the anatomy of the pit or fissure
   B. the precision of the technique
   C. the age of the material
   D. the amount of penetration
   E. the type of etchant utilized

122. Sealants should be applied
   A. as soon as possible following eruption
   B. at the age of 12
   C. at the age of 15
   D. after all permanent teeth have erupted
   E. to primary teeth only

123. Which of the following is continuous with the oral epithelium of the free gingiva and is covered with keratinized stratified squamous epithelium?
   A. col
   B. free gingival groove
   C. gingival sulcus
   D. attached gingiva

124. Calculus can attach to the tooth by way of
   A. attachment by means of an acquired pellicle
   B. direct contact between calcified intercellular matrix and tooth surface
   C. attachment to minute irregularities and undercuts in the tooth surface
   D. A and B only
   E. B and C only
   F. A, B, and C

125. Which of the following crystalline salts is most prevalent in dental calculus?
   A. octocalcium phosphate
   B. hydroxyapatite
   C. brushite
   D. whitlockite

126. A pathologic wearing away of the teeth through some abnormal mechanical process is called
   A. erosion
   B. attrition
   C. abrasion
   D. intrusion

127. Which of the following stains is composed of chromogenic bacteria and fungi?
   A. metallic stain
   B. green stain
   C. black line stain
   D. yellow stain

128. The type of mucosa that covers the inner surfaces of the lips and cheeks, floor of the mouth, underside of the tongue, soft palate, and alveolar mucosa is called
   A. specialized mucosa
   B. masticatory mucosa
   C. lining mucosa

129. Minute soft-tissue hemorrhagic spots of pinpoint to pinhead size are called
   A. ecchymoses
   B. petechiae
   C. exophytic
   D. punctate

130. A contra-angled sickle scaler would be indicated for use on which of the following teeth?
   A. mesial of #29
   B. mesial of #27
   C. distal of #8
   D. distal of #13
   E. A and D only
   F. B and C only

131. The best way to examine the dorsum of the tongue is to
   A. ask the patient to say "ah" and depress the tongue with the mouth mirror
   B. use a dental mirror for indirect vision
   C. extend the tongue fully by grasping with a dry gauze square and use direct vision
   D. palpate between the thumb and index finger

132. The submandibular lymph glands are best examined by
   A. using a dental mirror for indirect vision
   B. asking the patient to lift the tongue up and back
   C. direct vision
   D. bilateral palpation

133. The results of the extraoral and intraoral examination should be recorded in the patient's chart whenever
    A. findings are atypical
    B. findings are abnormal
    C. a lesion is found
    D. they are performed regardless of findings

134. The term *universal precautions* refers to
    A. a method of infection control in which all human blood and certain body fluids are treated as if known to be infectious
    B. previous precautions taken when treating a specific patient
    C. total care provided to patients

135. The utilization of an ultrasonic cleaner prior to instrument sterilization will
    A. increase penetration in parts of the instrument that harbor debris
    B. improve effectiveness for disinfection
    C. decrease the likelihood of the clinician contacting pathogenic microorganisms
    D. all of the above

136. Changes in the types of organisms occur within plaque as it matures. At which time do vibrios and spirochetes appear?
    A. 1 to 7 days
    B. 7 to 14 days
    C. 14 to 21 days
    D. 21 to 28 days

137. A sharp instrument increases efficiency by
    A. reducing slippage and trauma
    B. enhancing tactile sensitivity
    C. minimizing the number of strokes
    D. all of the above

138. Tactile sensitivity refers to
    A. the ability to distinguish relative degrees of roughness and smoothness on the tooth surface
    B. tooth hypersensitivity to touch
    C. the ability to touch

139. Which of the following are indicated for use on titanium implants?
    A. carbon steel instruments
    B. ultrasonic scaling instruments
    C. stainless steel instruments
    D. gold instruments
    E. plastic instruments

140. If a patient exhibits shortness of breath, dizziness, palpitation, or cold sweats following the administration of a local anesthetic, the patient
    A. is allergic to the anesthetic
    B. is probably apprehensive about dental treatment and reacting to the injection
    C. is possibly abusing illicit drugs
    D. has been given too much anesthesia

141. It is difficult to discriminate between calculus and the cementoenamel junction (CEJ) because
    A. the CEJ is not always smooth
    B. anatomic characteristics vary
    C. the type of tissue (enamel, cementum, dentin) at the CEJ can vary
    D. all of the above

142. Generalized gingival bleeding may be associated with which of the following conditions?
    A. infectious mononucleosis
    B. leukemia
    C. agranulocytosis
    D. cyclic neutropenia
    E. B and C only
    F. B and D only
    G. A, B, C, and D

143. The first step in managing a patient with cervical demineralization should be
    A. a thorough prophylaxis and fluoride treatment

B. instruction in sulcular brushing and daily use of fluoride

C. restoration of these areas

144. Which of the following conditions may be seen in a patient with cerebral palsy?

A. attrition and/or fractured teeth

B. periodontal disease

C. difficulty with mastication and swallowing

D. A and B only

E. B and C only

F. A, B, and C

145. A patient's record

A. begins with the initial examination and continues as long as the patient is under care

B. should be reviewed and updated at each appointment

C. must be legible

D. is confidential

E. all of the above

146. The first step in patient education is

A. disclosing the patient

B. developing rapport with the patient

C. demonstrating brushing and flossing

147. Which of the following conditions may be associated with improper flossing?

A. cuts of the papillae

B. destruction of the attachment fibers

C. abrasion

D. all of the above

148. Two weeks after treatment, the success of your root planing and oral hygiene instructions may be determined by

A. smooth roots

B. no bleeding upon probing

C. no plaque upon disclosing

D. no calculus

149. When establishing the recall frequency for patients, it should be based on which of the following?

A. the patients' desire

B. the maintenance of their oral health

C. the effectiveness of their oral hygiene

D. B and C only

E. A, B, and C

150. Dull instruments result in

A. operator fatigue

B. burnished calculus

C. reduced tactile sensitivity

D. A and B only

E. A, B, and C

151. When treating a patient suffering from hypertension, which of the following should be considered?

A. stress management

B. treatment planning

C. chair position

D. monitoring vital signs

E. drug side effects

F. A, B, and D only

G. A, D, and E only

H. A, B, C, D, and E

152. Your patient begins to complain of fatigue, nausea, and tachycardia, and you notice a fruity, acetone odor to his or her breath. The patient is probably suffering from

A. hypoglycemia

B. alcohol overdose

C. hyperglycemia

D. epilepsy

E. halitosis

153. Your patient has an increase in pulse and blood pressure, appears cold and clammy, and has chest pains radiating to the arm and neck. This attack lasts approximately 3 to 5 minutes. Which of the following conditions is related to these symptoms?
    A. myocardial infarction
    B. angina pectoris
    C. cardiac arrest
    D. congestive heart failure

154. A patient suffering from which of the following may exhibit symptoms such as weakness, dyspnea, rapid heart rate, difficulty breathing, or nocturia.
    A. right heart failure
    B. coronary thrombosis
    C. left heart failure
    D. angina pectoris

155. If your patient begins to experience a seizure, your response should be to
    A. discontinue treatment
    B. stay calm
    C. place the patient in a supine position
    D. monitor the patient's vital signs
    E. A and C only
    F. A, B, C, and D

156. Headache, confusion, impaired speech, respiratory difficulty, and unequal pupils are all symptoms of
    A. an allergic reaction
    B. a drug overdose
    C. a cerebrovascular accident
    D. hypertension

157. When treating a patient with Alzheimer's disease, which of the following should be considered?
    A. disorientation and mood swings
    B. the length of the appointment
    C. communication difficulty
    D. motor problems
    E. A and C only
    F. A, B, C, and D

158. When treating a patient suffering from congestive heart failure, which of the following should be considered?
    A. stress management
    B. appointment length
    C. chair position
    D. supplemental oxygen
    E. A, B, and C
    F. A, B, C, and D

159. Which of the following drugs can be associated with gingival hyperplasia?
    A. cyclosporine
    B. nifedipine
    C. diltiazem
    D. A and C only
    E. A, B, and C

160. When root planing, vertical strokes should be used first, followed by oblique strokes and horizontal strokes when applicable. Light pressure is utilized for root planing strokes to maximize tactile sensitivity.
    A. The first statement is true; the second statement is false.
    B. The first statement is false; the second statement is true.
    C. Both statements are true.
    D. Both statements are false.

161. Duraphat® (Colgate Oral Pharmaceuticals), 5% sodium fluoride varnish, is used for the treatment of:
    A. dentinal hypersensitivity
    B. dental caries prevention
    C. reducing demineralization and enhancing remineralization of incipient lesions
    D. A and B only
    E. A, B, and C

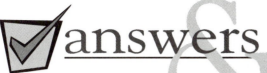

answers & rationales

1.

D. Before the patient is seated for an appointment, the dental chair should be at a low level with the back of the chair upright. The operator's height of operation is established by the height of the dental hygienist's elbow. The patient's head should be placed at the upper edge of the backrest or headrest on the side next to the clinician. Chair positioning relates directly to the type of dental chair. (5:73; 17:14–15)

2.

D. A convex surface is not a type of mirror surface. Dental mirror surfaces consist of plane, concave, flat, and front surface types. Front surface mirrors eliminate "ghost" images. (5:202)

3.

D. Transillumination is accomplished by reflecting the light from the dental light with the dental mirror through the surface being viewed. This technique is used to detect interproximal supragingival calculus and dental caries. (1:30–31; 6:4–5; 17:174)

4.

D. The modified pen grasp is the most useful grasp for periodontal instrumentation. The middle finger, index finger, and thumb all rest on the handle close to the junction of the handle and shank. The middle finger rests on the shank and the thumb and index finger are opposite each other on the handle. This grasp allows the clinician to roll the instrument to ensure proper adaptation to the tooth surface. It also aids the clinician in control of the instrument. (1:14; 5:520; 17:169–170)

5.

B. Instrument shanks vary greatly in length and angles. Instrument shank length and angle determine the accessibility of the instrument to specific areas of the mouth and in deeper periodontal pockets. Straight shanks are used in the anterior areas and longer, contra-angled shanks are used in the posterior areas. (1:12; 5:514–515; 6:15)

6.

C. The operating distance from the patient's mouth to the eyes of the operator should be approximately 14–16 inches. The operator's elbow should be close to his or her side. The patient's mouth should be adjusted to the operator's elbow height. (5:75)

7.

A. Normal adult body temperature is 37°C or 98.6°F. Normal pulse rate is 60 to 100 per minute. Normal rate of respiration is 14 to 20 per minute. The range of normal temperature is from 97°F to 99.6°F. Temperatures vary throughout the day, being lowest in the early morning and highest in the late afternoon. (8:35; 17:121–132)

8.

A. Time of day, hemorrhage, pathology, and application of external heat are all factors that influence body temperature. Other factors include starvation and physiologic shock. Normal human temperature is 37°C or 98.6°F. (5:106–107; 17:131–132)

9.

E. When taking a patient's temperature, the thermometer should be left in the patient's mouth for 3 minutes. Oral thermometers cannot be used for an unconscious patient. In this case axillary positions should be used. (5:107–109; 17:131–132)

10.

A. Normal respiration rate for adults is 14 to 20 per minute. For children, rates range from 18 to 30. Factors that may increase respiration include exercise, excitement, pain, hemorrhage, and shock. Sleep, pulmonary insufficiency, and certain drugs may decrease respiration. (5:111; 17:131)

11.

C. If a radial pulse cannot be found or taken, the temporal or facial arteries can be used as alternative sites for taking pulse rate. Exercise, stimulants, eating, strong emotions, and heart disease can increase pulse rates. Sleep, depressants, low vitality from prolonged illness, and fasting can decrease pulse rates. (5:110; 17:131)

12.

B. Humectants serve to retain moisture in commercial toothpastes. They comprise 20 to 40 percent of the total composition of commercial toothpastes. Commonly used humectants are sorbitol, glycerol, and propylene glycol. (5:387–388; 17:653)

13.

A. A therapeutic dentifrice has a drug or chemical agent added for a specific preventive or treatment action. Fluoride has been shown to be of the greatest benefit when added to the dentifrices. The American Dental Association (ADA) Council on Scientific Affairs evaluates dentifrices that claim therapeutic value. (5:388)

14.

D. The determination of the classification of occlusion is based on the principles of Edward H. Angle. He defined normal occlusion as the normal relation of the occlusal inclined planes of the teeth when the jaws are closed and based his system of classification on the relationship of the permanent first molars. (5:258–259; 17:298-300)

15.

B. Anodyne mouthwashes are prepared to relieve pain. Their essential ingredients consist of phenol derivatives and essential oils. Astringent mouth rinses are used for shrinking tissues. Buffering agents reduce oral acidity and dissolve mucinous films. Oxygenating agents are effective in debridement. Antimicrobial mouth rinses reduce the oral microbacterial count and inhibit bacterial activity. (5:385–386)

16.

B. A hypertonic sodium chloride solution contains 1/2 teaspoon salt added to 4 ounces of water. An isotonic solution contains 1/2 teaspoon $Na HCl_3$ to 8 ounces (1 cup) warm water. An $NaCO_2$ solution is made with 1/2 teaspoon $NaCO_2$ to 8 ounces (1 cup) of water. (5:385)

17.

A. A hypochlorite solution for cleaning dentures contains 2 teaspoons Calgon™, 1 tablespoon chlorine bleach, and 4 ounces water. Accumulations of stains and deposits on dentures vary between individuals in a manner similar to natural teeth. Denture pellicle forms readily after a denture is cleaned. (5:406)

18.

D. A line where two surfaces meet on an instrument is termed a cutting edge. The cutting edges are formed by the junction of the face and lateral surfaces. Parts of a blade include the face, lateral surfaces, back, tip or toe, and cutting edges. (5:514–516; 17:573)

19.

B. Chlorhexidine is the most effective chemical plaque control agent available. It has a bactericidal effect against a broad range of gram-positive and gram-negative bacteria and fungi. Chlorhexidine is effective because of its substantivity. It is rapidly absorbed to the tooth surface and to the acquired pellicle. It is released slowly and thus prolongs the bactericidal effect. (5:386–387)

20.

B. Light pressure is applied to locate a deposit. The term for this is exploratory stroke. The working stroke is employed to remove a deposit. (1:21; 17:573)

21.

B. The facial surface of a curette is opposite the back and between the lateral surfaces. The face of a curette blade is flat in cross-section. The back or undersurface of a curette is rounded. (5:516–517; 17:583)

22.

E. In scaling the line angles of a tooth, it is important to remember the following factors: 1) the tip or toe must be kept against the tooth surface to avoid laceration; 2) often a deposit is left if the blade is not extended to the gingival attachment (base of the sulcus); 3) one should be aware of the contour of the teeth and the relationship of the tip or toe of the instrument to the interdental papillae; and 4) a fulcrum must be established to help ensure control of the instrument. (5:522–525)

23.

C. Two opposite curette blades of area-specific curettes must be used to scale facial or lingual surfaces of any given anterior tooth because: 1) one blade will not adapt to both the mesial and distal of any given tooth surface; and 2) one side of the blade must be used from midline to mesial, and the other side of the blade from midline to distal. Area-specific curettes are paired, mirrored images of each other. Area-specific curettes for posterior use have greater curvatures of the shank. (5:516–517)

24.

E. In order for a curette blade to be properly activated against the tooth surface, the facial surface must be placed at an angle of at least 45° and not more

than 90° to the tooth surface. The ideal angulation is between 70° and 80°. These principles are the same for supragingival and subgingival scaling. (1:19)

25.

C. A sickle scaler with a curved blade is referred to as a curved sickle scaler. Curved sickle scalers have two cutting edges. The face and lateral edges form the cutting edge, which ends in a sharp point. (5:517–518)

26.

A. An instrument with multiple cutting edges lined up as a series of miniature hoes on a round, oval, or rectangular base, with multiple blades at 90° or 105° angles with the shank is a file. Files are used for removal of calculus, smoothing tooth surfaces, and root planing. Files are also used for smoothing down overextended or rough amalgam restorations. (1:299; 5:519–520; 17:578)

27.

D. A nib is not a major part of an instrument. A nib is the working end of a nonsharp instrument. Condensers, burnishers, and wooden points in porte polishers are examples of nibs. (5:514)

28.

D. The ultrasonic principle is based on the use of high-frequency sound waves. Ultrasonic instruments are indicated primarily for adult patients with gross calculus and periodontal pockets. Ultrasonic instruments are especially helpful in removing subgingival calculus, attached plaque, and endotoxins from the root surface, and unattached plaque from the sulcular space. (5:554–556; 17:548–553)

29.

E. Rapid abrasion, coarse abrasive polish, dry agents, and heavy pressure are all contraindicated when polishing. All of these factors increase frictional heat. Some loss of tooth structure occurs during polishing. (5:608–611; 17:657)

30.

A. A material composed of particles of sufficient hardness and sharpness to cut or scratch a softer material when drawn across its surface is an abrasive. Silex and flour of pumice are most often used in tooth polishing agents. Tin oxide is used for polishing amalgams. Jeweler's rouge is used to polish gold. (5:608–609)

31.

A. When taking an oral cytology smear, the scraped cells should be applied to the slide by wiping the tongue blade across the slide once. After preparing the slide, the cells must be fixed. Seventy percent alcohol is commonly used as a fixative. (5:126–127)

32.

B. Some loss of the fluoride-rich tooth structure does occur during polishing. The rate of abrasion can be controlled through speed, pressure, and amount of abrasive used. Fluoride should be applied after tooth polishing. (5:605)

33.

E. Fluoride applications are considered to be the most effective treatment for hypersensitive teeth. This includes self-applied fluoride by the patient. Sodium fluoride and stannous fluoride are commonly used to treat hypersensitive teeth. Acidulated phosphate fluoride is contraindicated for treatment of hypersensitivity due to the high acid pH. (5:600–601; 17:671)

34.

B. Diastolic pressure represents ventricular relaxation. Systolic pressure represents ventricular contraction. Normal adult blood pressure is 120/80. (5:112; 17:135–138)

35.

B. A blood pressure of 120/80 is considered normal. The top figure represents the systolic pressure. The bottom figure represents the diastolic pressure. Exercise, eating, stimulants, emotional disturbance, and menopause may increase blood pressure.

Factors that may decrease a patient's blood pressure include fasting, rest, depressants, quiet emotions, fainting, blood loss, and shock. (5:112; 17:135–138)

36.

A. The process by which all forms of life, including bacterial spores and viruses, are destroyed describes the process of sterilization. Sterilization can be achieved effectively through dry heat or autoclaving. Chemical vapor sterilization is used, but has more limitations. (5:60–61; 17:37)

37.

B. An instrument with a single, straight cutting edge, a blade that is at a 99° to 100° angle with the shank, a beveled cutting edge at a 45° angle to the end of the blade, and is used for removing large, tenacious, accessible supragingival calculus is a hoe. Hoes may be used to remove gross calculus that is 2 to 3 mm below the gingival margin. Lack of adaptability of the blade makes its use limited subgingivally. (1:299; 5:518–519)

38.

B. A tooth is most susceptible to a dental caries attack soon after eruption. A tooth is also the most susceptible to fluoride soon after eruption. Soon after eruption is often an excellent time to apply pit and fissure sealants. (5:238–240, 272–274, 480)

39.

A. Prolonged use of hydrogen peroxide for the treatment of necrotizing ulcerative gingivitis may produce a black hairy tongue. Hairy tongue may also be attributed to the use of antibiotics and systemic corticosteroids. With this condition, there is an elongation of the filiform papillae, which become matted and entrap bacteria, fungi, cellular debris, and foreign material. Discontinued use of the causative agent and careful daily brushing of the tongue should be of some benefit. Hydrogen peroxide is often recommended for acute gingival conditions. Salt water rinses can be used in place of hydrogen peroxide rinses. Geographic tongue is a condition of unknown cause. Clinically, the tongue will have small, round to irregular areas of dekeratinization and desquamation of the filiform papillae. The desquamated areas appear red with white to yellow elevated margins. Over time the patterns will change and appear to move across the tongue. Geographic tongue is also referred to as benign migratory glossitis. (4:112)

40.

B. A retrognathic profile is usually associated with Class II occlusion. Class I occlusion is associated with a mesognathic profile. Class III occlusion is associated with a prognathic profile. (5:258–259; 17:305–307)

41.

C. A prognathic profile is usually associated with Class III occlusion. Persons with prognathic profiles have normal maxillas and protruded mandibles. The buccal groove of the mandibular first permanent molar is mesial to the mesiobuccal cusp of the maxillary first permanent molar by at least the width of a premolar. (5:259; 17:305–307)

42.

D. Instruments receive the most wear from sharpening. A sharpening stone should be available at all times during scaling and root planing. The sharpening device must then be kept sterilized. (5:530–533)

43.

B. A mesial cavity in a mandibular right second premolar is classified as a Class II. Class II cavities are found in proximal surfaces of premolars and molars. (5:241)

44.

E. Subgingival calculus differs from supragingival calculus in location, density, and color. Subgingival calculus is harder and more dense than supragingival calculus. Subgingival calculus is usually heaviest on proximal surfaces and lightest on facial surfaces. (5:279)

45.

D. Dark green stain occasionally becomes embedded in surface enamel. Often the enamel under the stain is decalcified. Green stain results from oral uncleanliness and originates from chromogenic bacteria and fungi. (5:286–287; 17:651)

46.

E. A patient taking diphenylhydantoin sodium probably has epilepsy. Diphenylhydantoin sodium is used for controlling seizures. Often these patients have Dilantin-induced gingival fibromatosis. The condition is also called Dilantin hyperplasia or phenytoin-induced hyperplasia. (5:805–806; 8:285; 17:260–261)

47.

B. The most frequent error in the use of alginates for impressions is delaying the pouring of the cast. Undue dehydration or water loss from the alginate will distort the impression. Thus, the final cast will be inaccurate. (5:176)

48.

A. The best reason for using compressed air during an oral prophylaxis is to dry the calculus, making it more visible. Compressed air is an adjunct, of course, to visual examination and use of the explorer. Unstained supragingival calculus is usually white to creamy-yellow when dried with compressed air. (5:280)

49.

B. Repeated application of a topical fluoride will not cause enamel mottling because the tooth is already calcified and cannot be altered. The greatest amount of fluoride is taken up from topical preparations applied soon after eruption. Effectiveness of topical fluoride depends on its ability to deposit F_2 as fluorapatite in the tooth surface. (5:458–460)

50.

A. Oral irrigators (water spray devices) are useful for loosening debris from the gingival sulcus and dislodging debris from orthodontic appliances. Oral irrigators will disrupt bacterial plaque, but will not remove it. Use of oral irrigation is sometimes referred to as hydrotherapy. (5:381–383; 17:446–447, 618–622)

51.

1. A; 2. A; 3. B; 4. G; 5. G; 6. D; 7. E. The Gracey 1/2 and 3/4 are used for anterior teeth. The Gracey 5/6 is used for anterior and premolar teeth. The Gracey 7/8 and 9/10 are used for posterior teeth, buccal and lingual surfaces. The Gracey 11/12 is used for the mesial surfaces of posterior teeth. The Gracey 13/14 is used for the distal surfaces of posterior teeth. (1:206; 17:587–590)

52.

D. The effectiveness of topical anesthetic agents can be increased by drying the tissue before application and by isolating the area to prevent dilution. Drying the tissue helps keep the agent in the desired area, and it also ensures that the desired amount is being applied. If there is saliva in the area, the topical anesthetic will be carried away, lessening the amount applied and producing undesired anesthesia in other areas of the mouth. Topical anesthetics are effective only on soft tissue and are most effective on nonkeratinized soft tissue where they are more readily absorbed. Benzocaine, tetracaine, butacaine, and lidocaine are commonly used topical anesthetics. Topical anesthetics are used for localized relief. (5:507–510; 17:694–696)

53.

E. Improper technique, abrasive dentifrices, water contamination of the etched enamel, and a hard-bristle toothbrush are all factors that will decrease the retention and effectiveness of a pit and fissure sealant. Precise technique must be used without contamination. Contaminants that will cause the sealant to fail are saliva and water. (5:484, 487; 17:481–497)

54.

A. A chisel is best designed for removing supragingival calculus deposits in interproximal areas, particularly on anterior teeth. A chisel has a single, straight cutting edge. The end of the blade is flat and beveled at a 45° angle. (1:298)

55.

E. The pull stroke is best used with the hoe for the removal of calculus. A hoe has a single, straight cutting edge. The blade is turned at a 99° to 100° angle to the shank. The cutting edge is beveled at a 45° angle. (1:299)

56.

C. During mouth-to-mouth resuscitation or rescue breathing, repeat 12 times per minute for an adult, 20 times per minute for a child, and 20 times per minute for an infant. Maintain a hold under the patient's neck. At all times the airway must remain unobstructed. (5:904)

57.

B. Cardiopulmonary resuscitation is administered when breathing and heart action have stopped. Without both of these, oxygen cannot be carried to the cells and a deficiency occurs quickly. Within 4 to 6 minutes, there may be irreversible brain damage. CPR includes cardiac compressions and breaths. When CPR is being performed by one person, 15 compressions are delivered followed by two ventilations. When CPR is performed by two persons, the same ratio applies. (5:904–906; 17:112, 124)

58.

C. The Heimlich maneuver is performed in the event of an airway obstruction from a foreign body. The thrusts are given to provide pressure against the diaphragm that compresses the lungs, increasing pressure to the lungs, forcing air through the trachea and forcing the obstruction out. If the patient is sitting or standing, wrap the arms around the waist and make a fist. Hold the fist, thumb side down, above the navel and below the breastbone or xiphoid. Press the fist into the abdomen with quick upward thrusts. (5:907–908)

59.

D. On occasion, the dental patient will give a history of being "allergic" to local anesthetics. In most instances, careful questioning will show that syncope occurred following injection of a local anesthetic, but that no other untoward effects developed. This suggests that syncope was due to apprehension. Should a toxic reaction (hives, itching, edema, or flushed skin) occur, an antihistamine (orally, intravenously, or intramuscularly) and other supportive therapy should be administered. (5:506, 913–914; 8:365–367)

60.

D. Nitroglycerine (glyceryl trinitrate) in 0.3 to 0.6 mg tablets may be placed sublingually and administered several times to help prevent and ward off an attack of angina pectoris. The patient will usually give a history of the condition. Overdosage will cause a fall in blood pressure. Nitroglycerin normally reduces or eliminates discomfort dramatically within 2 to 4 minutes. Nitroglycerin is also available in a spray or patch. (5:856–857; 8:403)

61.

C. To date, chlorhexidine is the most effective chemical antiplaque and antigingivitis agent available. Listerine™, a phenolic compound, can be somewhat effective as an antiplaque, antigingivitis agent, but does not have the substantivity or the same bactericidal activity that chlorhexidine does. Hydrogen peroxide is an oxygenating agent and is effective in debridement, but does not have the bactericidal activity that chlorhexidine does. Zinc chloride is an astringent. (5:384–387)

62.

D. Vitamin D is the anti-Ricketts vitamin which is a fat-soluble vitamin. It is activated by exposure to sunlight. It is also considered a hormone, because in the presence of sunlight, skin cells are capable of synthesizing a sufficient supply of vitamin D for the body. The amount of sun exposure needed to produce vitamin D depends on the darkness of the skin. Light-skinned young people need 15 minutes a day, while dark-skinned people and the elderly need more sun exposure. (14:358–363)

63.

E. A push stroke may tear soft tissue and embed fragments of calculus and debris into the soft tissue, therefore, it is not recommended with these instruments. The pull motion is more widely used and safer. The two basic strokes are the exploratory stroke and the working stroke. The exploratory stroke is a light "feeling" stroke whereby the handle is grasped lightly. The working stroke may be a scaling or root planing stroke. With these strokes, the handle is grasped more firmly and lateral pressure is applied to the tooth surface in order to remove the calculus or necrotic cementum. Strokes may be directed vertically, horizontally, or obliquely. (1:21–22; 6:147–151)

64.

C. Myocardial infarction results from a sudden reduction or arrest of coronary blood flow. The symptoms include chest pains, cold sweat, weakness, shortness of breath, nausea, and lowered blood pressure. Elective dental and dental hygiene appointments should be postponed 3 months or longer, until the patient's physician has given consent. (5:857–858; 8:410)

65.

D. Discoloration of either primary or permanent teeth may occur as a result of tetracycline. The deposition occurs during prophylactic or therapeutic regimens instituted either in the pregnant female or postpartum in the infant. Tetracycline staining is often clinically confused with fluorosis. (4:518; 17:651–652)

66.

A. The term taurodontism refers to teeth that have elongated crowns or furcations that are apically displaced. These teeth will have pulp chambers with increased apical-occlusal height. Taurodontism can be an isolated incident in families or can be associated with syndromes, such as Down syndrome. Taurodontism is of little clinical significance and no treatment is required. (4:498–499)

67.

A. There are three tooth-designation systems in general use. The Universal System (also known as Continuous Numbers) utilizes the numbers 1 to 32 . The Quadrant System uses numbers 1 through 8. The Fédération Dentaire Internationale has adopted a two-digit figure system. (5:84–86; 17:235–236)

68.

C. A tooth in supraversion is elongated above the line of occlusion. A tooth in labioversion is in a position labial to normal. A tooth in lingoversion is in a position lingual to normal. (5:256)

69.

C. The source of minerals for subgingival calculus is the gingival sulcular fluid. The source of minerals for supragingival calculus is the saliva. The mode of attachment for calculus is the acquired pellicle. (5:280–281)

70.

A. Mucoceles (also called mucus extravasation phenomenon or mucous retention phenomenon) are considered to be related to mechanical trauma to the minor salivary gland excretory duct, resulting in its transection or severance. There is spillage of mucous into the surrounding connective tissue stroma. The most frequent site is the lower lip. Lesions may also be found on the buccal mucosa, ventral surface of the tongue, floor of the mouth, or retromolar region. (4:240–241)

71.

B. Iodophors are EPA registered and ADA accepted, biocidal within 5–10 minutes, and economical. They have been shown to be broad spectrum antimicrobials and have a prolonged or residual biocidal activity after application. They must be prepared daily, they may discolor some surfaces, and they may be inactivated by hard water. (7:121–127; 17:41–42)

72.

C. Chemical germicides manufactured for disinfection are regulated and registered by the Environmental Protection Agency. Sodium hypochlorite, iodophors, and synthetic phenols are EPA registered and ADA accepted as surface disinfectants. Alcohol has been shown to be ineffective as a disinfectant; therefore, it is not EPA registered. Quaternary ammonium compounds have been shown to be ineffective as disinfectants, but have

been shown to be effective cleaning agents. (7:118–127; 17:39–43)

73.

B. A macule is a circumscribed area not elevated above the surrounding skin or mucosa. It may be identified by its color, which contrasts with the surrounding tissue. Vesicles and bullae are classified as elevated blisterform lesions. Ulcers are classified as depressed lesions. (5:122–125)

74.

D. A vesicle is a small, circumscribed, fluid-filled lesion. It may contain serum or mucin and appear white. Papules and plaques are classified as nonblisterform lesions because they are solid and do not contain fluid. (5:123)

75.

C. The incubation period for hepatitis B is 2 to 6 months versus hepatitis A which is 15 to 50 days. The period of communicability varies and the presence of serum hepatitis B surface antigen (HBsAg) indicates communicability. (5:23, 26; 17:29–31, 65)

76.

D. Before any clinical procedure is performed, all equipment must be disinfected and/or sterilized as appropriate for the prevention of disease transmission. Prevention of cross-contamination begins at the very start of the appointment. The health status of dental patients is determined primarily by using the medical history. History taking should elicit information on the presence or absence of disease and identify patients at risk. Then, universal precautions should be utilized throughout the appointment. (5:87–88; 7:80; 17:23–67)

77.

E. Utilization of barriers, high-volume suction, and antiretraction valves have all been shown to lessen the chance of cross-contamination. The water lines to the handpiece and the air/water syringe tip should also be flushed before each patient to lessen the chance of contamination. (7:98–103; 17:23–67)

78.

B. The terminal or lower shank (portion closest to the working end) must be parallel to the surface being scaled in order to properly adapt the cutting edge. This places the cutting edge at the appropriate working angle of 70°. (1:208)

79.

C. The steam autoclave is an effective method of sterilization with a maximum sterilization period of 30 minutes. Advances in the equipment have allowed for the application of higher temperature and pressure for shorter cycle times (3–5 minutes, 10 minutes, or 15–20 minutes). The other methods of sterilization require sterilization cycles of 30 minutes, 1–2 hours, or 10–16 hours. (7:107–112; 17:23–67)

80.

C. In gingival curettage, the face of the blade should be positioned at a 70° angle with the soft tissue pocket wall or sulcular epithelium. The curette should be positioned at the bottom of the pocket, pressure applied with the finger on the outside of the pocket, with smooth even vertical strokes. The area should be flushed to remove debris and pressure applied to achieve close adaptation of the tissue to the tooth. (1:315; 5:525)

81.

D. The angle on the outside, between the instrument and the stone, is 100° to 110° (the internal angle is 70° to 80°). The stone and blade must remain in contact at the proper angle throughout the procedure or an irregularity will be ground into the cutting edge. (1:357; 5:534)

82.

D. An effective face mask will prevent passage of organisms, have minimal leakage, and filter particles. The shape, material, and degree of absorption of the mask will influence its efficiency. (5:45; 17:59–60)

83.

D. The goals of instrument sharpening are to restore and maintain a knife-like cutting edge, to preserve the original shape of the instrument, and to increase the working efficiency of the instrument. (1:343)

84.

A. The amide-type local anesthetics were introduced in the 1940s. Their widespread usage is due to the decrease in the frequency of allergic reactions versus the ester local anesthetics. (8:350; 17:681)

85.

D. The least desirable topical anesthetic is the spray or aerosol type because it is more concentrated than other types of topical anesthetics, increasing the potential for toxic reactions. Because of the spray, it is difficult to control the amount given and the area covered by the mist. There is also the possibility of inhalation by the patient. (6:339)

86.

B. Nitrous oxide–oxygen sedation produces a state in which the patient is conscious but relaxed. The advantages of this method of sedation include rapid effect due to the inhalation of these gases, easy regulation by altering the concentrations, and rapid reversal by having the patient breath pure oxygen at the completion of the dental procedure. (6:338–339; 17:699–715)

87.

E. Because topical anesthetics must be absorbed through the mucosa, they must be formulated in greater concentrations. The higher concentrations increase the potential for toxic reactions. Therefore, it is important to limit the amount used, the concentration used, and the area of application. (6:339; 17:694–696)

88.

A. Epinephrine is a vasoconstrictor added to local anesthetics to decrease the absorption of the anesthetic by the bloodstream, increasing the duration of the effect of the anesthetic and decreasing the toxicity of the anesthetic. (8:350–351; 17:682)

89.

C. Fine, flexible shanks are not appropriate for the removal of tenacious calculus. A curette with a rigid shank would be more appropriate. To reach calculus in a deep pocket on a molar, the curette of choice would be one with a long, multiangled shank. (6:15)

90.

A. Acquired pellicle is an amorphous, organic, tenacious membranous layer that forms on exposed tooth surfaces, restorations, and calculus. It is composed of glycoproteins from the saliva. (5:264–266)

91.

D. An unusually fast heartbeat or pulse rate is called tachycardia. This increase may be caused by exercise, stimulants, eating, strong emotions, extreme heat or cold, and some forms of heart disease. An unusually slow heart rate is called bradycardia and may be caused by sleep, depressants, fasting, quiet emotions, and low vitality from prolonged illness. While there is no absolute normal, the adult range for normal pulse rates is 60–100 beats per minute. Women have slightly higher normal pulse rates than men. (5:110)

92.

B. Ingestion of drinking water containing fluoride concentrations greater than 1 part per million during tooth development may result in enamel hypoplasia or fluorosis. The extent of the damage is dependent on the duration of ingestion, the timing of the ingestion (during development), and the intensity or concentration. Fluorosis ranges from white spots to mottled brown and white discolorations. There may also be pitting of the enamel. Enamel hypoplasia is caries resistant. (4:508)

93.

B. In order to insert a curette subgingivally, the face of the blade of the instrument must be flush to the tooth or at a 0-degree angle to the surface to be scaled. To establish the correct working angle, the shank of the instrument must be moved away from the tooth in order to open the angle of the blade to the tooth surface. The working angle should be more than 45° and less than 90°. (1:151; 6:143–144)

94.

G. The airabrasive polisher uses air and water pressure to propel fine particles of sodium bicarbonate in a warm spray. The spray must be kept in constant motion about 4 to 5 mm away from the tooth surface, angled away from the gingival margin. Precautions must be followed to minimize the contamination from aerosol production. The airabrasive is contraindicated in patients with respiratory conditions; a restricted sodium diet; a communicable disease; exposed cementum or dentin; soft, spongy gingiva; and nonmetallic restorations. (5:613–615; 17:658–660)

95.

B. The recommended standard regimen for patients able to take amoxicillin or penicillin is 2 grams of amoxicillin 1 hour before the appointment. For patients allergic to amoxicillin or penicillin, clindamycin or cephalexin are indicated. (19:1794–1801)

96.

D. The odontoblasts are cells of the pulp and the dentin. They form the organic matrix of the dentin and provide nutrition to the dentin and possibly play a role in the pain sensation of a tooth. They are also responsible for the formative, nutritive, and defensive functions of the pulp. The cells of the dentin should not be insulted by bacterial toxins, strong drugs, undue operative trauma (such as amalgam polishing), unnecessary thermal changes, or irritating restorative materials. (15:118, 146–150; 16:128–130)

97.

C. Dental professionals are routinely at risk while providing patient care. Many times clinicians fail to comprehend the potential for contamination. The health status of patients is determined by using the medical history. Patients may omit information during the taking of the medical history purposely or unknowingly. There may be negative conditions regarding their health that are undiagnosed or that they feel are not pertinent to their dental treatment.

They may also omit information out of fear. In order to protect yourself, you should treat all patients as though they are infectious. (7:71–89; 17:23–67)

98.

A. Instruments should be sharpened at the first sign of dullness to minimize the amount of metal removed. When sharpening an extremely dull instrument, a larger amount of metal must be removed, shortening the life of the instrument. It may be necessary to sharpen an instrument after each tooth during a difficult root planing appointment. (1:346; 17:604–615)

99.

D. Ending your series of sharpening strokes with a downward strike will prevent the formation of minute metal projections (wire edge) on the cutting edge. (1:350; 17:604–615)

100.

E. If sensitivity is experienced while using the ultrasonic scaler, you should evaluate the following: your pressure against the tooth, the water flow, the power setting, and your motion. Ultrasonic strokes should be applied lightly to the deposit; too much pressure will remove tooth structure. The handpiece and working end are cooled by the constant flow of water. Sensitivity and damage to the tooth may occur if there is an inadequate amount of water flowing through the handpiece. Constant motion of the instrument and the correct angulation of the tip to the tooth are also essential for correct operation of the ultrasonic scaler. (5:558–560)

101.

F. Patient education is more effective when given at the beginning of the appointment. If the instruction is delayed, the patient may be in a hurry to leave, the hygienist's time may also be limited, the gingiva and teeth may be sensitive, and there will be no calculus or plaque remaining on the teeth to show the patient what needs to be accomplished. Patients also place more importance on home care techniques when the hygienist is motivated and places great importance on home care. (5:336)

102.

B. Most fluoride is excreted through the kidneys, with a small amount excreted by the sweat glands. (5:456)

103.

B. Most fluoride is rapidly absorbed by the small intestine and stomach. Maximum blood levels are reached within 30 minutes of intake. In young children, about one-half of the fluoride intake deposits in calcifying bones and teeth. Fluoride is stored in mineralized tissues (99% of the body fluoride). The teeth store small amounts, with the highest levels on the tooth surface. (5:456)

104.

B. The pH of acidulated phosphate–fluoride gels is 3.0 to 3.5. Sodium fluoride (2%) has a basic pH of 9.2. Stannous fluoride (8%) has a pH of 2.1 to 2.3. (5:466)

105.

A. Fluoride is essential to the formation of sound teeth. It is deposited during the formation of the enamel. Sources of fluoride include drinking water and other ingested fluoride, such as tablets, drops, and foods. If there is an excess of fluoride during the mineralization stage, a defective enamel matrix can form. This can lead to dental fluorosis. (5:456)

106.

B. The use of the weekly rinse is the most common school-based program in the United States. Advantages are that it requires little time (about 5 minutes once weekly for an entire class); is inexpensive; is easy to learn and well accepted by participants; and can be carried out by nondental personnel. Responsibility for providing the correctly mixed solution and safe storage can be taken by school officials and a supervising dental hygienist. (5:470–471)

107.

B. School water fluoridation is a satisfactory method of bringing the benefits of fluoridation to children living in communities without fluoridated water supplies. (5:462)

108.

D. When determining the need for pediatric fluoride supplements, you need to consider the age of the patient, the amount of fluoride in the patient's drinking water, and the conscientiousness and motivation level of the patient or parents. Supervision must also be provided. The type of topical fluoride applied professionally is not a factor that you need to consider. (5:463–464)

109.

A. For a three-year-old in a nonfluoridated area, tablets should be prescribed. For children from birth to two years of age, fluoride drops are primarily used. The tooth contact of the chewable tablet provides the enamel surface with protective fluoride. (5:463–464)

110.

C. Chlorhexidine has been tested extensively and has been shown to be the most effective antiplaque and antigingivitis chemotherapeutic agent available. Chlorhexidine is active against a wide range of gram-positive and gram-negative organisms and fungi. It is rapidly adsorbed to teeth and pellicle and released slowly, thus prolonging the bactericidal effect. (5:386–387; 17:616–617)

111.

E. In selecting a toothbrush for a patient, the patient's manual dexterity, motivation and willingness, status of periodontal health, and the position of the patient's teeth should all be considered. All of these factors relate to the needs of the individual patient. (5:354)

112.

C. For most patients, dental floss is best used before brushing to assure that caries-susceptible proximal surfaces will be as free as possible from plaque and that the fluoride from the dentifrice used during brushing will be able to reach the proximal surfaces for caries prevention. (5:373)

113.

D. Uptake of fluoride depends on the amount of fluoride ingested (not delivered) and the length of time of exposure. Fluoride is a natural constituent of enamel. The surface has the highest concentration and the amount decreases rapidly toward the interior layers of the tooth. (5:458–459)

114.

B. The optimum fluoride level for water in temperate climates is 1 part per million (ppm). For warmer and colder climates, the amount can be adjusted from 0.6 to 1.2 ppm. (5:460–461)

115.

E. Stannous fluoride and neutral sodium fluoride are recommended for head and neck cancer patients to protect them from post-irradiation caries. Daily fluoride applications are recommended while the patient is receiving radiation therapy. Custom trays are made prior to the start of therapy and the patient places the fluoride gel from the tray in the mouth for four minutes a day. (5:469–470, 729)

116.

A. Stannous fluoride may discolor tooth-colored restorations and margins. There may also be staining of the teeth in demineralized areas, pits, fissures, and grooves. (5:288, 290)

117.

B. Subjective symptoms such as pain, tenderness, and itching are symptoms observed by the patient. Objective symptoms are frequently called signs. A sign is any abnormality that may indicate a deviation from normal or disease that is discovered by a professional while examining a patient. Examples of signs are changes in color, shape, or consistency of a tissue not observable by the patient. (5:83)

118.

B. A multiple fluoride preventive program is recommended for a patient with bulimia in an attempt to counteract dental erosion. A fluoride dentifrice, neutral sodium fluoride 0.05 percent rinse preparation, and a daily gel tray application with neutral sodium is recommended. (5:832–833)

119.

A. Sterilization can be accomplished at room temperature by way of ethylene oxide, a highly penetrative colorless gas. Many types of materials can be sterilized with little or no damage to the material itself. Ethylene oxide requires a long cycle time, is toxic and allergenic, and forms explosive mixtures with air. (5:63–64; 7:111–112)

120.

F. Bruxism is the clenching or grinding of the teeth when the patient is not chewing or swallowing. Bruxism may lead to acute pulpitis, wear facets, occlusal trauma, and muscle fatigue. Most people are not aware of the habit until it is brought to their attention. Opinions differ as to the primary cause, but occlusal prematurities, muscle tension, and emotional factors have been implicated. Bruxism can be treated through behavioral, emotional, and interceptive modalities. (2:779; 3:432–433)

121.

B. The length of time of retention of sealants depends almost entirely on the precision of the technique. Each step in the preparation of the tooth and the application of the sealant must be carefully performed. Improper technique is probably the major cause of early loss of a sealant from the tooth surface. (5:487)

122.

A. Applications of sealants should be made as soon as possible following eruption. When application is delayed, caries may start, and the surface no longer can be considered for sealant. When possible, sealants can be applied before full eruption, provided there is no tissue flap to interfere with application. (5:482–483)

123.

D. The attached gingiva is continuous with the epithelium of the free gingiva and is keratinized. The col is the depression between the lingual and facial papillae that conforms to the proximal contact area. It is not keratinized, making it more susceptible to disease. The gingival sulcus is the crevice between the free gingiva and the tooth. The free gingival groove is the demarcation between the free gingiva and the attached gingiva. (5:190–192)

124.

F. Calculus is more readily removed from some tooth surfaces than others. The ease of removal is related to the mode of attachment of the calculus to the tooth surface. Calculus can attach by means of the acquired pellicle, by mechanical locking into undercuts or minute irregularities in the tooth, or by direct contact between the intercellular matrix and the tooth surface. (1:5; 3:401; 5:281–282)

125.

B. At least two-thirds of the inorganic matter of calculus is crystalline, principally apatite. Predominating is hydroxyapatite, which is the same crystal present in enamel, dentin, cementum, and bone. Calculus also contains octocalcium phosphate, brushite, and whitlockite. (5:282)

126.

C. Abrasion is the mechanical wearing away of tooth substance by forces other than mastication. Erosion is the loss of tooth substance by a chemical process that does not involve known bacterial action. Attrition is the wearing away of a tooth as a result of tooth-to-tooth contact. Causes of abrasion include an abrasive dentifrice applied with vigorous horizontal toothbrushing, opening bobby pins, or holding items such as tacks or pins between your teeth. (3:498; 5:243–245)

127.

B. Green stain is composed of chromogenic bacteria and fungi. Black line stain is similar to calculus in that it is composed of microorganisms. Yellow stains are usually caused by food pigments. (5:286–288; 17:651)

128.

C. The lining mucosa covers the inner surfaces of the lips and cheeks, floor of mouth, underside of tongue, soft palate, and the alveolar mucosa. It is not firmly attached to the underlying tissue and it is not keratinized. The masticatory mucosa covers the gingiva and the hard palate, is firmly attached to the underlying tissue (except for the free margin of the gingiva), and is keratinized. The specialized mucosa covers the dorsum of the tongue. (5:188)

129.

B. Minute soft tissue hemorrhages appear intraorally, generally because of trauma or blood disease. Traumatic injury can result in leakage of blood into the surrounding connective tissue, producing red to purple lesions. Ecchymoses are soft tissue hemorrhages that are larger than pinpoint size. (4:157–159; 5:124, 866)

130.

E. Contra-angled or modified sickle scalers are paired instruments that are mirror images of each other to provide access to the interproximal surfaces of posterior teeth. One working end adapts to the facial and the other to the lingual. They are used to remove tenacious deposits in the posterior area prior to definitive scaling and root planing with curettes. (1:145; 5:518)

131.

C. To observe the dorsum of the tongue, hold the tongue with a gauze square, retract the cheek and move the tongue out, first to one side and then the other. (5:120)

132.

D. To examine the submandibular lymph nodes, you would place the fingers of both hands beneath the chin and palpate simultaneously. This method of palpation is called bilateral palpation and is used to examine corresponding structures on opposite sides of the body. (5:118–119)

133.

D. The oral examination is crucial to total patient care. The examination must be all-inclusive to include any detectable influences on the whole patient. The results of the oral examination should be recorded regardless of findings to provide information for continuing records for legal purposes and to provide a means of comparison over a series of appointments. (5:116–118; 6:4; 17:150, 155–156)

134.

A. The term *universal precautions* refers to the treatment of all blood and certain body fluids as if they are known to be infectious. (7:202, 231; 17:36)

135.

D. Ultrasonic cleaning prior to sterilization is safer than manual cleaning. Risk of injury to hands and of infection is not as great. The quality of cleaning is much better than by the hand-scrub technique. The removal of saliva and/or blood is significantly enhanced by this method. Ultrasonic cleaners should be operated with a cover to prevent aerosolization of contaminants. (5:59–60; 7:112; 17:20–21, 53–54)

136.

B. Plaque consists of a complex mixture of microorganisms that occur primarily as microcolonies. The population density is very high and increases as plaque ages. Changes in the types of organisms occur within plaque as it matures. Vibrios and spirochetes appear from day 7 to day 14. More gram-negative and anaerobic organisms appear. Also during this time, signs of inflammation are beginning to be observable. Early plaque consists of cocci, filaments, and slender rods. (5:267–270; 17:247–248, 455, 619)

137.

D. Instruments must be sharp if scaling and root planing are to be completed efficiently with minimal trauma to the tissues. A sharp instrument will require fewer strokes, provide greater control, and increase tactile sensitivity. (1:343–344; 5:530–531; 17:604–615)

138.

A. Tactile sensitivity refers to the ability to distinguish degrees of roughness and smoothness on the tooth surface. (6:93)

139.

E. Plastic instruments are indicated for use on titanium implants, as metal instruments scratch the titanium surface. Scratching a titanium implant surface with an unlike metal can create a battery or the production of ferric chloride (a caustic chemical) that can lead to implant failure. (9:364–368; 10:448–453; 11:447–466; 12:95–102; 13:491–495; 17:578–579)

140.

B. The most frequently observed adverse reactions are those associated with the administration of local anesthetics. The majority of these reactions are stress-related (psychogenic). Injection of local anesthetics with the patient in an upright position is most likely to produce a psychogenic reaction. Palpitations, headache, sweating, mild shaking, dizziness, and breathing difficulty are usually of psychogenic origin or are related to the administration of large doses of vasoconstrictors and are not allergic in nature. Allergic reactions normally involve itching or a rash on the skin, diarrhea or nausea, runny nose or watery eyes, wheezing or laryngeal edema, or tachycardia or hypotension. (5:914; 8:3, 104, 350, 353; 17:684, 692–694)

141.

D. The cementoenamel junction (CEJ) is not always smooth and can vary according to the type of tissue involved or because of alterations to the cemental surface. At the CEJ, cementum overlaps enamel in 60 to 65 percent of teeth; cementum and enamel meet directly in 30 percent of teeth; or the cementum and enamel may fail to meet in 5 to 10 percent of teeth, leaving a narrow zone of exposed dentin. (1:9; 5:229)

142.

G. Spontaneous gingival hemorrhage can occur with patients suffering from infectious mononucleosis, leukemia, agranulocytosis, or cyclic neutropenia. This bleeding (from the gingiva and other areas) is an important clinical sign suggesting a hematologic disorder. (3:475–479, 482; 4:77, 157–158)

143.

B. Demineralization means breakdown of the tooth structure with a loss of mineral content. Fluoride is readily taken into these demineralized areas. Both the Bass method and the modified Stillman method of toothbrushing are indicated for plaque removal from cervical areas, directly beneath the gingival margin, and interproximal areas. (5:356–360, 459–460)

144.

F. Patients with cerebral palsy have difficulty swallowing and chewing due to musculature dysfunction. Orally, they may exhibit problems with attrition, fractured teeth, dental caries, and periodontal disease. Cerebral palsy can occur at any age as a result of brain injury from a variety of causes. (5:781–783)

145.

E. A patient's record is a legal document that begins with the initial appointment the patient has in your office. These records must be reviewed and updated at each appointment and are maintained as long as the patient is under your care. Patient records are confidential and must be legible. (5:73, 314–315)

146.

B. Patient education must be tailored to the patient's needs and motivation. The first step must be to develop rapport with your patient and assess his or her needs. A preventive program involves a series of cooperative steps taken by the patient and the dental team. The information provided must be applicable to everyday living. (5:336–337; 6:330)

147.

D. Improper flossing may cause cuts or clefts of the papillae. Abrasion and destruction of the gingival attachment may occur when excess pressure is applied. (5:373–374)

148.

B. After root planing and oral hygiene instruction, the number of pocket microorganisms decreases substantially and there is a shift to aerobic, gram-positive organisms. The gingiva reflects these changes with a decrease in gingival inflammation. A lack of bleeding upon probing indicates removal of the irritants. (5:546)

149.

D. The recall frequency depends on the needs of each patient. The primary objectives are the prevention of new disease as well as the recurrence of disease. The appointment frequency depends on the patient's ability to control plaque, the rate of calculus formation, extent of previous treatment, restorative considerations, and systemic factors. Appointment intervals vary from 2 to 6 months. (5:642–644)

150.

E. It is impossible to efficiently and thoroughly remove calculus and root plane with dull instruments. With a dull instrument, the handle must be grasped much more firmly and more pressure applied to the tooth surface. Dull instruments result in fatigue due to heavy-handedness, burnished calculus, slipping, decreased tactile sensitivity, and inefficient use of time. (6:288–289)

151.

H. Hypertension means an abnormal elevation of blood pressure. It is a risk factor in many vascular diseases. Evaluation of blood pressure is essential in patient evaluation and treatment. When outlining a treatment plan and providing patient care, you must follow a stress reduction protocol to eliminate adverse effects on the patient's blood pressure. Postural hypotension (fainting, nausea, or dizziness) results when a person sits up quickly from a supine position. The patient's vital signs must be evaluated and recorded at all visits, and the patient referred to his or her physician if a problem is noted. Various side effects may be associated with medications prescribed for hypertension, and these side effects may affect your treatment plan and your patient care. Depression, fatigue, gastrointestinal disturbances, and xerostomia are possible side effects. (5:111–114, 852–854; 8:385–388; 17:102–103, 133–135)

152.

A. Hypoglycemia results when a patient has too much insulin or too little food in his or her system. The cause is lowered blood glucose with an excess of insulin. The symptoms may occur suddenly and include the following: fatigue, nausea, tachycardia, dizziness, sweating, headache, and the patient's breath may have a fruity, acetone odor. The treatment involves the administration of sugar or glucagon, depending on the patient's consciousness. (5:881–883; 8:241–242; 17:116, 122)

153.

B. Angina pectoris involves discomfort in the chest, which results from transient and reversible myocardial oxygen deficiency. Approximately 90 percent of angina attacks are related to coronary artery atherosclerosis. An attack may be precipitated by exertion, emotion, or a heavy meal. The symptoms are a feeling of weight on the chest, faintness, sweating, difficulty breathing, or clamminess. The attacks may last for seconds or minutes. (5:856–857; 8:401–402; 17:116, 122)

154.

C. Left heart failure alters output and causes respiratory difficulty because of the backup of fluid and blood into the lungs. The symptoms include weakness, fatigue, dyspnea, nocturia, increased blood pressure, increased heart rate, and anxiety or fear. The symptoms are more prominent at night and are relieved when the patient is sitting or in a semi-sitting position. (5:858)

155.

F. In the event your patient begins to experience a seizure, your first response is to discontinue treatment. You must also remain calm. Place your patient in a supine position, do not restrain the patient, clear away all equipment, loosen the patient's clothing, turn the patient's head to one side, and monitor the patient's vital signs. (5:807–808; 8:291–295)

156.

C. Cerebrovascular accident or stroke is a sudden loss of brain function resulting from interference with the blood supply to a part of the brain. Predisposing factors include atherosclerosis, hypertension, drug abuse, cardiovascular disease, diabetes, and oral contraceptive use. (5:775–776; 8:269–270; 17:117, 122)

157.

F. Alzheimer's disease is one of the nonreversible types of dementia. Dementia is severe impairment of the intellectual abilities (thinking, memory, and personality). There are four stages of impairment: early, middle, advanced, and terminal. Later symptoms include physical immobility, unawareness, and total helplessness. (5:687–688)

158.

F. Heart failure involves the inability or failure of the heart to pump blood at a rate necessary to meet the needs of the body tissues. The result is the collection of fluid in various body organs. In the treatment of a patient with congestive heart failure, stress reduction, appointment length, supplemental oxygen, and chair position should be considered. A medical consultation is recommended. Appointments should be scheduled in the morning and the length of the appointment should not exceed the patient's tolerance. Due to the patient's possible difficulty in breathing, the chair should be in a more semi-upright position and supplemental oxygen may be needed. (5:858–859; 8:42–43, 45, 208–216)

159.

E. Cyclosporine (an immunosuppressive), nifedipine, and diltiazem (calcium-blocking drugs) can all produce gingival hyperplasia as side effects of the drugs. Additionally, phenytoin can also produce gingival hyperplasia. (18:62–65)

160.

C. When root planing, vertical strokes should be used first, followed by oblique and then horizontal strokes. Light pressure should be utilized with root planing strokes to maximize tactile sensitivity. (5:553–554)

161.

E. Sodium fluoride varnishes have been proven to be effective in reducing dentinal hypersensitivity, in preventing dental caries, and in reducing demineralization and enhancing remineralization of incipient lesions. (20:333–334, 350)

5 Periodontics

DIRECTIONS Each of the questions below is followed by several suggested answers. Select the best answer in each case.

---

1. A periodontal pocket is a
   A. diseased gingival sulcus
   B. diseased gingival epithelium
   C. diseased gingival attachment
   D. all of the above

2. How many basic measurements are made on each tooth in periodontal charting?
   A. two
   B. four
   C. six
   D. eight
   E. ten

3. A pocket formed by gingival enlargement without apical migration of the junctional epithelium is which of the following?
   A. absolute pocket
   B. pseudopocket
   C. periodontal pocket
   D. true pocket

4. When measuring the depth of a periodontal pocket, the measurement is made from the base of the pocket or the attached periodontal tissue to
   A. the cementoenamel junction
   B. the height of the gingival margin
   C. a fixed point
   D. the unattached periodontal tissue

5. Which of the following conditions can possibly affect the accuracy of periodontal charting?
   A. bleeding, bone loss, and gingival enlargement
   B. gingival enlargement and gingival recession
   C. gingival recession, bone loss, and bleeding
   D. bone loss and bleeding
   E. ulcerated interdental papillae and bleeding

6. Most periodontal pocket depths up to what depth are usually related to a normal, healthy gingival sulcus?
   A. 3 mm
   B. 4 mm
   C. 5 mm
   D. 6 mm
   E. 7 mm

7. Which of the following BEST describes the objective of root planing?
   A. removal of factors that promote gingival inflammation

B. removal of diseased epithelial attachment
C. removal of diseased attached gingiva
D. removal of diseased sulcular epithelium
E. all of the above

8. Which of the following instruments is the most versatile for periodontal instrumentation?
   A. contra-angled sickle scaler
   B. curette
   C. chisel
   D. hoe
   E. file

9. Exposed cementum and dentin predispose the patient to
   A. acute dental caries
   B. hypersensitive teeth
   C. periodontal pockets
   D. gingival enlargement

10. Which statement BEST describes what periodontal disease and dental caries have in common?
    A. The etiology of both can always be directly attributed to poor oral hygiene.
    B. They are the most common chronic dental diseases.
    C. Both diseases are infections.
    D. Both diseases cause inflammation.
    E. All of the above.

11. A patient who manifests a peculiar inflammation of the marginal and attached gingiva and demonstrates ulcerated and necrotic epithelium that sloughs (or peels off) with air blasts probably has
    A. red mouth syndrome
    B. chronic desquamative gingivitis
    C. periodontitis
    D. necrotizing ulcerative gingivitis
    E. hyperplastic gingiva

12. Which of the following instruments is BEST suited for root planing?
    A. file
    B. chisel
    C. curette
    D. hoe
    E. scaler

13. Gingival curettage includes the removal of
    A. diseased sulcular epithelial lining
    B. necrotic cementum
    C. inflamed connective tissue
    D. A and B
    E. A and C

14. Which of the following local factors is (are) implicated in the etiology of periodontal disease?
    A. calculus
    B. mouth breathing
    C. smoking and/or drug use
    D. tooth malposition
    E. faulty restorations
    F. all of the above

15. Incidental gingival curettage is performed during
    A. scaling and root planing
    B. polishing
    C. ultrasonic scaling
    D. all of the above

16. Which of the following groups of gingival fibers arises from the alveolar crest and inserts coronally into the lamina propria?
    A. dentogingival fibers
    B. alveologingival fibers
    C. transseptal fibers
    D. circular fibers
    E. dentoperiosteal fibers

17. Which of the following is NOT a function of the periodontal ligament?
    A. supportive
    B. formative
    C. nutritional
    D. sensory
    E. regenerative

18. Which of the following does NOT occur in the periodontal ligament as a result of aging?
    A. hypercalcification
    B. decrease in vascularity
    C. decrease in fibroplasia
    D. increase in elastic fibers
    E. decrease in mitotic activity

19. When bacteria invade through some break in the gingival tissue, the result can be
    A. a periapical abscess
    B. a periodontal abscess
    C. a gingival abscess
    D. a radicular cyst

20. The gingival cyst occurs as a painless, bluish-gray nodule in the gingiva and has the appearance and consistency of a mucocele. On a dental radiograph it
    A. cannot be detected
    B. appears radiopaque and well circumscribed
    C. appears radiolucent and well circumscribed

21. An enlargement of the marginal gingiva with the formation of a lifesaver-like gingival prominence describes
    A. Stillman's cleft
    B. gingival cyst
    C. gingival abscess
    D. fistula
    E. McCall's festoon

22. A patient who evidences the typical signs of traumatic occlusion is likely to have radiographs that demonstrate which of the following?
    A. widening of the periodontal space
    B. angular bone destruction
    C. thickening of the lamina dura
    D. all of the above

23. Calculus is harmful to gingival and periodontal tissues for all of the following reasons EXCEPT which?
    A. It provides a haven for plaque and is irritating.
    B. It provides a permeable surface that can store toxic irritants.
    C. Calculus is covered by plaque.
    D. It is a mechanical irritant.

24. Which of the following periodontal factors cannot be determined through a radiographic evaluation alone?
    A. height or contour of bone located on the facial or lingual surfaces of the teeth
    B. presence or absence of periodontal pockets
    C. presence or absence of occlusal trauma
    D. A and C only
    E. all of the above

25. Which of the following structures is nonkeratinized?
    A. attached gingiva
    B. hard palate
    C. interdental papillae
    D. sulcular epithelium

26. Which of the following gingival conditions would NOT respond to definitive curettage?
    A. fibrous gingival tissue

B. spongy gingival tissue
C. relatively shallow pockets
D. suprabony pockets

27. In root planing, as the surface becomes smoother, the strokes should be
    A. longer, with reduced pressure
    B. shorter, with reduced pressure
    C. the same, with even pressure
    D. longer, with even pressure
    E. shorter, with even pressure

28. Which of the following is the LEAST important diagnostic aid in recognizing the early stage of gingival disease?
    A. gingival color
    B. depth of the gingival crevice
    C. stippling of the gingival tissue
    D. hemorrhaging of the gingival tissue

29. The severity of periodontal disease is determined by the
    A. probing depths
    B. degree of mobility
    C. amount of bleeding
    D. shape of the gingiva

30. Periodontal dressings
    A. maintain patient comfort
    B. control surgical bleeding
    C. provide some splinting of mobile teeth
    D. all of the above

31. Furcation involvement is BEST detected by which of the following methods?
    A. use of an explorer
    B. use of a Nabers probe
    C. use of radiographs
    D. use of a curette
    E. all of the above

32. The depression between the lingual and facial papillae that conforms with the proximal contact area is termed
   A. col
   B. papilla
   C. sulcus
   D. embrasure

33. Which of the following factors would influence instrument selection?
   A. tissue state
   B. length of the clinical crown
   C. sulcular or pocket depth
   D. amount of calculus
   E. accessibility of the areas involved
   F. all of the above

34. Phase I of periodontal therapy includes
   A. treatment of dental emergencies
   B. removal of overhangs
   C. patient education
   D. extraction of hopeless teeth
   E. all of the above

35. The term peri-implantitis BEST describes which of the following clinical conditions?
   A. inflammatory response in the peri-implant tissues
   B. bone loss around an osseointegrated implant
   C. gingivitis associated with an osseointegrated implant
   D. suppuration around an osseointegrated implant

36. The acidity of infected tissue inhibits the action of
   A. subgingival irrigation
   B. local anesthetics
   C. fluoride
   D. antimicrobial mouth rinses

37. The organism(s) most commonly associated with the etiology of juvenile periodontitis include
   A. Actinobacillus actinomycetemcomitans
   B. Capnocytophaga sputigena
   C. Actinomyces viscosus
   D. A and B only
   E. A and C only
   F. A, B, and C

38. Which attachment apparatus of the periodontium is LEAST affected by occlusal trauma?
   A. gingival attachment
   B. periodontal ligament
   C. alveolar bone
   D. cementum

39. Which of the following oral hygiene aids is appropriate for cleaning a Class II furcation?
   A. toothpick in a holder
   B. end tuft brush
   C. interdental brush
   D. oral irrigator

40. Which of the following are removed during root planing?
   A. cementum
   B. dentin
   C. calculus
   D. A and C only
   E. A, B, and C

41. Bleeding upon probing in the presence of periodontal disease is caused by which of the following histologic changes?
   A. fibrosis associated with chronic inflammation
   B. edema

C. ulceration of the sulcular epithelium

D. infiltration of cells and fluid associated with inflammatory exudate

42. Suprabony pockets are most commonly associated with
   A. horizontal bone loss
   B. vertical bone loss

43. A major difference between juvenile periodontitis (JP) and prepubertal periodontitis (PPP) is that
   A. prepubertal periodontitis does not produce severe bone loss
   B. prepubertal periodontitis affects primary teeth and permanent teeth
   C. juvenile periodontitis produces only mild bone loss

44. Periodontitis is preceded by gingivitis. All untreated gingivitis does not necessarily proceed to periodontitis.
   A. The first statement is true; second statement is false.
   B. The first statement is false; second statement is true.
   C. Both statements are true.
   D. Both statements are false.

45. Progression of periodontal disease appears to be a cyclic process with periods of exacerbation and quiescence. This explains why chronic periodontitis may exist for many years without rapid bone loss and without certain loss of teeth.
   A. The first statement is true; second statement is false.
   B. The first statement is false; second statement is true.
   C. Both statements are true.
   D. Both statements are false.

46. In the presence of periodontal disease, the spread of inflammation into the deeper structures of the periodontium follows which of the following pathways?
   A. bony
   B. perivascular
   C. intraepithelial

47. Which of the following antibiotics has been used in the treatment of *A. actinomycetemcomitans* infections in localized aggressive periodontitis (formerly known as localized juvenile periodontitis)?
   A. Doxycycline
   B. Minocycline
   C. Penicillin VK
   D. A only
   E. A and B

48. Which of the following controlled-release delivery systems for site-specific antimicrobial therapy is nonresorbable and requires later removal by the clinician?
   A. Actisite®
   B. Perio Chip®
   C. Atridox®
   D. none of the above

49. The Perio Chip®, a gelatin chip, contains 2.5 mg of which of the following antimicrobials used in adjunctive periodontal maintenance?
   A. triclosan
   B. chlorhexidine gluconate
   C. tetracycline
   D. doxycycline hyclate

50. Atridox® is composed of 10% doxycycline hyclate in what type of formulation?
   A. liquid
   B. powder
   C. paste
   D. gel

51. Which of the following products utilizes a subantimicrobial-dose doxycycline as its active ingredient to inhibit collagenase activity in the treatment of periodontal disease?

A. Periogard™

B. Peridex™

C. Periostat®

D. Periocline®

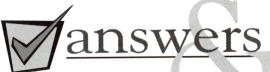

answers & rationales

1.

A. A periodontal pocket is a diseased gingival sulcus. A pocket forms as a result of disease or degeneration which causes the junctional epithelium to migrate apically along the cementum. Periodontal pockets are also referred to as true pockets or absolute pockets. Periodontal pockets can be classified as suprabony or infrabony (the base of the pocket is coronal to the crest of the alveolar bone or the base of the pocket is apical to the crest of the alveolar bone). (5:227)

2.

C. Six basic measurements are made in periodontal charting on each tooth: mesial, broad surface, and distal on buccal or facial aspect; and mesial, broad surface, and distal on lingual aspect. In addition to charting pocket depths, other periodontal problems should also be charted. These include recession, furcation involvement, mucogingival involvement, and width of the attached gingiva. (5:212–213; 9:270)

3.

B. A pseudopocket is a pocket formed by gingival enlargement without apical migration of the junctional epithelium. It does not involve the loss of bone. Pseudopockets are also referred to as gingival pockets, false pockets, or relative pockets. All gingival pockets are suprabony (the base of the pocket is coronal to the crest of the alveolar bone). (5:227)

4.

B. Pocket depths measure the depth of the sulcus from the base of the pocket to the height of the gingival margin. Probed attachment level refers to the measurement of the position of the attached periodontal tissue at the base of the sulcus to a fixed point. Pocket depth and attachment level are important in the evaluation of the patient's periodontal status. (1:32–35, 60; 5:206–210)

5.

B. Gingival enlargement and gingival recession can affect the accuracy of periodontal charting. Gingival enlargement may represent a pseudopocket or gingival pocket, in which there may be no bone loss or involvement of the deeper periodontal structures. On the other hand, in the presence of gingival recession, the operator may get a very low reading upon probing (1 to 2 mm), which in ordinary circumstances would represent healthy conditions. However, in the case of recession, the gingiva could be in very poor condition. This point should emphasize the necessity of determining bone level and the height of the gingiva and charting them both on the periodontal chart. (1:4–5)

6.

A. Most periodontal pocket depths up to 3 mm are usually related to a normal, healthy gingival sulcus. Periodontal pockets are divided into gingival and periodontal types. They are further categorized by their position in relation to alveolar bone. Healthy sulci are shallow and may be only 0.5 mm. The average depth of the healthy sulcus is about 1.8 mm. (3:201–205; 5:190, 227; 6:35)

7.

A. The objective for successful root planing involves removal of factors that promote gingival inflammation (plaque, calculus, altered cementum) and irregular, roughened root surfaces. The technique for root planing is basically the same as for scaling. The difference between scaling and root planing should be the degree of resulting smoothness. (1:4–5; 5:553–554; 9:535)

8.

B. Curettes are the most widely used and most effective and versatile of the periodontal instruments. The design of the curette allows it to be inserted subgingivally with less chance of trauma to the tissue. The curve of the blade of the curette adapts to the curved surfaces of the teeth. Most curettes are smaller and thinner than other scaling instruments, allowing for increased tactile sensitivity and ease in insertion. The universal curette can be adapted to all surfaces of the teeth. The Gracey curettes are the most commonly used area-specific curettes. Their design features permit maximum access to certain areas of the oral cavity. They are particularly useful in planing deep periodontal pockets. (1:148, 206; 6:131–132)

9.

B. Exposed cementum and dentin predispose the patient to hypersensitive teeth. Hypersensitive teeth can be treated with fluoride or iontophoresis. The patient can help control it with plaque control, diet, nonabrasive dentifrices, and self-applied fluorides. (5:595–601; 9:667–669)

10.

B. Periodontal disease and dental caries are the two most common chronic dental diseases. Both are caused primarily by the presence of dental plaque. Preventive measures can eliminate both of these oral diseases extensively. (4:537)

11.

B. A patient who manifests a peculiar inflammation of the gingiva and demonstrates ulcerated and necrotic epithelium that sloughs off with air blasts probably has chronic desquamative gingivitis. Chronic desquamative gingivitis has no known etiology. It occurs most frequently in women. (3:166; 9:260)

12.

C. A curette is the instrument of choice for root planing procedures. Curettes with rigid shanks are best used for heavy deposits. Curettes are also employed in soft-tissue curettage. (1:207)

13.

E. Gingival curettage includes the removal of diseased sulcular epithelium and inflamed connective tissue. Scaling removes calculus. Root planing removes residual calculus and altered cementum. (1:313)

14.

F. Local factors implicated in the etiology of periodontal disease are: calculus, mouth breathing, smoking and/or drug use, tooth malposition, and faulty restorations. The American Academy of Periodontology has classified periodontal disease into four types. Type I is gingivitis, Type II is early periodontitis, Type III is moderate periodontitis, and Type IV is advanced periodontitis. (4:538–539)

15.

A. Incidental gingival curettage occurs during scaling and root planing. This incidental or inadvertent curettage includes the debridement of the lining of the sulcus or pocket. Incidental gingival curettage is caused by the outer or unused side of the curette blade. (1:313)

16.

B. The alveologingival fibers arise from the alveolar crest and insert coronally into the lamina propria of the gingiva. The transseptal fibers of the periodontal ligament extend interproximally between adjacent teeth. Transseptal fibers are accessory fibers. The dentogingival fibers arise in the cementum and extend apically into the junctional epithelium. The circular fibers encircle the teeth. The dentoperiosteal fibers extend from the tooth and pass over the alveolar crest and blend with fibers of the periosteum of the alveolar bone. (2:42–43; 3:29–32)

17.

E. The periodontal ligament serves the physical, formative, nutritional, and sensory functions. It is composed of dense connective tissue. Its primary function is to support the tooth in the alveolus. (2:57; 3:34–38)

18.

A. The results of aging on the periodontal ligament include increase in elastic fibers and decrease in vascularity. Mitotic activity also decreases and there is a decrease in fibroplasia. The periodontal ligament may or may not widen with age. Also, with age, the amount of mucopolysaccharides and collagen fibers in the periodontal ligament decreases. (3:82–83)

19.

C. Gingival abscesses occur when bacteria invade through some break in the gingival tissue. They can occur as a result of mastication, oral hygiene procedures, or dental treatment. The gingival sulcus is rarely involved at the onset. (2:123-125)

20.

A. The origin of the gingival cyst is probably from remnants of the dental lamina or as a result of traumatic implantation of surface epithelium into gingival connective tissue. The overlying epithelium is intact and smooth. The lesion may appear white to blue. (4:129–132)

21.

E. A festoon ("McCall's festoon") is an enlargement of the marginal gingiva with the formation of a life-saver-like gingival prominence. Frequently, the associated total gingiva is very narrow. Also, apparent recession is usually present. (5:196)

22.

D. In the absence of local irritants severe enough to produce periodontal pockets, trauma from occlusion may cause excessive loosening of teeth. Thus, the periodontal ligament may widen. Vertical alveolar defects may occur in the alveolar bone without pockets. (2:267–271)

23.

D. Calculus is mineralized plaque; therefore, it causes irritation to the tissue. Submarginal calculus is always covered by active plaque, which is in direct contact with the sulcular epithelium. Its permeable surface serves as an excellent storage place for bacteria. (5:277–278)

24.

E. The following are periodontal factors that cannot be determined through radiographic evaluation alone: presence or absence of periodontal pockets, height or contour of bone located on the facial or lingual surfaces of the teeth, and presence or absence of occlusal trauma. (11:137)

25.

D. Sulcular epithelium is a continuation of the oral epithelium covering the free gingiva, but it is not keratinized and therefore is more susceptible to the pathogenic potential of dental plaque. The sulcular epithelium makes up the outer boundary of the gingival sulcus. The attached gingiva, hard palate, and interdental papilla are all keratinized. (5:190–192)

26.

A. Definitive curettage is curettage that is expected to have a direct role in the elimination of inflammation and the reduction of the pocket to maintainable levels. Gingival tissue with firm, fibrous consistency contains fibrotic, collagenous elements that do not permit shrinkage of a pocket wall. (5:517; 6:429)

27.

A. Smooth strokes with even lateral pressure that overlap and cross each other are used in root planing. As the surface becomes smoother, longer strokes with reduced pressure will help to remove small lines, scratches, or grooves. Vertical, then oblique strokes are used. Many strokes are needed before the root feels glassy, smooth, and hard. (5:553)

28.

C. Inflammation, bleeding upon probing, and pocket depths are the most important diagnostic aids or signs of gingival or periodontal disease. Gingiva may or may not be stippled whether healthy or inflamed. The presence or absence of stippling is not diagnostic. (3:107; 6:31)

29.

A. Pocket formation and probing depths represent the severity of periodontal disease. Mobility and bleeding are also associated with periodontal disease, but the depth of periodontal pockets determines the severity of the condition. (6:31, 35-36)

30.

D. Periodontal dressings are placed over surgical wounds following periodontal surgery and gingival curettage. They serve a variety of purposes including providing protection, maintaining patient comfort, splinting of mobile teeth, controlling bleeding, and shaping or molding the flap. (3:763; 5:590–592; 9:625–640)

31.

B. The presence of furcation involvement is best detected by use of special curved probes such as a Nabers-1 or a Nabers-2 probe. (11:135–136)

32.

A. The col is the depression between the lingual and facial papillae. It is not keratinized and susceptible to disease. Most periodontal infection begins in the col area. (5:191–192)

33.

F. When selecting the appropriate instrument, you must consider the length of the clinical crown, pocket depth, amount of calculus, accessibility of the area to be scaled, and the tissue state. Longer shanks with more acute bends are necessary to scale or plane posterior areas with deeper pocket depths. Curettes with fine flexible shanks would not be indicated for a patient with tenacious calculus. Large, bulky blades are inappropriate in patients with firm, non-retractable tissue. (1:148, 209; 5:513–515; 6:163–164)

34.

E. A dental treatment plan involves various phases. Phase I therapy is also called initial therapy. It may involve any or all of the following: patient education and establishment of therapist–patient alliance, treatment of dental emergencies, oral hygiene instructions, scaling and root planing, caries control, removal of overhangs and other inadequate restorations, endodontics, extraction of hopeless teeth, temporary stabilization, occlusal adjustment, and reevaluation. Reevaluation is done throughout all phases of treatment. Phase II therapy is called surgical and restorative therapy. It includes periodontal surgery and/or final restorative treatment. Phase III is the maintenance phase. In this phase, long-term follow-up care is provided. (6:329–331)

35.

A. Peri-implantitis is similar to chronic adult periodontitis and is preceded by gingivitis characterized by gingiva that is edematous, enlarged, red, and/or hyperplastic. If peri-implantitis is untreated, the inflammation will increase in severity, resulting in bleeding upon probing, increased probing depths, mobility, fistulas, osteitis, and radiographic signs of bone loss. (7:22–26; 8:330–334)

36.

B. The pH of normal tissue is approximately 7 (neutral) as compared to an infected area, where the pH is more acidic (about 5). The more acidic pH interferes with the ability of the anesthetic to effectively stabilize the nerve membrane and block impulse conduction. The result is decreased and delayed anesthesia in the area. Infiltration anesthesia is also not recommended because of the risk of spreading infection. (9:599)

37.

D. Juvenile periodontitis is a periodontal condition usually affecting permanent first molars and incisors of adolescents. The most prevalent organisms associated with this condition are Actinobacillus actinomycetemcomitans and Capnocytophaga sputigena. The periodontal breakdown progresses rapidly and often appears to become arrested. (3:307; 4:551; 9:215, 219–220)

38.

A. The gingival attachment is least affected by occlusal force. Occlusal trauma does not cause gingival changes or pocket formation. The periodontal ligament may be crushed, hemorrhage, and in the chronic phase, it becomes wider. The cementum tears and fractures in the acute phase. In the chronic phase, there may be cemental hyperplasia or dentinal resorption. With occlusal trauma, there is resorption of the alveolar bone. (2:422–423; 3:266, 270–271; 5:261–262)

39.

A. A toothpick in a holder is indicated for plaque removal at or just under the gingival margin for concave tooth surfaces and for exposed furcations. In a Class II furcation, the bone has been destroyed to an extent that the area between the roots has moderate involvement, but instruments or oral hygiene aids may not pass through the area between the roots. (5:379)

40.

E. Root planing removes calculus embedded in cementum, toxic cementum and dentin, and plaque. The result is a smooth glassy root surface and removal of irritants that cause inflammation. (1:4–5)

41.

C. Gingival bleeding in the presence of periodontal disease is due to the ulceration of the sulcular epithelium. Additionally, capillaries become engorged and extend near the gingival surface. (10:28)

42.

A. Horizontal bone loss refers to a generalized reduction in height of the alveolar crest in which the crestal bone is generally at right angles to the root surface. Suprabony pockets are associated with horizontal bone loss. (10:28–29; 11:77)

43.

B. Prepubertal periodontitis (PPP) affects primary teeth soon after their eruption but can also affect the permanent dentition. Juvenile periodontitis (JP), on the other hand, usually affects permanent teeth, especially the anterior teeth and first molars. Patients with JP often have widened interproximal spaces. (10:31)

44.

C. Periodontitis is preceded by gingivitis; however, not all untreated gingivitis will proceed to periodontitis. (10:32)

45.

C. Progression of periodontitis appears to be a cyclic process with periods of exacerbation and quiescence. Attachment loss worsens during the periods of exacerbation; however, if attachment loss is not severe, the patient may have chronic periodontitis for years without suffering tooth loss. (10:32–33; 11:76)

46.

B. In the presence of periodontal disease, the spread of inflammation into the deeper structures follows a perivascular pathway because the vascular channels offer less resistance than the fibers of the periodontal ligament. (10:32–33)

47.

E. Tetracyclines as a group are bacteriostatic, inhibiting growth and multiplication by inhibiting protein synthesis. Doxycycline and minocycline have been used to treat Aa infections in localized aggressive periodontitis (formerly known as localized juvenile periodontitis) and refractory periodontitis. (12:360)

48.

A. Actisite® is an ethylene vinyl acetate flexible fiber impregnated with 12.7 mg of tetracycline HCl. It is placed subgingivally into the periodontal pocket, where the tetracycline is released slowly over 7 to 10 days. It is nonresorbable and must be removed at a follow-up appointment. (12:365)

49.

B. The active ingredient in PerioChip® is 2.5 mg of chlorhexidine gluconate. (12:366)

50.

D. Atridox® is a biodegradable gel delivered via a syringe system to the diseased pocket for use in the treatment of chronic periodontitis to promote attachment level gain, to reduce pocket depths, and to reduce bleeding on probing. (12:367)

51.

C. Periostat® capsules (20 mg twice daily) have proven effective in the inhibition of collagenase activity in individuals with periodontal disease. (12:369–370)

6 Community Dental Health

DIRECTIONS Each of the questions below is followed by several suggested answers. Select the best answer in each case.

---

1. The Ramfjord teeth commonly used to simplify dental indexes include

    A. the maxillary right first molar, left central incisor, left first bicuspid, and the mandibular left first molar, right central incisor, and right first bicuspid

    B. the maxillary right first molar, left central incisor, left first molar, and the mandibular left first molar, left central incisor, and right first molar

    C. the division of the mouth into sextants from the upper right third molar to the first bicuspid, cuspid to cuspid, left first bicuspid to third molar and the lower right third molar to the first bicuspid, cuspid to cuspid, and left first bicuspid to third molar

    D. the use of any six surfaces of any six teeth as long as operationally defined by examiner

2. Fluoridation is the adjustment of the fluoride ion content in
   A. a gel solution
   B. a water supply
   C. an aerosol spray
   D. an ingestible tablet

3. If the major purpose of an epidemiologist's research is to determine caries susceptibility as opposed to immediate treatment needs, the BEST caries index to use is
   A. DMFT
   B. DMFS
   C. CPITN
   D. TSIF

4. Fluorides are stored in skeletal tissues. Even when concentrations reach 8 ppm, no impairment in general health can be detected.
   A. The first statement is true; second statement is false.
   B. The first statement is false; second statement is true.
   C. Both statements are true.
   D. Both statements are false.

5. Water fluoridation ranks as a very successful primary oral health measure because
   A. it demonstrates to the public that caries and tooth loss are not inevitable
   B. its greatest benefit is to halt dental caries in the earliest possible stage
   C. its clinical efficacy and effectiveness are well established in the dental literature
   D. all of the above

6. Based on results of recent fluoride studies, prenatal fluoride supplements are recommended by both the ADA and AMA in

communities where water supplies are fluoridated. The results demonstrated a reduction of caries in primary teeth by 20 percent.
   A. Both statements are true.
   B. Both statements are false.
   C. The first statement is true; second statement is false.
   D. The first statement is false; second statement is true.

7. Controversy surrounding fluoridation of the drinking water has once again resurfaced. Opponents feel that fluoridated drinking water is a
   A. violation of individual rights
   B. risk factor for bone cancer
   C. risk factor for Down's syndrome
   D. all of the above

8. The human body possesses a prompt and efficient excretory mechanism for fluorides; however, this does not minimize the danger of long-term accumulation of fluorides which can be toxic.
   A. The first statement is true; second statement is false.
   B. The first statement is false; second statement is true.
   C. Both statements are true.
   D. Both statements are false.

9. Dental health surveys overestimate dental needs more so than private practitioners because
   A. they are conducted under ideal conditions
   B. they utilize standardized examiners
   C. they reflect a congruence between need and demand for care
   D. the statement is false; dental needs are underestimated

10. A special characteristic of the Root Caries Index (RCI) as compared to other dental indexes is
    A. a carious lesion is only included in the count when it appears below the cementoenamel junction
    B. a carious lesion is included in the count when it appears above or below the gingival margin
    C. it is unique in that it includes the concept of teeth at risk
    D. it is based on 28 permanent teeth, excluding third molars

11. For epidemiological studies, the BEST available index for the measurement of periodontitis is the
    A. Sulcus Bleeding Index
    B. Periodontal Index
    C. Community Periodontal Index of Treatment Needs
    D. indirect method of scoring loss of periodontal attachment (LPA)

12. If the dental hygienist is asked to present a community dental health presentation for a deaf audience, the dental hygienist should
    A. switch the lights on and off to attract the group's attention, give written information for reinforcement, and immediately begin the program.
    B. enlist the support of an interpreter, review the program with him or her, and ask the interpreter to interject appropriate comments when necessary
    C. present using sign language with written materials to augment the presentation
    D. switch the lights on and off to attract the group's attention, allow the audience to read handouts before initiating the program, and use sign language or an interpreter

13. The Klein and Palmer Index can be recorded as DMFT or DMFS. The DMFS would be the recommended choice in which of the following situations?
    A. Radiographs are not available.
    B. Time is a limiting factor in the screening process.
    C. The examiner is not highly skilled in the detection of caries.
    D. There is a need to detect sensitive changes in caries incidence.
    E. All of the above.

14. Females have been found to have higher DMF scores than males. One could also conclude from these findings that females are more caries susceptible than their male counterparts.
    A. Both statements are true.
    B. Both statements are false.
    C. The first statement is true; second statement is false.
    D. The first statement is false; second statement is true.

15. The OHI-S measures which of the following?
    A. dental caries
    B. debris
    C. gingival bleeding
    D. B and C only

16. A treatment category of II on the Community Periodontal Index of Treatment Needs (CPITN) indicates that
    A. bleeding was observed upon probing or pressure
    B. calculus was felt during probing and 3.5–5.5 mm pockets were recorded
    C. improved oral hygiene and scaling are necessary
    D. this index does not include treatment categories

17. The proportion of persons within a population suffering from a particular condition at a given point in time is known as
    A. need for care
    B. epidemiology
    C. frequency
    D. incidence
    E. prevalence

18. The MOST common cause of tooth loss in adult life prior to age 60 is
    A. dental caries
    B. periodontal disease
    C. accidents
    D. acquired immunodeficiency syndrome

19. The effectiveness of a dental health program can be measured by
    A. the degree to which it meets program objectives
    B. the number of participants involved
    C. the cost of the program
    D. the length of the program
    E. all of the above

20. Which of the following age groups is (are) MOST subject to rampant dental caries?
    A. young children with poor oral hygiene, adults with gingival recession
    B. young children with poor oral hygiene
    C. adults with gingival recession
    D. rampant caries are not age-related

21. Which of the following indices is used to measure oral debris?
    A. Plaque Index
    B. Gingival Index
    C. Decayed, Missing, and Filled Surfaces of Teeth (DMFS)
    D. Decayed, Missing, and Filled Teeth (DMFT)

22. Edentulism is closely related to oral hygiene practices of the patient. Partial edentulism is more closely related to the dentist's/patient's attitude toward extraction of his or her own teeth as the primary method of dental care.
    A. Both statements are true.
    B. Both statements are false.
    C. The first statement is true; second statement is false.
    D. The first statement is false; second statement is true.

23. Dental fluorosis is defined as
    A. hypermineralization of the enamel caused by overingestion of fluoride immediately after tooth eruption
    B. hypermineralization of the enamel caused by overingestion of fluoride during tooth development
    C. hypomineralization of the enamel caused by overingestion of fluoride immediately after tooth eruption
    D. hypomineralization of the enamel caused by overingestion of fluoride during tooth development

24. Sensitivity, a characteristic of a diagnostic test, should determine if a high proportion of individuals who are tested for a disease and found positive
    A. will not subsequently develop the disease
    B. will subsequently develop the disease
    C. has little place in oral epidemiology even though a positive test was determined
    D. will seek treatment once notified of the results

25. When a patient comes to a dental office, the first procedure is an examination. The first step in a public health procedure is

A. analysis

B. survey

C. diagnosis

D. treatment

26. The MOST important determinants of dental utilization are

   A. socioeconomic status, dentate status, and gender

   B. socioeconomic status and gender

   C. dentate status and gender

   D. undetermined at this time

27. What percentage of United States children exhibit some form of fluorosis today?

   A. 7–15%

   B. 20–25%

   C. 25–33%

   D. 40–50%

28. Fluoridation has several mechanisms for caries inhibition. Included are enhancement of remineralization of enamel, inhibition of glycolysis, incorporation of fluoride into the enamel hydroxyapatite crystal, and bacteriocidal action.

   A. Both statements are true.

   B. Both statements are false.

   C. The first statement is true; second statement is false.

   D. The first statement is false; second statement is true.

29. Which of the following caries indexes applies to primary dentition?

   A. DMF

   B. DEF

   C. DMFS

   D. def

   E. OHI-S

30. Which of the following indexes should be used to estimate MOST severe periodontal disease?

   A. OHI

   B. OHI-S

   C. PI

   D. GI

31. In 1989, fluoridation of the public water supply was estimated to cost on the average

   A. 20 cents per person per year

   B. 51 cents per person per year

   C. $20 per person per year

   D. $51 per person per year

32. There are 10 million HIV positive patients worldwide. A new case occurs every 15–20 seconds.

   A. First statement is prevalence of HIV; second statement is incidence.

   B. First statement is incidence of HIV; second statement is prevalence.

   C. The above statements describe an endemic.

   D. The above statements describe mortality rates related to HIV.

33. Medicare, Title XVIII of the Social Security Act, pays for dental as well as medical care for patients aged 65 and over. All types of dental care are included in this coverage.

   A. Both statements are true.

   B. Both statements are false.

   C. The first statement is true; second statement is false.

   D. The first statement is false; second statement is true.

34. Medicaid, Title XIX of the Social Security Act, approaches public-supported dental care by providing
    A. dental care for mothers and children receiving Aid to Families with Dependent Children benefits
    B. emergency dental treatment for everyone regardless of ability to pay
    C. dental care (screening, diagnosis, treatment) to needy children up to at least 20 years of age
    D. emergency dental care to needy children up to at least 20 years of age

35. The most important concept of Winslow's definition of public health is
    A. the art and science of preventing disease
    B. promoting mental and physical efficiency
    C. promotion through organized community effort
    D. health is not merely the absence of disease or infirmity

36. Prevention is the major objective of public health programs because it entails
    A. ethics
    B. teamwork
    C. cost efficiency
    D. all of the above

37. Primary prevention covers those measures taken before any disease appears. Secondary prevention is synonymous with early disease control.
    A. The first statement is true; second statement is false.
    B. The first statement is false; second statement is true.
    C. Both statements are true.
    D. Both statements are false.

38. The minimum population level that is necessary to support a public health department is
    A. 4,000–5,000
    B. 7,500–10,000
    C. 10,000–15,000
    D. 35,000–50,000

39. Which level of the health department offers direct services to the individual?
    A. local
    B. state
    C. national
    D. international

40. Education plays an important role in public health because
    A. preventive measures are taught and learned
    B. it decreases the need for government intervention
    C. the programs allow for cost-efficiency
    D. a teamwork approach is necessary

41. The term morbidity, used in epidemiology, refers to
    A. death
    B. disease and disability
    C. reasons as to why disease and death occur in a population
    D. loss of subjects

42. Milestones in dental public health in the early twentieth century were characterized by all of the following EXCEPT which?
    A. The Dental Department of the U.S. Public Health Service was founded in 1919.
    B. G.V. Black led discussion on fluoride at the Colorado State Dental Association in 1908.
    C. Fones opened a training school for dental nurses in New Zealand.
    D. Irene Newman became the first dental hygienist in 1906.

43. Health Maintenance Organizations (HMOs) are similar to preferred provider organizations (PPOs) in that they both are nontraditional methods for delivering and financing dental care. PPOs, however, are more of a financing arrangement than a structure.
   A. Both statements are true.
   B. Both statements are false.
   C. The first statement is true; second statement is false.
   D. The first statement is false; second statement is true.

44. Currently, a public health problem is defined as a health issue that
   A. results in public demand for immediate intervention by the government
   B. causes or potentially causes widespread morbidity and/or mortality
   C. has caused widespread morbidity and/or mortality
   D. involves a perception on the part of the public, public health authorities, and the government that a public health problem is occurring
   E. B and D only

45. Various ways in which epidemiological studies can be used include
   A. collecting data to describe normal body processes such as temperature
   B. measuring distribution of diseases in populations
   C. conducting and evaluating clinical trials
   D. all of the above

46. Endemic refers to the
   A. cause of the disease
   B. occurrence of disease beyond normal expectancy

C. expected level of disease found within a particular locality
D. sudden outbreak of disease

47. Many factors such as climate, familial and genetic patterns, and socioeconomic status have been studied to determine their relationship to dental caries. Since the advent of fluoridation of public water supplies, socioeconomic status has been proven to be a powerful determinant of caries status in the community.
   A. Both statements are true.
   B. Both statements are false.
   C. The first statement is true; second statement is false.
   D. The first statement is false; second statement is true.

48. Dietary histories of all patients entering the hospital with insulin-dependent diabetes mellitus (IDDM) are compared to the dietary histories of patients whose DMF scores are low and also to patients whose DMF scores are high to determine the relationship between diet and caries. This is an example of what type of study?
   A. cohort
   B. prospective
   C. retrospective
   D. both A and B

49. Nutritional status does directly influence prevalence of caries. Dietary factors do not.
   A. Both statements are true.
   B. Both statements are false.
   C. The first statement is true; second statement is false.
   D. The first statement is false; second statement is true.

50. The epidemiology of periodontal disease is much more difficult to study than dental caries because of
   A. involvement of more than one structure, greater accumulation later in life, problems with quantitative assessment, and inability to correctly assess impairment in tooth function
   B. greater accumulation later in life, problems with quantitative assessment, and inability to correctly assess impairment in tooth function
   C. involvement of more than one structure, greater accumulation later in life, and problems with quantitative assessment
   D. reversible shifts in gingivitis, problems with quantitative assessment, and inability to correctly assess impairment in tooth function

51. Patients who suffered increased coronal caries are at a greater risk for root caries. It was estimated in a 1985–1986 U.S. survey that over half of the dentate employed adult population and seniors studied exhibited at least one carious root surface lesion.
   A. Both statements are true.
   B. Both statements are false.
   C. The first statement is true; second statement is false.
   D. The first statement is false; second statement is true.

52. Susceptibility to periodontitis increases with age, but not as part of the aging process. Dentate or partially dentate elderly persons are at an extreme risk for total tooth loss.
   A. Both statements are true.
   B. Both statements are false.

C. The first statement is true; second statement is false.
D. The first statement is false; second statement is true.

53. Severe caries is operationally defined in groups of children as a DMFT of 7.0. Five percent of children in the United States today will fall into this category.
   A. Both statements are true.
   B. Both statements are false.
   C. The first statement is true; second statement is false.
   D. The first statement is false; second statement is true.

54. Gingivitis precedes periodontitis. Areas of the mouth affected by gingivitis will most likely become affected in later years by periodontitis.
   A. Both statements are true.
   B. Both statements are false.
   C. The first statement is true; second statement is false.
   D. The first statement is false; second statement is true.

55. DMF surfaces have an advantage over DMF tooth counts because they are
   A. more economical
   B. concerned with permanent dentition
   C. a simple, expedient index
   D. a more sensitive measurement

56. Prevalence is used to measure dental caries when
   A. radiographs are available
   B. animal studies are performed to determine progression of lesion
   C. caries rates and tooth loss are expected to be high
   D. caries rates are expected to be low

57. As a dental hygienist, your role in the community concerning tobacco use should be to
    A. ask, advise, assist, and arrange for all patients to stop using tobacco
    B. not personally use any form of tobacco
    C. conduct diligent oral exams on both patients who report and those who do not report tobacco use
    D. all of the above

58. Adults ingest approximately how many milligrams of fluoride daily?
    A. 1–3
    B. 10–30
    C. 100–200
    D. 250–500

59. When organizing and providing dental care services, *need* may be defined as
    A. the particular frequency or desired frequency of dental care from a population
    B. a normative, professional judgment as to the amount and kind of services required to attain and maintain health
    C. the quantity of dental care services available
    D. the number of dental care services actually consumed by a given population

60. Dental public health, or community dental health, is BEST defined as
    A. health care provided to maintain the health of the poor
    B. rendering health care services and deducing the nature of health problems
    C. protecting people's health through privately funded agencies
    D. activity directed toward the improvement and protection of the health of a population group

61. Evaluation of a community-based dental care program is
    A. an ongoing process
    B. important to provide qualitative and quantitative documentation of the program
    C. not an important consideration during the planning phase
    D. A and B only
    E. A, B, and C

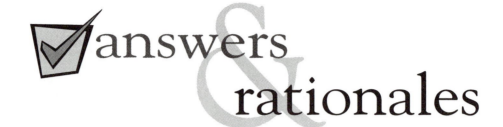

answers & rationales

1.

A. The Ramfjord teeth, by definition, are those included in answer A. (8:294)

2.

B. Fluoridation is the controlled adjustment of the fluoride ion content of a domestic water supply to the optimum concentration that will provide maximum protection against dental caries. (1:297)

3.

A. The results of the DMFT index yields a group's caries susceptibility without use of radiographs. However, the DMFS measures carious, missing, or filled surfaces and often incorporates use of radiographs. The CPITN and the TSIF are not used for measurement of caries. Use of radiographs in diagnosis of DMF surfaces is of far greater importance for determining immediate treatment need, whereas visual exams without radiographs can estimate caries susceptibility. (2:350)

4.

C. Fluoride is taken up at the tooth surface from both fluoridated drinking water and topical application. Some is deposited harmlessly within the skeletal system, even at 8 ppm. (2:157)

5.

A. According to Burt, increased public awareness resulting from caries prevention activities of water fluoridation has had a major impact as to how the public views tooth loss. Public acceptance of water fluoridation was essential for initiation and continuation of this public health program. (1:297–299)

6.

B. According to Burt, results of many studies have shown no benefit of use of prenatal fluoride supplements. (1:304)

7.

D. In the January 1990 issue of *Science*, the fluoride controversy reemerged with arguments launched concerning water fluoridation's relationship to cancer. Burt disputes charges that fluoridation is unsafe. (1:310; 3:276–277)

8.

A. The human body possesses an efficient excretory mechanism for fluorides. No damage to the human body has been reported from fluoridation of domestic water supplies. (1:284–285)

9.

D. Dental health surveys often underestimate dental treatment due to complicating factors. Criteria used to diagnose caries may vary; incongruencies occur between patients' perceived needs and practitioners' ideas of need; surveys look at short-term findings while practitioners must be concerned with long-term outcomes for patients; and treatment philosophies change rapidly. (1:182–183)

10.

C. The Root Caries Index (RCI) is unique as compared to DMF and other indexes because it takes into account "teeth at risk." A tooth is considered to be at risk of dental root caries if enough gingival recession has occurred to expose the cementum to the oral environment. (1:181–182)

11.

D. The indirect method of scoring loss of periodontal attachment (LPA) utilizes a fixed point, the cementoenamel junction (CEJ), in partial calculation of the index. The first step is a traditional measure of pocket depth, the second measure is the measurement from gingival crest to the CEJ, and the final calculation is step one minus step two. Other indexes utilizing the first step only may give inaccurate readings because the level of the gingiva is not always static. (1:186)

12.

D. For a community presentation for deaf audiences, flashing lights on and off is necessary to attract the group's attention. Interpreters are used to interpret only and probably have little knowledge concerning a dental hygiene–related topic. Allow ample time for the audience to review handouts prior to the beginning of the presentation because deaf individuals depend on reading for communication, and also must rely on their sight to follow the presenter and/or interpreter. (4:10–11)

13.

D. The Klein and Palmer Index can be recorded as "S" for surface and "T" for tooth. Surface counts are more sensitive than tooth counts. DMFS requires the use of radiographs, is more time-consuming, and requires that the examiner be highly skilled in the use of the index. (2:324)

14.

C. While the first statement is true and may be explained by earlier tooth eruption patterns in females and utilization of dental care, current research demonstrates that it is erroneous at this time to assume from these findings that females are more caries-susceptible than males. (1:219)

15.

B. The OHI-S measures plaque and calculus on six surfaces of six teeth. Caries and gingival bleeding are not determined by this index. (5:146–147)

16.

C. The Community Periodontal Index of Treatment Needs (CPITN) is an index of treatment needs rather than an index for determining periodontal status. These are the four treatment categories: 0 = no treatment necessary; I = improved oral hygiene needed; II = improved oral hygiene and scaling needed; and III = improved oral hygiene, scaling, and complex treatment needed. (1:187–188)

17.

E. Prevalence, by definition, is the situation described in the stem of this question; incidence refers to the number of new cases over a certain amount of time; epidemiology is the study of distribution of disease/death in a population; and frequency is simply a count. (5:142)

18.

A. Periodontal disease, for many years, was thought to be the major cause of tooth loss. Recently, research has revealed that dental caries is the primary cause of tooth loss at almost all ages, with the exception of the very old. (1:208–209)

19.

A. The results of a program are measured against the objectives developed during planning. Effectiveness deals with the attainment of objectives. Efficiency deals with cost-effectiveness. (1:40–41)

20.

A. Rampant caries may be seen in children with poor oral hygiene or adults with xerostomia and gingival recession. (6:115)

21.

A. The Plaque Index is used to determine accumulation of plaque and oral debris. The Gingival Index is used to determine, as the name indicates, bleeding and gingival health. DMFS and DMFT are caries indices. (1:188–189)

22.

B. Just the opposite is true. While edentulism reflects attitude toward treatment by both patient and dentist, partial edentulism seems to be more closely related to oral hygiene. (1:203)

23.

D. Fluorosis occurs when excessive amounts of fluoride are ingested during tooth development. (1:259)

24.

B. By definition, sensitivity is a proportion of positive tests with subsequent disease. It should not be confused with the term *specificity,* which, by definition, is the proportion of negative tests without subsequent disease. (1:175)

25.

B. When a patient comes to the dental office or clinic, the dentist first performs a careful examination. The first step in modern public health procedures is identical to that used by the dental clinician, only here it is the community that must be examined. It is called a survey instead of an examination. (1:37)

26.

A. The future use of dental services will most likely be linked to the patient's gender (female), high socioeconomic status, and presence of most all natural teeth. (1:19–20)

27.

B. Dean, in his early work with fluoridation, reported that 7 to 16 percent of children exhibited some form of fluorosis. However, this figure has increased in children today, with various studies reporting from 22 to 25 percent. (1:282–286)

28.

A. It was thought for many years that the mechanism of fluoride was limited to incorporation of fluoride into the enamel hydroxyapatite crystal. According to Burt, the mechanism for the effectiveness of fluoride in the prevention of dental caries is multifactorial. (1:290)

29.

D. Lowercase letters are used for measuring caries susceptibility in primary dentition. OHI-S is a debris index, and a primary dentition counterpart is not reported in the dental literature. (1:178–179, 188)

30.

C. The OHI and OHI-S are debris indexes and do not measure severity of periodontal disease. The GI index is confined to measurements within the gingiva. The Periodontal Index (PI) is used to measure presence and severity of periodontal disease. (1:186, 188)

31.

B. The estimated cost in 1989 per person per year was 51 cents. However, costs have been shown to vary from 12 cents to $5.41 per person per year. (1:307)

32.

A. Prevalence is the number of existing cases at a certain point in time. Incidence refers to the number of new cases over a specific period of time. (5:142)

33.

C. Medicare does cover medical care for this population. Dental benefits are limited to those dental problems such as fractures and oral cancer that require hospitalization. (1:106–107)

34.

C. The Medicaid program instituted in 1968 required states to provide dental screening, diagnosis, and treatment for needy children up to at least age 20 years. (1:109)

35.

C. Winslow's definition utilizes the concept of organized community effort. All individuals within the population, whether fatally ill from the disease, susceptible, or disease-resistant, are encompassed. The entire community is taken into account. (1:34)

36.

D. It is more ethical to prevent disease than to cure disease. Teamwork is necessary to handle large groups efficiently, and delegation of responsibilities to auxiliary personnel is utilized. Cost-efficiency plays a major role because prevention is cheaper than the cure. (2:6)

37.

C. Primary prevention deals with the prepathogenic state of disease and involves health promotion and specific protection. Secondary prevention occurs in early pathogenesis. This involves early diagnosis and prompt treatment. (2:13)

38.

D. To be well supported by available tax funds, the 35,000 to 50,000 population is targeted. The essence of public health is dealing with large groups. Due to this fact, public health officials are educated with this orientation. Often it is more cost-efficient for two small counties to combine to form the target population. (2:19)

39.

A. The local health department provides such direct functions as home visits, dental clinics, and supervision of local water supplies. The state and national levels perform supervisory and administrative functions. The international level often works with worldwide health promotion and prevention. (2:19)

40.

B. Prevention, cost-efficiency, and teamwork are fundamental principles of public health. However, in a democratic society where government regulation is small, it is important for the public to understand why they must undertake proper health measures by their own volition. The individual must learn why such regulations are of value in order to increase compliance. (Wearing a seat belt is mandatory in some states, yet many people refuse to wear a seat belt. When one learns how many lives are saved yearly, then one is more inclined to comply.) (2:25)

41.

B. Morbidity refers to the amount of disease or disability in a population. Death rates are synonymous with mortality. Epidemiology has been termed the diagnostic procedure in mass disease. (2:6, 26)

42.

C. T.A. Hunter urged the founding of the training schools for dental nurses in New Zealand. In 1905, Alfred Fones trained Ms. Irene Newman in dental prophylaxis procedures. At that time, Dr. Fones was Chairman of the Legislative Committee of the Connecticut Dental Association. He introduced a bill to allow assistants to perform prophylaxes under direct supervision. (2:46–49)

43.

A. These two forms for delivery and financing of dental care became a more accepted part of health care in the 1980s. Often discussed together, they do differ because PPOs typically involve contracts between insurers and a number of practitioners. Patients are allowed to select from whom they will receive dental care depending upon whether or not the practitioner participates in the PPO arrangement. Participants of HMOs are much more limited in selection of practitioners. (1:102–103)

44.

E. Blackerby originally defined a public health problem as 1) a condition or situation that caused widespread death and/or disease, 2) where a body of knowledge existed that could relieve the situation, and 3) the body of knowledge was not being applied. Today, the definition has been expanded to include public and governmental perception of such a problem. (1:35)

45.

D. Collecting data to describe normal body processes such as temperature, measuring distribution of diseases in populations, and conducting and evaluating clinical trials are appropriate uses of epidemiological studies. (1:159–160)

46.

C. Endemic refers to the expected level of disease that occurs within a particular locality. (2:113)

47.

A. After assessment and evaluation of many global studies to determine predictive and risk factors for dental caries, socioeconomic status was determined to be a powerful determinant factor of caries status in any community. (1:221–223)

48.

C. Retrospective studies look at events or experiences in patients' pasts to determine if inferences can be drawn concerning etiologic factors of a disease under study. Cohort studies, also known as prospective studies, look at a group of patients free of disease and follow them to a given point into the future to determine causes of disease. (1:161–162)

49.

B. Recent studies indicate that nutritional factors, defined as absorption of nutrients, have no bearing on caries development. However, dietary factors, relating to how patients select foods that they eat, have a clear influence on caries development. (1:224–225)

50.

A. Due to involvement of both gingiva and bone, periodontal disease is more difficult to study. The increased accumulation with age contributes to the difficulty. Problems with establishing a reliable and valid quantitative instrument for measuring periodontal disease and assessing tooth function impairment also increase the difficulty of studying periodontal disease. (2:167–169)

51.

A. It has now been determined that patients with gingival recession who experienced high coronal caries

rates will most likely experience high root surface caries rates. (1:228–230)

52.

B. Post-1980 studies have indicated that elderly dentate or partially dentate patients are actually less susceptible to periodontitis. Highly susceptible individuals exhibit signs/symptoms of disease when they are young. (1:243–244)

53.

C. By definition, severe caries is now classified by a DMFT score of 7.0 or above. Twenty percent of U.S. children still suffer from severe caries today. (1:217)

54.

C. Basic, clinical, and epidemiological research from the 1970s on have revealed that while gingivitis precedes periodontitis, only a fraction of the sites affected by gingivitis will later suffer periodontitis. (1:237)

55.

D. A more sensitive measure for dental caries is DMFS. It reaches its greatest usefulness when dental radiographs are incorporated. In cases of high caries attack rates where almost no unaffected teeth remain, the DMFS well demonstrates a more accurate caries count than DMFT because only the whole tooth is taken into account in the latter index. (2:324)

56.

D. Prevalence is useful when caries counts are low. It is useful in ancient skull studies where many teeth are lost due to reasons other than caries. It is best utilized when one or two carious teeth are the criterion for differentiating affected individuals from unaffected individuals (those with no history of dental disease). (2:324)

57.

D. As role models, as well as health professionals in the community, dental hygienists have a responsibility to support cessation of all forms of tobacco use as well as to be aware of tobacco-associated general and oral health problems. (7:xi, 31)

58.

A. Adults ingest 1–3 mg of fluoride daily and have for many years. Acute fluoride poisoning occurs in adults when 250–500 mg are ingested over a 24-hour period. (1:288–289)

59.

B. Need can be defined as a normative, professional judgment as to the amount and kind of services required to attain and maintain health. Demand is the particular frequency or desired frequency of dental care from a population. Supply is defined as the quantity of dental care services available. Utilization is the number of dental care services actually consumed by a given population. (9:53)

60.

D. Dental public health is best defined as a concern for and activity directed toward the improvement and protection of the health of a population group. It is not limited to the health of the poor, to rendering health services, or to deducing the nature of health problems. Also, it is not defined by the method of payment for health services or by the agency supplying those services. (9:38)

61.

D. Evaluation is an ongoing process and actually is thought about in the planning phase when objectives and goals are being developed. It is also important that you are able to provide qualitative and quantitative documentation of the program to the target population, administrators, funding agency, and public on an ongoing basis. (9:172, 198)

7 Dental Morphology and Occlusion

DIRECTIONS Each of the questions below is followed by several suggested answers. Select the best answer in each case.

---

1. In normal occlusion, the buccal cusps of maxillary teeth occlude

   A. with the lingual surface of mandibular teeth

   B. with the buccal surface of mandibular teeth

   C. in the central sulci of mandibular teeth

   D. cusp tip to cusp tip

2. In ideal occlusion, the buccal cusps of maxillary teeth occlude with

   A. grooves and embrasures of mandibular teeth

   B. grooves only of mandibular teeth

   C. marginal ridges and embrasures of mandibular teeth

   D. marginal ridges only of mandibular teeth

3. The mandibular permanent second molar differs from the mandibular permanent first molar in the number of
   A. cusps
   B. roots
   C. lingual grooves
   D. marginal ridges

4. An individual tooth may be recognized by which of the following landmarks?
   A. cusps
   B. marginal ridges
   C. pits
   D. developmental grooves
   E. all of the above

5. The largest cusp of the maxillary permanent first molar is the
   A. distobuccal
   B. mesiobuccal
   C. distolingual
   D. mesiolingual

6. The height of contour of the buccal surface of the mandibular permanent first molar is at the
   A. junction of the occlusal and middle thirds
   B. center (in an occlusocervical direction)
   C. junction of the cervical and middle thirds
   D. cervical third of the tooth

7. The most distinguishable difference between the maxillary first and second permanent premolars is in
   A. the size of the crown
   B. the curvature of the facial surface
   C. the number of roots
   D. the length of the lingual cusp

8. With the exception of the third molars, the greatest variation in occlusal anatomy is found on
   A. maxillary second molars
   B. mandibular second molars
   C. mandibular second premolars
   D. mandibular first premolars

9. The permanent tooth that has the longest crown is the
   A. maxillary lateral incisor
   B. maxillary central incisor
   C. mandibular canine
   D. maxillary first molar

10. The anterior tooth MOST likely to have a bifurcated root is the permanent
    A. maxillary canine
    B. mandibular canine
    C. maxillary central incisor
    D. mandibular lateral incisor
    E. mandibular central incisor

11. Overbite is currently referred to as
    A. overhang
    B. overclosure
    C. malocclusion
    D. vertical overlap
    E. horizontal overlap

12. The occlusal anatomy of the mandibular primary first molar resembles that of the
    A. mandibular primary second molar
    B. mandibular permanent first molar
    C. mandibular second premolar
    D. maxillary first premolar
    E. its anatomy is unlike any other tooth in the mouth

13. A tooth occasionally exhibits a lingual groove that extends from the enamel onto the cemental area of the root. This is MOST likely to be the permanent
    A. maxillary canine
    B. maxillary third molar
    C. maxillary central incisor
    D. maxillary lateral incisor
    E. mandibular second premolar

14. The MOST reliable distinguishing feature of the mandibular third molar is the
    A. fused and compressed root system
    B. short, bulbous outline of the crown
    C. marginal ridge forming a smooth circle
    D. marked distal inclination of the root trunk
    E. great morphologic resemblance to the first molar

15. The primary function of the dental pulp is to
    A. form dentin
    B. protect the periodontium
    C. assure root-end closure
    D. prevent multiple foramina

16. Within a tooth, the entire space occupied by dental pulp is properly referred to as the
    A. pulp cavity
    B. pulp chamber
    C. intradental space
    D. interdental space
    E. pulp canals
    F. interproximal space

17. Bone surrounding the root of the tooth and providing attachment for principal fibers of the periodontal ligament is the
    A. alveolar bone proper
    B. bone trabeculae
    C. cancellous bone
    D. compact bone

18. Which teeth have the MOST variable crown shape of all permanent teeth?
    A. maxillary lateral incisors
    B. maxillary third molars
    C. mandibular lateral incisors
    D. mandibular second premolars
    E. mandibular third molars

19. The characteristic common to all mandibular first premolars when viewed from the occlusal aspect is
    A. the middle buccal lobe makes up the majority of the tooth
    B. the buccal ridge is flat
    C. the marginal ridges are underdeveloped
    D. the lingual cusp is large

20. Which of the following anterior teeth occlude with only one opposing tooth?
    A. maxillary central incisor
    B. mandibular central incisor
    C. maxillary lateral incisor
    D. mandibular lateral incisor
    E. mandibular canine

21. Mamelons are
    A. developmental grooves on the labial surface of maxillary cuspids
    B. sulci on the facial surface of mandibular molars
    C. three rounded protuberances found on the incisal ridges of newly erupted incisal teeth
    D. protuberances on the occlusal surface of mandibular cuspids

22. The mandibular second molar is different from the mandibular first molar in which of the following aspects?
    A. The mandibular second molar has four well-developed cusps, while the first molar has five cusps.
    B. The second molar has two well-developed roots which are shorter than the first molar roots.
    C. The second molar is smaller than the first.
    D. All of the above.

23. Which of the permanent incisors is MOST frequently concave on the lingual surface?
    A. maxillary central
    B. maxillary lateral
    C. mandibular lateral
    D. mandibular central

24. The size of the pulp cavity is influenced by the tooth's
    A. age
    B. functional activity
    C. history
    D. all of the above

25. The mandibular second premolar MOST closely resembles the mandibular first premolar
    A. from the buccal aspect
    B. from the occlusal aspect
    C. in that both have bifurcated roots
    D. in that the lingual cusp is of the same size

26. In an ideal intercuspal position, tips of the lingual cusps of a three-cusped mandibular second premolar
    A. lie in the central groove of the maxillary second premolar
    B. contact the lingual cusp of the maxillary second premolar
    C. contact the buccal cusp of the maxillary second premolar
    D. are free of contact

27. The mental foramen is located closest to the
    A. mandibular canine
    B. mandibular second premolar
    C. mandibular first molar
    D. maxillary first premolar
    E. maxillary third molar

28. In comparison with the mandibular permanent canine, the maxillary permanent canine in the same mouth
    A. has a shorter root
    B. is wider mesiodistally
    C. is narrower mesiodistally
    D. has a less pronounced cingulum

29. The compensating curvature (curve of Spee) which the maxillary arch assumes from anterior to posterior is usually
    A. convex
    B. concave
    C. a triangle
    D. parallel to the plane of occlusion

30. The lingual embrasures are ordinarily larger than the facial embrasures. The reason for this is that
    A. most teeth are wider on the lingual side than on the facial side
    B. most teeth are narrower on the lingual side than on the facial side and their contact points are located in the facial third of the crowns
    C. the contact points are located in the lingual third of the crowns
    D. the arch curve is extreme in this region

31. Which of the permanent teeth appear first in the mouth?
    A. first molars
    B. mandibular central and lateral incisors
    C. maxillary central incisors
    D. mandibular canines

32. The mesiobuccal cusp of the maxillary permanent first molar occludes with the mandibular permanent first molar in the
    A. central occlusal fossa
    B. lingual groove
    C. distobuccal groove
    D. mesiobuccal groove

33. That surface of the tooth that lies next to the lips or cheek (in either anterior or posterior teeth) is most correctly designated as the
    A. buccal surface
    B. facial surface
    C. labial surface
    D. lingual surface

34. Which of the following permanent anterior teeth has the greatest crown–root length?
    A. maxillary canine
    B. mandibular lateral incisor
    C. maxillary central incisor
    D. maxillary lateral incisor

35. The permanent anterior tooth MOST often missing is the
    A. mandibular canine
    B. maxillary central incisor
    C. maxillary lateral incisor
    D. mandibular central incisor
    E. mandibular lateral incisor

36. The posterior permanent tooth MOST likely to have a pronounced concavity on its mesial surface is the
    A. maxillary first premolar
    B. maxillary second premolar
    C. mandibular first molar
    D. mandibular first premolar
    E. mandibular second premolar

37. The mesial contact area of a maxillary permanent lateral incisor is usually located
    A. in the incisal third of the crown
    B. at the junction of the middle and incisal thirds of the crown
    C. at the junction of the middle and cervical thirds of the crown
    D. at the middle of the middle third

38. The permanent maxillary tooth that has the longest length of the crown is the
    A. lateral incisor
    B. central incisor
    C. canine
    D. first molar

39. The maxillary permanent first molar viewed from the occlusal has which of the following shapes?
    A. square
    B. rectangular
    C. obtuse
    D. rhomboid

40. The sensory nerve supply to the jaws and the upper maxillary arch and the lower mandibular teeth is derived from the
    A. masseter nerve
    B. temporal nerve
    C. external pterygoid nerve
    D. trigeminal nerve

41. From the occlusal aspect, what is the primary distinguishing feature or difference between the permanent maxillary first premolar and the maxillary second premolar?
    A. shape of the crown
    B. mesio-distal diameter of the crown
    C. bucco-lingual diameter of the crown
    D. a well-defined developmental groove in the enamel of the mesial marginal ridge of the maxillary first premolars

42. The hard tissue forming the largest portion of the tooth is the
    A. enamel
    B. cementum
    C. dentin
    D. alveolus

43. Of the following dental structures, which is (are) found on both anterior and posterior permanent teeth?
    A. mamelons
    B. oblique ridges
    C. marginal ridges
    D. cingulum
    E. transverse ridges

44. Permanent incisors, canines, and premolar teeth are ALL
    A. similar in heights of contour
    B. identified by one facial and three lingual lobes
    C. succedaneous
    D. anterior teeth

45. Which of the following permanent molars frequently exhibits a small fifth cusp attached to the lingual surface of the mesiolingual cusp?
    A. maxillary second molar
    B. maxillary first molar
    C. mandibular first molar
    D. mandibular second molar

46. The first primary tooth to erupt is
    A. the maxillary central incisor
    B. the maxillary lateral incisor
    C. the mandibular central incisor
    D. the mandibular lateral incisor

47. Which of the following teeth in the primary set resemble the permanent premolars?
    A. primary canine
    B. primary first molar
    C. primary second molar
    D. all of the above
    E. none of the above

48. A comparison of primary and permanent teeth will show which of the following differences in form?
    A. The crowns of primary anterior teeth are wider mesiodistally in comparison with their crown length than are the permanent teeth.
    B. The roots of primary anterior teeth are narrower and longer than those of permanent teeth.
    C. Cervical ridges positioned buccally on the primary molars are more pronounced than on permanent teeth.
    D. All of the above.

49. Which is the largest permanent tooth in the mandibular arch?
    A. first molar
    B. second molar
    C. third molar

50. From a developmental viewpoint, all mandibular molars have how many major cusps, as compared to how many major cusps on maxillary molars?
    A. 5;3
    B. 4;6
    C. 3;4
    D. 4;5
    E. 5;4

51. The first evidence of calcification of the primary lateral incisor is seen at approximately which of the following ages?
    A. 2 months in utero
    B. 4 months
    C. 6 months
    D. 4 1/2 months in utero
    E. 1 1/2 years

52. The primary first and second molars first show evidence of calcification at approximately which of the following ages?
    A. 5–6 months in utero
    B. 5–6 years
    C. 3–4 months in utero
    D. 4 1/2 months in utero
    E. 1 year

53. The permanent maxillary lateral incisor erupts at approximately which of the following ages?
    A. 5–6 years
    B. 6–7 years
    C. 8 years
    D. 8–9 years
    E. 9–10 years

54. The roots of the permanent third molars are completely formed at which of the following ages?
    A. 10–12 years
    B. 13–14 years
    C. 14–16 years
    D. 18–25 years

55. The mandibular permanent second bicuspid shows evidence of crown completion at which of the following ages?
    A. 3–4 months in utero
    B. 2 1/2–3 years
    C. 4–6 years
    D. 6–7 years
    E. 8–10 years

56. The maxillary central incisors erupt at approximately which of the following ages?
    A. 5 years
    B. 6 years
    C. 7–8 years
    D. 9 years

57. A 15-month-old child would have all of the following teeth erupted except the
    A. primary central incisor
    B. primary lateral incisor
    C. primary canine
    D. primary first molar
    E. primary second molar

58. Each tooth has approximately three or more centers of formation. The formation of each center proceeds until there is a coalescence of all of them. Each of these centers is called
    A. a tubercle
    B. a cusp
    C. a lobe
    D. a cuticle
    E. an enamel pearl

59. Deciduous teeth are exfoliated by which of the following processes?
    A. Pressure from the permanent tooth pushes the primary tooth out.
    B. The primary tooth undergoes resorption from the crown apically to the root.
    C. The primary tooth undergoes resorption from the apical portion of the root upward.

60. A cingulum is normally located
    A. at the incisal third of the lingual surface of anterior teeth
    B. at the middle third of the lingual surface of anterior teeth
    C. at the cervical third of the lingual surface of anterior teeth
    D. at the cervical third of the lingual surface of posterior teeth

61. A small enamel projection located in the cingulum area of maxillary or mandibular anterior permanent teeth is called

A. an enamel pearl

B. a tubercle

C. a supernumerary tooth

D. a marginal ridge

62. Lingual fossae are generally found on the

A. lingual surface of mandibular premolars

B. lingual surface of maxillary premolars

C. lingual surface of anterior teeth

D. lingual surface of mandibular molars

63. The permanent maxillary canine can be distinguished from the permanent mandibular canine by which of the following characteristics?

A. The mandibular canine has a less prominent cingulum.

B. The cusp of the mandibular canine is not so well developed, nor is its tip normally as sharp as the maxillary canine.

C. The lingual surface of the mandibular canine is generally smoother and lacking in anatomic detail.

D. All of the above.

64. The mixed dentition period ends

A. at about age 6

B. at age 12

C. with the exfoliation of the last primary tooth

D. with the eruption of the first permanent molars

65. All of the primary teeth have normally begun their development

A. in utero

B. 6 months after birth

C. 12 months after birth

D. 18 months after birth

66. A small nodule of enamel with a tiny core of dentin, found most frequently in the furcation area of maxillary molars, is called

A. a talon cusp

B. a tubercle

C. accessory ridges

D. an enamel pearl

67. When looking directly into a patient's mouth from the front, the second tooth from the midline to the left, in the stationary jaw member, is the

A. mandibular left canine

B. mandibular right lateral incisor

C. mandibular left central incisor

D. maxillary right lateral incisor

E. maxillary left canine

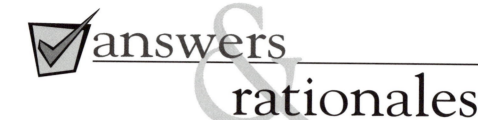

answers & rationales

1.

B. The buccal cusps of the maxillary teeth occlude with the buccal surfaces of the mandibular teeth in normal occlusion. The maxillary posterior teeth are slightly buccal to the mandibular posterior teeth. The tip of the mesiobuccal cusp of the maxillary first molar is aligned directly over the mesiobuccal groove on the mandibular first molar. The distal buccal surface is more lingual than the mesiobuccal, allowing the distobuccal cusp to occlude properly with the lower first molar. (3:364–366)

2.

A. In ideal occlusion, the buccal cusps of the maxillary teeth occlude with the grooves and embrasures of the mandibular teeth. Ideal occlusion may be considered to be theoretical or a practical goal for diagnosis and treatment. (1:441–445)

3.

A. The permanent mandibular second molar has four cusps. The permanent mandibular first molar has five cusps. The mandibular molars are larger than any other mandibular teeth. (1:242, 274)

4.

E. In order to study an individual tooth, one must be able to recognize all landmarks of importance by name. Dental anatomical landmarks include: lobe, pit, cusp, developmental groove, supplemental groove, sulcus, fossa, oblique ridge, transverse ridge, triangular ridge, tubercle, cingulum, ridge, and marginal ridge. (1:8–11)

5.

D. The mesiolingual cusp is the largest cusp of the maxillary permanent first molar. The maxillary first molar is normally the largest tooth in the maxillary arch. This tooth has four large functioning cusps and one supplemental cusp. (1:242)

6.

C. The height of contour of the buccal surface of the mandibular permanent first molar is at the junction of cervical and middle thirds. From the buccal aspect, the crown of the mandibular first molar is roughly trapezoidal. (1:276–286)

7.

C. The most distinguishable difference between the permanent maxillary first and second premolar is the number of roots. The maxillary first permanent premolar has two roots. The maxillary second premolar has a single root. (1:194–195)

8.

C. With the exception of the third molars, the greatest variation in occlusal anatomy is found on the mandibular second premolars. These teeth have two common occlusal forms. The three-cusp type appears square. The two-cusp type appears round. (1:231–240)

9.

C. The mandibular canine has the longest crown, approximately 11 mm in length. The maxillary canine has a crown length of approximately 10 mm.

The mandibular canine crown is narrower mesiodistally than the maxillary canine. (1:182)

10.

B. The anterior tooth most likely to have a bifurcated root is the permanent mandibular canine. This variation is not rare. (1:184)

11.

D. Overbite is that characteristic of the teeth in which the incisal ridges of the maxillary anterior teeth extend below the incisal ridges of the mandibular anterior teeth when the teeth are placed in centric occlusal relation. Dental professionals refer to the relative degree of overbite or vertical overlap. The presence of horizontal overlap in the molar areas prevents cheek biting. (1:432)

12.

E. In reference to occlusal anatomy, the mandibular primary first molar has characteristics unlike any other tooth in the mouth, primary or permanent. It has two strong roots, one mesial and one distal. (1:74)

13.

D. From a lingual aspect of the maxillary lateral incisor, it is not uncommon to find a deep developmental groove at the side of the cingulum. This is usually found on the distal side, which may extend up on the root for part or all of its length. The linguoincisal ridge is well developed and the lingual fossa more concave than the central incisor. (1:145)

14.

D. The average mandibular third molar has two roots, one mesial and one distal. These roots are usually shorter, generally with a poorer development than the roots of the first or second molars, and their distal inclination in relation to the occlusal plane of the crown is greater. This is the most reliable distinguishing feature of this third molar. (1:274, 299–301)

15.

A. The dental pulp is the soft-tissue component of the tooth. It is a connective tissue originating from the mesenchyme of the dental papilla and performs multiple functions throughout life. It is the formative organ of the dentin and the source of nutrition and maintenance of the dentin. (1:43, 308–309)

16.

A. Within a tooth, the entire space occupied by the dental pulp is properly referred to as the pulp cavity. The silhouette of the pulp tissue represents the entire pulp cavity, which is divided into a pulp chamber with branching pulp canals. (1:308–312)

17.

A. The alveolar bone/alveolar bone proper is the thin, compact bone that forms the wall of the tooth socket or the alveolus. The only space between the root cementum and this alveolar bone is that occupied by the periodontal ligament, which suspends and attaches each tooth to the bone. The alveolar bone proper provides the attachment for the principal fibers of the periodontal ligament. The principal fibers of the periodontal ligament are the oblique fibers, interradicular fibers, transseptal fibers, horizontal fibers, and apical fibers. (1:319)

18.

B. Maxillary third molars have the most variable crown shape of all permanent teeth, followed by mandibular thirds. These anomalies can range in shape from a small peg-shaped crown to a multicusped, malformed version of either the first or second molar. (3:236)

19.

A. The middle buccal lobe makes up the majority of the tooth. A lobe is one of the primary sections that form the crown. Cusps and mamelons are representative of lobes. (1:11, 38, 92)

20.

B. The permanent mandibular central incisor occludes with only one opposing tooth, the upper permanent central incisor. (1:428–432)

21.

C. A mamelon is any one of the three rounded protuberances found on the incisal ridges of the newly erupted permanent incisor teeth. They are very prominent in newly erupted teeth, but usually disappear with normal incisal wear. (1:11, 91)

22.

D. Normally, the second molar is smaller than the first molar by a fraction of a millimeter in all dimensions. The mandibular molars perform the major portion of the work of the lower jaw. They are the largest in bulk and have the best anchorage. The two roots of the second molar are well developed and shorter than the first molar roots. (1:274, 297)

23.

B. The permanent maxillary lateral incisor is more concave on the lingual surface than any other incisor tooth. The linguoincisal ridge is well developed, and the lingual fossa is more concave and circumscribed than that found on the central incisor. (1:145)

24.

D. All of these statements are correct. The size of the pulp cavity is influenced by the age of the tooth, its functional activity, and its history. (1:308)

25.

A. The mandibular second premolar most closely resembles the mandibular first premolar from the buccal aspect only. Although the buccal cusp is not as pronounced, the mesiodistal measurement of the crown and its general outline are similar. The tooth is larger and has better development in other respects. (1:231)

26.

D. In an ideal intercuspal position, tips of the lingual cusps of a three-cusped mandibular second premolar are free of contact. (1:435)

27.

B. The mental foramen is located closest to the apex of the root of the mandibular second premolar. This landmark is on the external aspect of the mandible. This position is not always permanent, and the foramen may be located between the first and second premolars. (1:374)

28.

B. In comparison with the mandibular permanent canine, the maxillary permanent canine in the same mouth is wider mesiodistally. Canines are the longest teeth in the mouth. Their roots are usually longer than any other roots. (1:182–184)

29.

A. The compensating curvature (curve of Spee), which the maxillary arch assumes from anterior to posterior, is usually convex. (1:88–89, 422)

30.

B. The lingual embrasures are ordinarily larger than the facial embrasures because most teeth are narrower on the lingual side than on the facial side and because their contact points are located in the facial third of the crowns. These contact area locations and the buccal and lingual embrasures are seen when the dental arch is examined from the occlusal view. (3:290)

31.

A. The usual order in which the permanent teeth appear is as follows: 1) first molars, 2) mandibular central and lateral incisors, 3) maxillary central incisors, 4) maxillary lateral incisors, 5) mandibular canines, and 6) first premolars. (1:25)

32.

D. The mesiobuccal cusp of the maxillary permanent first molar occludes with the mandibular permanent first molar in the mesiobuccal groove. (1:441–442)

33.

B. When labial and buccal surfaces are spoken of collectively they are called facial surfaces. Facial surfaces oppose the cheeks and lips. Conversely, lingual surfaces face the tongue. (1:7)

34.

A. The canines exhibit the greatest combined crown plus root length in each arch, and their roots are very firmly anchored in alveolar bone. Because of this bony support and the length of the root, the canines are usually the most steadfast teeth in the mouth. (2:252)

35.

C. The permanent maxillary lateral incisor is the tooth in each maxillary quadrant of the permanent dentition that is second from the midline. Contact is shared with the permanent central incisor on the mesial, while the distal contact is with the primary canine until its exfoliation at about age 12, and then with the permanent canine. It resembles the central incisor in all aspects, but on a smaller scale. The maxillary lateral incisors display greater variation in form than any other permanent tooth, except the third molars. Maxillary laterals sometimes are congenitally missing. (2:372–376)

36.

A. The posterior permanent tooth most likely to have a pronounced concavity on its mesial surface is the maxillary permanent first premolar. Immediately cervical to the mesial contact area, centered on the mesial surface, is a marked depression called the mesial developmental depression, which continues up to and includes the cervical line. The concavity continues apically beyond the cervical line, joining a deep developmental depression between the roots, which ends at the root bifurcation. (1:207)

37.

B. The mesial contact area of a maxillary permanent lateral incisor is usually located at the junction of the middle and incisal thirds of the crown. The development of this tooth can vary considerably in form. If its form variation is too great, it is considered a developmental anomaly. (1:140; 2:372–376)

38.

B. The average length of the maxillary central incisor (permanent) is 10.5 mm. This tooth has the longest crown length of any tooth in the maxillary arch. The length of its root is approximately 13 mm. (1:128–133)

39.

D. The maxillary permanent first molar is rhomboidal in shape when viewed from the occlusal aspect. The outline following the four major cusp ridges and the marginal ridges indicates this to be especially true. The maxillary first molar crown is wider mesially than distally and wider lingually than buccally. (1:256)

40.

D. The sensory nerve supply to the jaws and teeth is derived from the maxillary and mandibular branch of the fifth cranial nerve, also known as the trigeminal nerve. The trigeminal nerve has two branches, the maxillary and the mandibular. Its ganglion is the gasserian, located at the apex of the petrous portion of the temporal bone. (1:387)

41.

D. The maxillary first premolar has a well-defined developmental groove in the enamel of the mesial marginal ridge. The marginal groove is continuous with the central groove of the occlusal surface of the crown and divides the surface evenly buccolingually. This groove is not present on the occlusal aspect of the maxillary second premolar. The central developmental groove is shorter and more irregular on the maxillary second premolar. (1:208–209, 216–217)

42.

C. Dentin is the hard tissue that forms the main body of the tooth. It surrounds the pulp cavity and is covered by the enamel in the anatomical crown and by the cementum in the anatomical root. The dentin constitutes the bulk, or majority, of the total tooth tissues but, because of its internal location, is not directly visible in a normal tooth. (2:250; 3:182–183)

43.

C. Marginal ridges are linear elevations that are convex in cross-section and are found at the mesial and distal terminations of the occlusal surface of posterior teeth. They are also found on anterior teeth, but are less prominent. Oblique ridges are special types of transverse ridges which cross the occlusal surfaces of maxillary molars of both dentitions in an oblique direction from the distobuccal to mesiolingual cusps. A cingulum is a large, rounded eminence on the lingual surface of all permanent and primary anterior teeth. A transverse ridge is a combination of two triangular ridges that transversely cross the occlusal surface on a posterior tooth to merge with each other. (2:259–261, 433)

44.

C. The permanent teeth that are succedaneous teeth include the incisors and canines, which replace their primary counterparts, and the premolars, which replace the primary molars. Therefore, the only permanent teeth that are not succedaneous are the molars. (2:278)

45.

B. Frequently there is a small fifth cusp attached to the lingual surface of the mesiolingual cusp of the maxillary first molar. This fifth cusp is usually 2 mm cervical to the tip of the mesiolingual cusp. The fifth cusp varies greatly in shape and size. It may be a conspicuous, well-formed cusp or, at the other extreme, it may be barely discernible or absent, or there may even be a depression in this location. (3:137)

46.

C. The first primary tooth to erupt is the mandibular central incisor. This tooth usually erupts at 8 months of age. The root is fully formed and calcified at 18 months of age. (1:25)

47.

E. No primary teeth resemble permanent premolars. However, primary molars are replaced by premolars. Deciduous teeth are usually completely erupted by 27 months of age. (1:48)

48.

D. 1) The crowns of primary anterior teeth are wider mesiodistally in comparison with their crown length

than are the permanent teeth. 2) The roots of primary teeth are narrower and longer than those of permanent teeth. 3) The cervical ridges positioned buccally on the primary molars are much more pronounced, especially on first molars, maxillary and mandibular. (1:48–50; 2:276–285)

49.

A. The largest tooth in the mandibular arch is the mandibular first permanent molar. The largest primary tooth is the mandibular second molar. The mandibular central incisor is the smallest permanent tooth and the mandibular lateral incisor is the smallest primary tooth. (1:60, 77, 150, 274; 2:463)

50.

E. From a developmental viewpoint, all mandibular molars have five major cusps, whereas maxillary molars have four major cusps. Maxillary molars are smaller than mandibular molars. (1:241, 274)

51.

D. The first evidence of calcification of the primary lateral incisor is seen at approximately 41/2 months in utero. Hard tissue formation occurs in all primary teeth by the eighteenth week in utero. All primary teeth have usually erupted by 27 months of age. (1:25–26)

52.

A. The primary first and second molars first show evidence of calcification at 5 to 6 months in utero. Their roots are completely formed by 3 years of age. Girls' teeth usually erupt earlier than boys'. (1:25–26)

53.

E. The permanent maxillary lateral incisor erupts at approximately 8 to 9 years of age. In girls, eruption occurs at about 8 to 8.8 years; in boys, slightly later (8.4 to 9.1 years). (1:25, 141)

54.

D. The roots of the permanent third molars are completely formed by 18 to 25 years of age. Third molars are the teeth most likely to be malformed.

They are also commonly associated with dentigerous cysts. (1:25, 267, 275)

55.

D. The mandibular permanent second premolar shows evidence of crown completion at 6 to 7 years of age. The mandibular permanent first premolar shows evidence of crown completion at 5 to 6 years of age. The maxillary premolars show crown completion at the same approximate time as the mandibular premolars. (1:25)

56.

C. The maxillary central incisors erupt at approximately 7 to 8 years of age. The maxillary lateral incisors erupt at 8 to 9 years of age. Mandibular incisors are usually both erupted by 8 years of age. (1:25)

57.

E. At 15 months, a child will have all primary teeth erupted except the primary second molars. The primary second molars erupt at 27 to 29 months of age. The permanent teeth begin eruption at 6 years of age. (1:26)

58.

C. A lobe is one of the primary sections of formation in the development of the crowns. Cusps and mamelons are representative of lobes. Maxillary molars have three lobes and mandibular molars usually have four lobes. (1:11, 241, 274; 2:427)

59.

C. Before the permanent tooth can come into position, the primary tooth must be exfoliated; this is brought about by the phenomenon called resorption of the primary root. The permanent tooth in its follicle attempts to force its way into the position held by its predecessor. The pressure brought to bear against the primary root evidently causes resorption of the root, which continues until the primary crown has lost its anchorage, becomes loose, and is finally exfoliated. (1:36)

60.

C. A cingulum is a large rounded eminence on the lingual surface of all permanent and primary anterior teeth which encompasses the entire cervical third of the lingual surface. (2:259)

61.

B. A tubercle is a small enamel projection in the cingulum area of maxillary or mandibular anterior permanent teeth. Frequently, the projection has a pulp horn so that radiographically it may be mistaken for a supernumerary tooth superimposed over an anterior tooth or dens in dente. Removal is often necessary because of its interference in jaw closure with centric occlusion. Because the pulp horn is present, endodontic treatment is usually required when it is removed. (3:242–243)

62.

C. Lingual fossae are generally found on the lingual surface of anterior teeth. The crowns of the incisors exhibit a concavity that covers roughly the incisal half of the lingual surface. The remainder of the lingual surface is occupied by a general convexity which is defined as a cingulum. (2:259)

63.

D. The lingual outline of the permanent mandibular canine is similar to that of the maxillary canine, except the cingulum convexity is less prominent. The cusp of the mandibular canine is not so well developed, nor is its tip normally as sharp as in the maxillary canine. The lingual surface of the mandibular canine is generally smoother and lacking in anatomic detail when compared to the maxillary canine. The cingulum does not extend so far incisally, and the marginal ridges are not so prominent. (2:393–399)

64.

C. Mixed dentition period is the period during which both primary and permanent teeth are present, and lasts from approximately 6 years to 12 years of age. This period ends and the permanent dentition period begins around age 12, with the exfoliation of the last primary tooth, normally the maxillary canine. (2:278, 296)

65.

A. For the primary dentition, the crowns of all 20 teeth begin to calcify between 4 and 6 months in utero and on the average take 10 months for completion. It is about 6 months later on the average before the mandibular crowns emerge and 9 months after crown completion before the maxillary teeth reach the oral cavity. The primary roots are completed on the average 14 months after emergence for the mandibular dentition and 15 months after emergence for the maxillary teeth. Only 3 years after the roots are complete, they begin to resorb as the permanent teeth begin their occlusal migration. (3:31)

66.

D. Enamel pearls are small nodules of enamel with a tiny core of dentin. They are found most frequently in the furcation area of maxillary molars. They appear radiographically as small, round radiopacities. Being covered with enamel, they prevent the normal connective tissue attachment and consequently may channel disease (periodontal problems) into this region. (3:238, 242)

67.

D. The maxillary right lateral incisor (#7) is the tooth in the maxillary right quadrant of the permanent dentition that is second from the midline. Contact is shared with the permanent central incisor on the mesial, while the distal contact is with the primary canine until its exfoliation at about age 12, and then with the permanent canine. (2:372–377)

CHAPTER

8 Radiology

DIRECTIONS Each of the questions below is followed by several suggested answers. Select the best answer in each case.

---

1. Dental x-ray machines that use more than 70 kVp are required to have a total filtration of at least
   A. 0.5 mm of aluminum
   B. 1.5 mm of aluminum
   C. 2.0 mm of aluminum
   D. 2.5 mm of aluminum

2. A radiograph that is too light in density may be caused by
   A. overdeveloping the film
   B. using an exhausted developer
   C. using high kilovoltage
   D. too much radiation exposure time

3. Periapical or bitewing radiographs that exhibit the error of overlapping proximal structures are a result of
   A. incorrect vertical positioning
   B. incorrect vertical positioning of the cone
   C. incorrect horizontal positioning of the cone
   D. incorrect vertical angulation, but correct horizontal angulation

4. The radiopacity that frequently obliterates the apices of maxillary molars when using the bisecting angle technique for intraoral radiography is the
   A. zygoma and the zygomatic process of the maxilla
   B. orbital process of the zygomatic bone
   C. palatine bone and the zygoma
   D. maxillary sinus and nasal fossa
   E. maxillary tuberosity and zygoma

5. Yellow-brown stains on radiographs can result from all of the following EXCEPT
   A. unclean processing tanks
   B. insufficient fixing
   C. insufficient washing
   D. overfixing

6. When making bitewing radiographs, the vertical angle utilized should be
   A. approximately 5° downward
   B. approximately 5° upward
   C. 0°
   D. adjusted for the curve of Spee

7. The paralleling technique using the extension cone, compared with the bisecting angle technique, involves
   A. greater vertical angulation
   B. greater object-to-film distance
   C. shorter developing time

D. shorter anode-to-film distance
E. all of the above

8. If the operator wants to change from the long-scale contrast film technique to a short-scale contrast film technique and maintain the same density, what should be done?
   A. Decrease the kVp and the mA.
   B. Decrease the kVp and increase the mA.
   C. Increase the kVp and mA.
   D. Increase the kVp and decrease the mA.
   E. Increase the kVp and use the same mA.

9. When using the bisecting angle technique, directing the x-ray beam perpendicular to the long axis of the teeth causes
   A. an overlapping of tooth images
   B. a reduction of tooth images
   C. a foreshortening of tooth images
   D. an elongation of tooth images
   E. a decreased penumbra formation

10. Image magnification may be minimized by
    A. using a long cone
    B. using a short cone
    C. placing the film as far from the tooth as possible
    D. shortening the exposure time

11. Radiographic examinations should be made on patients
    A. at least every 2 years
    B. at various intervals depending on their dental history
    C. at least every 3 years
    D. whenever professional judgment dictates

12. All of the following statements describe the latent radiographic image EXCEPT which?
    A. It may be visible prior to developing and fixing.

B. It is produced by the interaction of x-ray photons with silver halide salts.

C. It may be called the invisible radiographic image.

D. It is a minute speck of metallic silver.

13. On intraoral radiographs, dark areas around the necks of teeth are sometimes misinterpreted as carious lesions. These areas result from
    A. attrition
    B. abrasion
    C. the mach band effect
    D. cervical burnout
    E. all of the above

14. Oral structures of greater density may require increased penetration by x-ray photons. This may be accomplished by
    A. increasing the mA
    B. increasing the exposure time
    C. increasing the kVp
    D. decreasing the exposure time

15. A processed film that is clear and has no image may be a result of which of the following errors?
    A. placing the film in the fixer prior to its development
    B. a saliva leak into the film packet
    C. reversing the film packet in the mouth
    D. exposing the film to white light prior to processing

16. In processing radiographs, which of the following is a function of the fixing solution chemicals?
    A. Softens the emulsion.
    B. Causes silver deposits at the sites of exposed crystals.
    C. Develops the exposed silver halide salts.
    D. Removes the undeveloped silver halide salts.
    E. All of the above.

17. Which of the following cells are LEAST sensitive to radiation (radioresistant)?
    A. epithelial cells of the gastrointestinal tract
    B. lymphocytes
    C. erythrocytes
    D. nerve cells
    E. fibroblasts

18. Black lines on a film may be produced by
    A. fixer spills onto the film prior to processing
    B. high temperature
    C. static electricity
    D. air bubbles

19. Panoramic radiographs are very useful for many reasons, but they may NOT accurately depict which of the following?
    A. interproximal caries
    B. presence of foreign bodies
    C. the relationship of one intraoral structure to another
    D. fractures of the mandible

20. Intensifying screens used when extraoral radiographs are made
    A. aid in decreasing radiation exposure to the patient
    B. contain silver bromide crystals
    C. increase radiographic sharpness
    D. reduce film fog

21. The function of the raised dot on a dental film is to identify the
    A. side of the film that should be next to the tongue
    B. side of the film that should be toward the line of occlusion
    C. side of the film that should be facing the x-ray beam
    D. maxillary or mandibular teeth, depending on how the film is placed in the mouth

22. Cone cutting (partial image) on a radiograph is caused by
    A. pointed plastic cone of radiation
    B. underexposure
    C. improper coverage of the film with the primary beam of radiation
    D. placing the film in reverse to the beam of radiation
    E. all of the above

23. Patient protection from useless radiation may be increased by the use of an aluminum filter and a restricting collimator because the filter reduces the amount of soft radiation that reaches the facial tissue and the collimator reduces the size of the tissue area that is exposed.
    A. Both statements and reasons are correct and related.
    B. Both statements and reasons are correct but not related.
    C. The statements are correct, but the reasons are not.
    D. The statements are not correct, but the reasons are accurate.
    E. Neither the statements nor the reasons are correct.

24. Which of the following type films can be used intraorally and extraorally?
    A. occlusal film
    B. periapical film
    C. bitewing film
    D. screen film
    E. panorex

25. Anatomical landmarks seen on mandibular posterior radiographs include all of the following EXCEPT the
    A. submandibular fossa
    B. external oblique ridge
    C. mental foramen
    D. mandibular foramen
    E. mandibular canal

26. When radiographs are made on patients in a dental office, leaded (protective) aprons should be used on
    A. female patients in the childbearing years
    B. children
    C. apprehensive patients
    D. all patients
    E. those patients who request them

27. Film fog affects the contrast of an intraoral film because it
    A. decreases film density, resulting in a light radiograph
    B. increases film density, resulting in an overall gray radiograph
    C. produces phosphorous crystals on the film
    D. produces white speckles on the film

28. Increasing kVp causes the resultant radiograph to have
    A. more latitude
    B. decreased density
    C. a longer scale of contrast
    D. a shorter scale of contrast

29. Anatomic landmarks seen on maxillary posterior periapical radiographs include all of the following EXCEPT
    A. coronoid process
    B. hamular process
    C. zygomatic arch cross section
    D. infraorbital foramen

30. Presently, the maximum permissible dose (MPD) for whole-body exposure for occupationally exposed radiation workers is
    A. 0.05 Sv (Sievert) per week
    B. 0.05 Sv per year
    C. 0.05 Sv per 13-week period
    D. 5 rem (roentgen equivalent in man) maximum per 13-week period

31. The HVL (half-value layer) is the amount of
    A. lead necessary to reduce the radiation to zero
    B. copper in the target needed to conduct away the heat
    C. absorber needed to attenuate the radiation beam by half and is used to denote the quality of the beam
    D. opening in the lead diaphragm needed to collimate the beam to its proper size

32. Other than showing the interproximal surfaces of the posterior teeth without overlap, the purpose of bitewing radiographs is to
    A. determine the relationship of the maxilla to the mandible
    B. examine the occlusion of the patient
    C. see a more nearly accurate level of the intercrestal bone
    D. detect the presence of calculus

33. On viewing a radiograph, the operator finds that the lower half is acceptable, but the upper half is clear. What is the most probable cause of this error?
    A. The developer was too low in the tank.
    B. The fixer was too low in the tank.
    C. The developer was too weak.
    D. The film was not fixed properly.

34. If a horizontal fracture of a tooth root is expected, which should be done to confirm your suspicion on a radiograph?
    A. Use a variety of horizontal angulations.
    B. Use a variety of vertical angulations.
    C. Increase the density of the radiograph.
    D. Decrease the density of the radiograph.

35. Which of the following describes a radiographic image that has many gradations of gray, from totally white to completely black?

A. overexposed
B. underexposed
C. long-scale contrast
D. short-scale contrast

36. To reduce radiation exposure when taking radiographs, the operator should
    A. stand behind a suitable barrier
    B. stand at least 4 feet away from the patient and 125 degrees away from the central beam
    C. use speed D film
    D. stand behind the head of the x-ray unit

37. Of all the periapical views included in a paralleling technique full-mouth series of radiographs, which region is closest to satisfying all the principles of shadow casting and parallel placement of the film?
    A. the maxillary molar view
    B. the maxillary premolar view
    C. the mandibular molar view
    D. the mandibular premolar view

38. All of the following landmarks occur in the anterior region of the maxilla EXCEPT the
    A. nasal fossae
    B. hamular process
    C. median palatal suture
    D. nasal septum
    E. incisive foramen

39. Which of the following is a radiolucent restorative material?
    A. amalgam
    B. acrylic
    C. silver points
    D. gold

40. Which of the following combinations of structures appear radiolucent in a radiograph?
    A. nasal fossae, mental foramen, periodontal ligament space
    B. nasal fossae, incisive canal, genial tubercle
    C. hamular process, nutrient canal, nasal septum
    D. maxillary sinus, internal oblique ridge, mental foramen

41. Which of the following extraoral projections is most useful in the diagnosis of maxillary sinus conditions?
    A. lateral skull projection
    B. Water's view
    C. posteroanterior projection
    D. lateral oblique projection

42. For localizing objects in the mandible, in the buccolingual dimension, the film technique of choice is a
    A. panoramic film
    B. right-angle or cross-sectional occlusal film
    C. topographical projection occlusal technique film
    D. lateral oblique projection

43. A lateral oblique of the mandible (Lateral Jaw) radiograph is most frequently used for observing structures in
    A. both the maxilla and mandible for early periodontal disease detection
    B. the posterior teeth for periapical disease
    C. areas such as the symphysis of the mandible for possible fractures
    D. posterior areas of the mandible and/or maxillae that are too large to be depicted on a periapical film

44. If an exposure time of 30 impulses produces the proper density for an intraoral film at a focal spot film distance of 8 inches, what exposure time would be required to produce the same density at a 16-inch distance?
    A. 60 impulses
    B. 90 impulses
    C. 120 impulses
    D. 150 impulses

45. In panoramic radiography, the focal trough is the
    A. slit where excess radiation is filtered
    B. area that is in focus when the mA and kVp are adjusted
    C. zone of sharpness
    D. area that is collimated

46. In the rare event someone who works in a dental office has no shielding available and cannot leave the room, he or she should stand at least how many feet from the x-ray machine?
    A. 3
    B. 4
    C. 5
    D. 6
    E. 7

47. Given the scenario in question 46, in what position should the person stand in relation to the primary beam?
    A. between 90° and 180°
    B. behind the patient's head
    C. between 90° and 135°
    D. between 135° and 180°

48. Which of the following is the BEST attenuator of an x-ray beam?
    A. aluminum
    B. zinc
    C. lead
    D. tin
    E. tungsten

49. An anatomical landmark located in the mandibular bicuspid area when superimposed on or adjacent to the apex of a tooth could easily be mistaken for periapical pathology. That landmark is the
   A. submandibular fossa
   B. mental foramen
   C. mental fossa
   D. mandibular canal

50. Which of the following is the periapical lesion that is LEAST likely to be seen on radiographs?
   A. an acute alveolar abscess
   B. a chronic alveolar abscess
   C. a cyst
   D. a granuloma

51. Duplicating film is a type of photographic film that appears similar to x-ray film but is exposed by the action of
   A. infrared light
   B. ultraviolet light
   C. infrared and ultraviolet light
   D. ultraviolet and visible light

52. Digital imaging systems used in dentistry replace film with an alternative sensor known as a (an)
   A. PID (position indicating device)
   B. CCD (charged-couple device)
   C. TLD (thermoluminescent dosimeter)
   D. MRI (magnetic resonance imaging)

53. The vertical bitewing radiographic technique uses
   A. seven #2 films in the molar, premolar, canine, and midline regions
   B. seven #2 films in the molar, premolar, lateral incisor, and midline regions
   C. four #2 films in the molar and premolar regions

D. four #2 films in the molar, premolar, canine, and midline regions

54. Regarding quality assurance in dental radiography, the ALARA concept stands for
   A. as low as radiographically acceptable
   B. as limited as reasonably acceptable
   C. a lower area of radiographic accessibility
   D. as low as reasonably achievable

55. Quality assurance testing of the x-ray machine includes which of the following?
   A. collimation
   B. filitration
   C. output
   D. clearing time
   E. all except C
   F. all except D

56. Processing solutions should be monitored and changed every
   A. day
   B. week
   C. 2 weeks
   D. 4 weeks

57. Which form of radiation is known to cause ionization of body tissue cells?
   A. microwaves
   B. radar
   C. x-ray
   D. radio

58. The majority of x-rays produced by dental x-ray machines are formed by
   A. Bremsstrahlung radiation
   B. characteristic radiation
   C. coherent scattering
   D. photoelectric effect

59. Gloves should be worn during the exposing of dental radiographs in order to protect the skin from contact with
   A. blood and saliva
   B. mucous membranes
   C. contaminated equipment and surfaces
   D. all of the above

60. Radiation injury during tooth development can lead to
   A. hypocalcification
   B. tooth bud destruction
   C. complete anodontia
   D. radiation caries
   E. hyperplastic enamel

61. A herringbone pattern on a dental radiograph is indicative of
   A. poor washing technique
   B. overdevelopment
   C. inadequate fixation
   D. film placed backward
   E. inadequate development

62. Reticulation of a dental radiograph is indicative of
   A. inadequate fixation
   B. moisture contamination of the film packet
   C. excessive exposure
   D. weak developing solution
   E. sudden temperature changes during fixation

63. Storage of dental radiographs in too warm a place can cause
   A. reticulation
   B. light fogging of the radiograph
   C. staining of the film
   D. discoloration of the radiograph at a later date

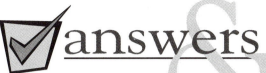
answers & rationales

1.

D. The peak voltage of an x-ray machine determines the total amount of filtration required. Below 70 kVp, the total filtration should be 1.5 mm of aluminum. When the kilovoltage is above 70 kVp, the recommended amount is 2.5 mm of aluminum. (1:28, 33, 34)

2.

B. A weakened developer will not fully develop the latent image in the usual time, and the density of the radiograph will be too light. A rough indication of an exhausted developer solution can be obtained by matching a good density radiograph with one taken at a later time. Less density in the more recent radiograph indicates an exhausted developer. A film positioned backward in the patient's mouth will also result in a lack of density due to the attenuation of the primary beam by the lead backing of the film. Additionally, a kVp, mA, exposure time that is too low or a target film distance (TFD) that is too great results in a film that is too light. (1:124–126, 132–136, 138; 2:245–246; 3:172)

3.

C. Incorrect horizontal angulation produces the same result in the bisecting, paralleling, or bitewing techniques. The radiograph will show overlapping of the proximal images of adjacent teeth. To correct this error, the central ray of the x-ray beam should be directed horizontally through the contact points of the proximal surfaces of the teeth. This direction for posterior teeth is usually somewhat anterior–posterior. (1:385; 2:50–51, 66, 68, 131, 133; 3:2, 30, 40, 54, 82, 86, 164, 180, 184, 190; 4:169)

4.

A. Less vertical angulation in the maxillary molar region will avoid superimposing the shadow of the zygomatic arch on the teeth. The apices of molar teeth are better visualized when superimposition of the zygomatic arch does not occur. The paralleling technique utilizes less vertical angulation than the bisecting angle technique; therefore, a better view is reproduced. (1:239; 2:50, 133–135; 3:2–12, 104–110, 114, 120, 122, 140, 144; 4:169)

5.

D. Film must be fixed in a fresh solution for an adequate length of time, i.e., 10 minutes, then washed in running water for 20 minutes. Failure to do either of these procedures will result in a lack of removal of processing chemicals. Remaining chemicals on the film will result in discoloration of the image. Additionally, if all the exposed crystals are not removed during processing, they will oxidize over a period of time and stains will result. (1:126–127, 133, 136; 2:21–30; 3:2, 80, 180, 182, 190, 192)

6.

A. As a result of the slope of the palate, a correctly placed bitewing film will not be parallel to the saggital plane, but will be slanted such that a downward (plus) angle of 5° is needed if the beam is to be at right angles to the film and the vertical plane. (1:248–251; 2:72–73)

7.

B. The paralleling technique positions the film farther away from the teeth so that the film is parallel to the long axis of the teeth. The paralleling technique must be used with the long cone to counteract the loss of image sharpness produced when the film is moved away from the crown of the teeth. Less vertical angulation is used than with the bisecting angle technique, and thus similar buccal and lingual portions of teeth appear closer to each other in the radiograph. (1:15, 17, 89, 117, 201–228; 2:76–81)

8.

B. The term *density* is used to denote the overall blackening of the film. Density increases with both the kVp and mA. Contrast is the variation of density or "shades of gray." The basic factors affecting contrast are the kVp, filtration, and the temperature of the developing solution. Higher kVp produces more penetrating x-rays and lengthens the scale of radiographic contrast. Thus, to maintain the same density with a change to short-scale contrast (high contrast), decrease the kVp and increase the mA. (1:103–105; 2:40)

9.

D. In the bisecting angle technique, when the x-ray beam is not perpendicular to the bisector, underangulation results and produces a longer radiographic image (elongation). When the x-ray beam is directed perpendicular to the long axis of the tooth, the beam strikes the bisector at an acute angle, not at a 90° angle. This elongation produces a tooth with a distorted image. (1:15, 17, 89–90, 116, 228–246; 2:77–78; 4:169)

10.

A. The paralleling technique requires a target-to-object distance that is as long as possible to remain practical. The technique also requires that the x-rays strike the object and recording surface at right angles, with the x-ray film placed parallel to the long axis of the tooth. The paralleling technique requires wide separation of tooth and film. This lack of contact between tooth and film would produce distortion if a short target-to-film distance cone were used; magnification of the image on the film would occur. There is a reduction in magnification when the extended distance cone is used. (1:15, 17, 89, 117, 201–228; 2:76–81)

11.

D. Currently there are no specified lengths of time between which radiographs should be made on various types of patients in various age groups. The old description of "routine radiographs" has no place in today's practice of radiation reduction. The decision for radiographic examinations is therefore based on professional judgment as far as dental radiography is concerned. (1:81–83; 2:124–130)

12.

A. The silver halide crystals are charged whenever they absorb x-ray photons. The result of radiation absorption is precipitation or formulation of a speck of silver in each affected crystal. This speck of silver consists of only a small amount of the total silver contained in the entire crystal. Collectively, these specks of silver are called the latent image. For the radiographic image to be seen, the film must be processed. (1:97, 121–126; 2:21)

13.

D. The area of the tooth between the enamel-covered crown and the portion of the root superimposed upon by alveolar bone attenuates fewer photons than the areas superior and inferior to it. As a result, a dark area referred to as cervical burnout is seen on the radiograph. (1:174; 3:136; 4:116–117)

14.

C. Photons move through space in a straight line and have a wave pattern. The greater the energy a photon has, the shorter the photon's wavelength. In the x-ray region of the electromagnetic spectrum, the shorter the wavelength of the photon (a high kVp), the easier it is for the photon to pass through matter. Long wavelength, low-energy (a low kVp) photons are called "soft x-rays." Oral structures of greater density require increased penetration or a high kVp. (1:21–24; 2:1–5)

15.

A. Film will become clear if it is placed in the fixer prior to its development. This type of clear film is identical to an unexposed (to radiation) film that is processed. (1:97, 100; 2:16–17)

16.

D. The function of the fixing solution is to remove the undeveloped silver halide salts. If the crystals (salts) are not removed, the image will be obscured. A second function of the fixing solution is to harden the emulsion which was softened by agents in the developing solution. (1:126–127, 133, 136; 2:21–26, 246–247; 3:2, 80, 180, 182, 190)

17.

D. The cells that are the most sensitive to the biologic effects of radiation have been found to be those that are least differentiated, immature, and are experiencing or will experience mitotic activity. Conversely, cells of nervous tissue and mature bone, which are well differentiated, are the least sensitive. (1:50, 2:109–110)

18.

C. A film packet should never be opened forcefully, especially when the darkroom air is dry. This could produce static electricity, which appears characteristically as dark streaks on the processed radiographs. The film should be held by the edges to prevent crimping or fingernail pressure, which appears as a crescent-shaped dark area. Bending a film can also produce a black line because the emulsion is sensitized to energy. (2:26–27)

19.

A. Despite their many advantages (broad coverage, anatomical relationships, the speed and ease with which they are made, and the exposure reduction when compared to a complete mouth survey), panoramic radiographs, as a result of magnification, distation, and interproximal overlap, frequently are not usable for determining the existence and/or extent of interproximal caries. (1:314–336; 2:160–185; 3:112–126)

20.

A. Intensifying screens consist of tiny calcium tungstate crystals bonded in a uniform layer on a firm x-ray penetrable base material. These screens are generally used in pairs with a double-emulsion base. This method of recording the image of an object requires much less radiation to the patient compared with when the x-ray film alone is used. (1:85, 101–103, 325; 2:19–20)

21.

C. Every radiograph has an embossed or raised dot to help indicate the film orientation. When the film packet is placed in the mouth, the raised portion of the dot faces the x-ray machine. This assists in aligning films for proper placement into film mounts. (1:98, 140; 2:106)

22.

C. If the central ray is not directed at the center of the film, cone cutting will result. The unexposed or white part of the film will not be in the path of radiation. *Cone cut* is the term commonly used to describe a radiograph made when the primary beam of an x-ray does not completely cover the film. (1:144, 152; 2:78–79; 3:96–100, 176, 180, 184)

23.

A. Useless, soft radiation may be removed by aluminum filters placed over the beam's exit port. This reduces facial tissue exposure. Collimation decreases the size or area of facial tissue by constricting the diameter of the primary x-ray beam. (1:35, 85–89; 2:10, 115–117, 249–250)

24.

A. Occlusal films can be used intraorally in a topographic occlusal view and also in a cross-sectional occlusal view. Extraoral projections using occlusal film are also possible in some instances. Three extraoral projections using the occlusal film are the maxillary and mandibular third molars and a tangential projection of the anterior region. Additionally, occlusal films may be used for lateral oblique views of the mandible ("lateral jaw" views) for children. (1:99, 254–260; 2:140–141; 3:96–98, 100)

25.

D. The submandibular fossa, mental foramen, and mandibular canal appear as radiolucencies, and the external oblique ridge as a radiopaque border. The mandibular foramen is not seen, however, because x-ray photons do not go directly through its lumen. (1:191–192, 194, 301, 328, 337; 2:94–107; 3:46–62, 66–70, 74)

26.

D. If proper exposure parameters are utilized, the amount of radiation reaching the gonadal areas of patients receiving intraoral radiographs is extremely small. If, however, the very smallest amount is to be delivered, the use of a lead apron is recommended for all patients. (1:88–89; 2:117–118)

27.

B. A common darkroom error is fogged film. These radiographs have an overall gray appearance because of diminished ability to see contrast. This may be caused by light leaks in the darkroom or improper safelighting, film storage, or processing solution temperatures. (1:35, 108, 124, 129, 138; 2:44–45; 4:166)

28.

C. Increased kVp produces more useful photons in terms of penetration and thus an increase in density. Radiographic contrast is also affected by kilovoltage. The lower the kVp, the greater the contrast and the shorter the scale of contrast; the higher the kVp, the longer the scale of contrast. (1:28, 30–32; 2:40–47)

29.

D. The coronoid process of the mandible, the hamular process from the medial pterygoid plate, and the cross section of the zygomatic arch are seen on maxillary posterior radiographs. The infraorbital foramen is never seen, however. (1:189, 195, 337; 2:93–107; 3:2–12; 4:52, 61–63)

30.

B. The maximum permissible doses (MPDs) are recommended limits of radiation exposure. They are set below levels at which biologic damages have been observed. These limits are recommended for persons who are engaged in occupations that necessitate a proximity to radiation. (1:75–76; 2:124–125)

31.

C. If a certain thickness of material reduces the intensity of an x-ray beam by 50 percent, the beam is said to have a half-value layer (HVL) of the thickness used, measured in terms of the absorbing material. In diagnostic radiography, aluminum is the absorber of choice. The half-value, measured in millimeters of pure aluminum, is the thickness of aluminum that reduces the intensity or energy of a beam of radiation by 50 percent. This measurement indicates the average quality or penetrating ability of the x-ray beam. (1:33, 147–148; 2:11–12)

32.

C. In addition to assisting in the early detection of interproximal caries, bitewings most accurately depict the most nearly true intercrestal bone level. This is the result of the very small vertical angle used when bitewing radiographs are made. (1:98, 248–253, 384–386; 2:18–19, 72–75; 3:88–94)

33.

A. The primary function of the fixer is to remove the undeveloped silver halide crystals from the film emulsion. If the developer is too low in the tank, the top part of the films on the film hanger will be only partially immersed; therefore, the upper parts of the films will not be developed when placed in the fixer. The undeveloped crystals in the upper parts of the films will be dissolved away, leaving a clear band. (1:126–127, 133, 136; 2:26–30)

34.

B. Because the x-ray photons may not strike the line of fracture at one vertical angle, several different vertical angulations should be utilized. (1:724–725; 2:1–3, 7, 12)

35.

C. The variation of densities or "shades of gray" is referred to as contrast. Low-contrast radiographs have many gradations and less density difference. High-contrast is short scale and has fewer "shades of gray" or density levels. (1:105–108; 2:21, 40–42, 198)

36.

A. Standing behind a suitably constructed barrier will reduce the radiation to the operator to zero. Common usage has resulted in the recommendation of lead barriers. There are other suitable materials, such as steel, concrete, bricks, tile, or plaster when adequate thickness is used. (2:120–123)

37.

C. When using the paralleling technique, it is usually necessary to use a relatively long tooth-to-film distance because of anatomic considerations. However, this violates one of the rules of shadow casting, namely that the distance from the object to the recording surface should be as short as possible. In the mandibular molar view, however, low muscle attachment allows the film packet to be placed quite close to the teeth and parallel to their long axes. Therefore, this approaches the ideal. (1:15, 17, 89, 117, 201–228; 2:76–81)

38.

B. The maxillary midline area depicts several radiographic landmarks. The nasal fossae, median palatal suture, and incisive foramen are radiolucent. The nasal septum is radiopaque. The hamular process is also radiopaque but is a part of sphenoid bone and is never seen on maxillary anterior radiographs. (1:179–180, 182–183, 337; 2:91, 100; 3:24–44, 96; 4:31–35, 63)

39.

B. The radiopacity of dental materials is contingent on atomic weight. Materials with low anatomic weight, such as acrylic, are radiolucent. Materials with high atomic weight, indicating a greater density, are radiopaque. (1:18–21; 2:94–96)

40.

A. Radiolucent structures appear on a radiograph as relatively dark areas. Cavities and spaces will form radiolucent images because of their lack of density. Structures of greater density such as teeth and bone will appear radiopaque. (1:105; 2:40–43)

41.

B. The Water's view is a projection that enlarges the middle third of the face and is useful in the diagnosis of maxillary sinus and other pathologic conditions involving this part of the face. The posteroanterior skull projection is not effective for studying the maxillary sinus because of the superimposition of other cranial structures. The lateral skull is not effective because it superimposes the right and left sides. The lateral oblique projection is used primarily to survey the mandible. (1:306; 2:150–156; 3:140)

42.

B. For localizing in the buccolingual dimension, a right angle or cross-sectional occlusal technique is used. The central ray of the x-ray beam is directed from under the mandible so that it is perpendicular to the center of the film packet. It is necessary to tip the headrest of the chair back and have the patient extend his or her head and neck posteriorly. (1:254–260; 2:143–144)

43.

D. Lateral Jaw or lateral oblique of the mandible radiography is the term used to describe extraoral lateral projections of the mandible and/or the maxilla. At best, this projection entails a certain degree of oblique angulation. Any region examined by this technique will have well-proportioned images and will depict a larger area than the periapical technique. (1:299–300; 2:143–149; 3:104–110)

44.

C. The inverse square law indicates that the intensity of a beam is 1/4 as great at 16 inches as it would be at 8 inches. Thus, four times as much exposure would be required if all other exposure factors remained the same. (1:36; 2:3)

45.

C. The tomogram or panograph is a radiograph that shows a sharp image of a layer of tissue with the layers above and below it being blurred. The width or thickness of the sharp layer (zone of sharpness or focal trough) varies with the angle of movement of the x-ray beam. A large angle produces a narrow focal trough; a small angle results in a wide focal trough. (1:319; 2:160–163; 3:306–312)

46.

D. In this unlikely event, it is recommended that the office worker stand at least 6 feet from the source of radiation. This takes advantage of the inverse square law regarding the intensity of the beam of radiation. (1:92; 2:3, 120–123)

47.

C. The recommended position of between 90° and 135° is the result of the consideration that most of the scatter radiation will be absorbed by the head of the patient. (1:92; 2:12)

48.

C. The best attenuator (absorber) of x-radiation of the energies used in diagnostic radiology is the one with the most mass per unit volume. Of the materials listed here, lead is best and is the most frequently used shielding material. (1:88, 98, 146; 2:117–118)

49.

B. The mental foramen may be superimposed or adjacent to the apex of mandibular bicuspid teeth and look much like a periapical lesion. A comparison of its appearance on the contralateral side will frequently rule out the possibility of its being a lesion. (1:191, 328, 337; 2:96–99, 106, 152–153; 3:58–62, 66, 72, 104–112, 114, 120, 124; 4:48–49)

50.

A. For a periapical lesion to be seen radiographically, there must have been a certain amount of tissue destruction. In the cases of chronic lesions, this will have occurred; but in the case of an acute lesion, this will not have occurred. (1:465–471; 2:207)

51.

C. Duplicating film appears similar to x-ray film but is exposed by the action of infrared and ultraviolet light, rather than x-rays. Only one side of the film is coated with emulsion. (5:172)

52.

B. A charged-couple device (CCD) is a solid-state electronic plate used to transmit signals directly into a computer in digital imaging systems. (5:10)

53.

A. Recently, some periodontists have recommended the use of vertical bitewing radiographs for patients with periodontal disease. This series consists of seven #2 films as vertical bitewing radiographs in the molar, premolar, canine, and midline regions. (5:271)

54.

D. The ALARA concept stands for "as low as reasonably achievable." This is the conservative view that the minimum amount of radiation should be used to get the job done. (5:212)

55.

F. Collimation, filtration, output, beam alignment, timer accuracy, and tube head stability are all quality control tests for dental x-ray machines. A test for fixer solution strength is called a clearing time test. (5:219)

56.

D. Processing solutions should be changed every 4 weeks or as recommended by the manufacturer. (5:217)

57.

C. Any radiation that produces ions is called ionizing radiation. The concern in dental radiography is that possible changes can occur in the cellular structures of the tissues as the ions are produced by the passage of x-rays through the cells. (5:20)

58.

A. Bremsstrahlung radiation is produced when high-speed electrons are stopped or slowed down by the tungsten atoms of the dental x-ray tube. Characteristic radiation accounts for only a very small part of the x-rays produced in an x-ray machine. Coherent scattering and photoelectric effect are types of interactions of x-rays with matter. (5:26–28)

59.

D. As part of a health care professional's practice of universal precautions, gloves should be worn to avoid contact with possibly infectious body fluids, i.e., blood and saliva, and the mucous membranes of a possibly infectious person. (5:153–154)

60.

B. Radiation in children can affect the odontogenic cells. A tooth bud may be completely destroyed if irradiated before mineralization has started. The damage may not appear for several years after radiation exposure. Head and neck irradiation therapy can also cause osteoradionecrosis. (6:729)

61.

D. A herringbone pattern indicates placement of the packet in the mouth backward with foil next to the teeth. Film exposed prior to processing can produce radiation fog. (6:167)

62.

E. Reticulation is produced by sudden temperature changes during processing. This occurrence is usually due to changes during processing, particularly from warm solutions to very cold water. Reticulation produces a puckered or pebbly surface. (6:167)

63.

D. Discoloration at a later date after storage of a completed radiograph may be due to incomplete processing or rinsing, storage in too warm a place, or storage near chemicals. Imbalance or deterioration of processing solutions can lead to fogging. Unintentional exposure to light can also produce fogging. (6:167–168)

9 Oral Histology and Embryology

DIRECTIONS Each of the questions below is followed by several suggested answers. Select the best answer in each case.

1. The epithelium of the oral mucous membrane may be
   A. keratinized
   B. parakeratinized
   C. nonkeratinized
   D. all of the above

2. Which of the following types of oral mucosa is NOT keratinized under normal conditions?
   A. buccal mucosa
   B. vermillion border of the lips
   C. incisive papillae
   D. hard palate
   E. gingiva

3. The right and left medial nasal folds and the intervening tissue are termed the
   A. primitive nares
   B. maxillary process
   C. mandibular process
   D. frontonasal process

4. The anterior two-thirds of the tongue develops from the
   A. third arch mesenchyme
   B. copula
   C. hypobranchial eminence
   D. tuberculum impar and adjacent tissue

5. The cheeks are formed
   A. from the hypobranchial eminence
   B. by fusion of the maxillary and mandibular processes
   C. from the copula
   D. from the tuberculum impar

6. The deep cleft between the growing maxillary and mandibular processes is the
   A. anterior naris
   B. primitive mouth
   C. frontonasal process
   D. olfactory pit

7. In the development of the face, which of the following play(s) a major role?
   A. lateral nasal process
   B. maxillary process
   C. mandibular process
   D. frontonasal process
   E. all of the above

8. The premaxilla contains tooth buds of the
   A. incisors and cuspids
   B. incisors, cuspids, and bicuspids
   C. incisors
   D. incisors, cuspids, bicuspids, and molars

9. The premaxilla has a single center of ossification which is
   A. in the anterior part of the palate (primary palate)
   B. in the posterior part of the palate
   C. in the palatine bone
   D. in Meckel's cartilage

10. The salivary glands arise from
    A. the ectodermal germ layer
    B. the endodermal germ layer
    C. ectodermal and endodermal germ layers
    D. oral mesenchyme

11. The two mineralized connective tissues of the periodontium are cementum and alveolar bone. The two fibrous connective tissues are the periodontal ligament and the lamina propria of the gingiva.
    A. The first statement is true; second statement is false.
    B. The first statement is false; second statement is true.
    C. Both statements are true.
    D. Both statements are false.

12. The passageway connecting the olfactory pit with the roof of the primitive oral cavity fuses and forms the
    A. premaxilla
    B. maxillary process
    C. primary palate
    D. pharyngeal roof
    E. eustachian tube orifice

13. The orthodontic movement of the teeth is enhanced by the fact that
    A. cementum does not resorb
    B. secondary cementum does resorb
    C. cementum does resorb
    D. secondary cementum will replace resorbed cementum

14. Which of the following structures separates the stomodeum (primitive mouth) from the foregut (primitive pharynx)?
   A. third arch cartilage
   B. cervical sinus
   C. Reichert's cartilage
   D. Meckel's cartilage
   E. buccopharyngeal membrane

15. Cells that resorb bone and tend to be large and multinucleated are
   A. odontoblasts
   B. osteocytes
   C. fibrocytes
   D. osteoclasts
   E. odontoclasts

16. Cells found in the periodontal ligament that can undergo proliferation under certain pathologic conditions to produce cysts and tumors of the jaws are
   A. cementoblasts
   B. epithelial rests
   C. Hertwig's epithelial root sheath
   D. macrophages
   E. mast cells

17. The lamina propria that supports the oral epithelium does so by interlocking with epithelium through
   A. epithelial rests
   B. rete pegs
   C. rete ridges
   D. A and B
   E. A, B, and C

18. Keratinized oral epithelium has four layers. Which of the following is NOT a layer of keratinized oral epithelium?
   A. basal layer
   B. laminal layer
   C. spinous layer
   D. granular layer

E. cornified layer

19. The major part of the alveolar ridge of the upper jaw develops from the
   A. third branchial arch
   B. lateral nasal process
   C. maxillary part of the first branchial arch
   D. maxillary part of the second branchial arch

20. The buccopharyngeal membrane is formed
   A. when the stomodeum ectoderm contacts the endoderm of the foregut
   B. from the primitive gut
   C. from the fifth branchial arch
   D. from the tuberculum impar

21. The first indication of tongue development is seen as a median elevation known as the
   A. tuberculum impar
   B. lingual notch
   C. copula
   D. hypobranchial eminence

22. Of the following, which is NOT a stage in the development of the tooth germ?
   A. bud
   B. cap
   C. bell
   D. ring

23. The area of the foramen cecum of the tongue is produced embryonically because the
   A. tuberculum impar is a retrogressing tongue component
   B. thyroglossal duct invaginates from this region
   C. apex of the V-shaped row of vallate papillae terminates in this region

D. bilateral pattern of the anterior two-thirds of the tongue fails to develop

D. A and B

E. A and C

24. The source of salivary lipase in the oral cavity is the
    A. parotid salivary gland
    B. submaxillary salivary gland
    C. von Ebner's glands
    D. sublingual salivary glands
    E. circumvallate papillae

25. Bitter and sour taste sensations of the tongue are mediated by the intermediofacial nerve by the chorda tympani. Sweet and salty tastes of the tongue are mediated by the glossopharyngeal nerve.
    A. The first statement is true; second statement is false.
    B. The first statement is false; second statement is true.
    C. Both statements are true.
    D. Both statements are false.

26. The first evidence of tooth development occurs when
    A. the dental lamina is formed as a segmented band (one for each deciduous tooth)
    B. a downgrowth of epithelium grows into the mesenchyme forming each dental arch
    C. the embryo is 20 mm long, and it manifests itself as an epithelial proliferation
    D. an epithelial thickening occurs over each developing arch, with the thickening having continuity around the arch

27. The remnants of the epithelial sheath of Hertwig are called the epithelial rests of Malassez. The fate of these is that they may
    A. undergo calcification
    B. form into cementicles
    C. become fibrous

28. Hertwig's epithelial sheath is derived from the
    A. inner dental epithelium and stratum intermedium
    B. inner dental epithelium and stellate reticulum
    C. outer dental epithelium and stellate reticulum
    D. outer dental epithelium and stratum intermedium
    E. inner dental epithelium and outer dental epithelium

29. After the tooth is formed, the dental papilla becomes
    A. the dental sac
    B. dentin
    C. the dental pulp
    D. bone

30. Hunger-Schreger bands are best demonstrated by
    A. transmitted light
    B. diffracted light
    C. reflected light
    D. polarized light

31. The rhythmical formation of enamel matrix is called
    A. calcification
    B. apposition
    C. mineralization
    D. cell division

32. The incremental lines of Retzius are
    A. globules of dentin
    B. lines of enamel apposition
    C. lines of dentin apposition
    D. lines of cementum apposition

33. The hardest tissue in the human body is
    A. dentin
    B. enamel
    C. bone
    D. cementum

34. The primary enamel cuticle is formed by
    A. external enamel epithelium
    B. ameloblasts just prior to tooth eruption
    C. fusion of oral epithelium and reduced enamel epithelium
    D. ameloblasts at the outer edge of the enamel
    E. fusion of oral epithelium and external enamel epithelium

35. Enamel lamellae, shown in Figure 9-1,
    A. are composed of poorly calcified rod segments
    B. arise in erupted teeth where the cracks are filled with organic material (saliva)
    C. may develop in planes of tension
    D. consist of degenerated cells
    E. all of the above

36. An age change that takes place in the enamel is that
    A. enamel becomes harder, therefore more caries-resistant
    B. organic content is decreased, thus the enamel often appears darker
    C. enamel surface changes in composition, thus becoming less acid-soluble
    D. inorganic content is increased, therefore the enamel becomes less permeable to acids

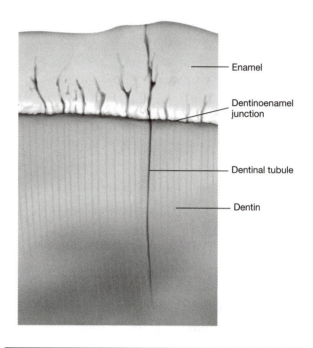

FIGURE 9-1. Transverse ground section through a lamella reaching from the surface into the dentin. (*Redrawn from Melfi RC, Alley KE:* Permar's Oral Embryology and Microscopic Anatomy, *10th ed. Philadelphia: Lippincott Williams and Wilkins, 2000.*)

37. In the normal human enamel, incremental lines are termed the
    A. lines of Gnarle
    B. bands of Hunter
    C. lines of Retzius
    D. bands of Schreger

38. Intercalated ducts
    A. collect secretions of terminal secretory units of salivary glands
    B. empty salivary secretions into striated ducts
    C. are thin branching tubes of variable length that connect terminal secretory units to the next larger ducts
    D. all of the above

39. The region where gnarled enamel is found to the greatest extent is
   A. at the cementoenamel junction
   B. on the anterior teeth
   C. under the tips of cusps
   D. on the perikymata

40. The ameloblasts enter their formative stage
   A. prior to the formation of any dentin
   B. after the first layer of dentin has been formed
   C. prior to the reversal of functional polarity of the cells
   D. immediately after reversal of functional polarity but prior to any dentin formation

41. Structures confined to the enamel rod are
   A. Hertwig's sheath
   B. cross-striations
   C. incremental lines
   D. enamel cuticles

42. The enamel tufts, as shown in Figure 9-2, are
   A. odontoblastic processes
   B. gnarled enamel
   C. enamel rods and interprismatic substances
   D. enamel cuticles

43. The tooth pulp is initially called the dental papilla. The dental papilla controls early tooth formation.
   A. The first statement is true; second statement is false.
   B. The first statement is false; second statement is true.
   C. Both statements are true.
   D. Both statements are false.

44. Mineral-poor ectodermal structures in enamel include
   A. tufts
   B. lamellae
   C. spindles
   D. A and B
   E. A and C

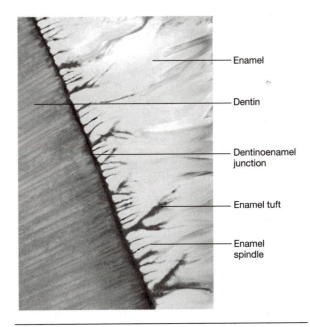

FIGURE 9-2. Transverse ground section through a tooth under low magnification. Numerous tufts extending from the dentinoenamel junction into the enamel. (*Redrawn from Melfi RC, Alley KE:* Permar's Oral Embryology and Microscopic Anatomy, *10th ed. Philadelphia: Lippincott Williams and Wilkins, 2000.*)

45. The secondary cuticle is the last secreted product of the ameloblasts because it is calcified.
    A. Both statement and reason are correct.
    B. Both statement and reason are correct but not related.
    C. The statement is correct, but the reason is not.
    D. The statement is not correct, but the reason is an accurate statement.
    E. Neither statement nor reason is correct.

46. As a general rule, enamel rods in the middle one-third of the enamel run
    A. at right angles to the long axis of the tooth
    B. parallel to the long axis of the tooth
    C. at 90 degrees to a line drawn tangent to the external surface of the tooth
    D. at 45 degrees to a line drawn tangent to the external surface of the tooth

47. Interglobular dentin, shown in Figure 9-3, is
    A. hypercalcified
    B. decalcified
    C. hypocalcified
    D. normally calcified

48. Comparing the dentinal tubules near the pulp with those near the dentinoenamel junction in a newly erupted tooth, those near the pulp are
    A. farther apart and of larger caliber
    B. farther apart and of smaller caliber
    C. closer together and of larger caliber
    D. closer together and of smaller caliber

49. Dentin is a type of connective tissue
    A. with the same structural feature as bone
    B. best considered as dead tissue rather than living tissue
    C. that is softer than enamel but harder than bone
    D. that, except for location, is identical with cementum
    E. that contains numerous, easily demonstrated nerve endings, making it very sensitive

50. The most highly mineralized region of the dentinal matrix has been demonstrated to be
    A. interglobular dentin matrix
    B. intertubular dentin matrix
    C. peritubular dentin matrix
    D. circumpulpal dentin

51. Deposition of calcium salts into dentinal tubules produces
    A. transparent dentin
    B. secondary dentin
    C. irregular dentin
    D. dead tracts

52. All of the following structures may be found in the dentin except

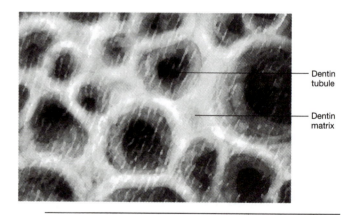

Dentin tubule

Dentin matrix

FIGURE 9-3. Interglobular dentin (decalcified section). The dentinal tubules pass uninterrupted through the uncalcified and hypocalcified areas. (*Redrawn from Melfi RC, Alley KE: Permar's Oral Embryology and Microscopic Anatomy, 10th ed. Philadelphia: Lippincott Williams and Wilkins, 2000.*)

A. Tomes's fibers

B. lines of Owen

C. globular dentin

D. von Ebner's lines

E. striae of Retzius

53. External resorption of dentin is repaired by

A. dentin apposition

B. cementum apposition

C. bone apposition

D. loose connective tissue

54. The narrow layer of minute areas of interglobular dentin near the dentinocementum junction is known as

A. sclerotic dentin

B. zone of Weil

C. lamellae

D. Tomes's granular layer

55. Terminal branches of dentinal tubules are found

A. somewhat adjacent to the dentinoenamel junction

B. somewhat adjacent to the odontoblasts

C. equally throughout dentin

D. in enamel

56. A histologic feature that readily distinguishes dentin of the root from crown dentin is the presence of

A. odontoblasts

B. mantle dentin

C. reparative dentin

D. Owen's contour lines

E. Tomes's granular layer

57. Primary dentin is considered to be vital because it

A. contains Tomes's processes and tissue fluid

B. is capable of forming secondary dentin

C. transmits stimuli from the enamel

D. is less calcified than enamel

58. Sclerotic dentin differs from primary dentin in that it

A. is more sensitive to stimulation than primary dentin

B. has relatively less organic material than primary dentin

C. has less inorganic salt and is harder than primary dentin

D. is demonstrable in decalcified sections, whereas primary dentin can be studied in both decalcified and ground sections

59. Nerve fibers of the central part of the dental pulp are mostly

A. unmyelinated

B. myelinated with no nodes

C. myelinated with long internodes

D. myelinated with short internodes

60. One function of tooth pulp is the

A. repair of resorbed cementum

B. production of reparative dentin

C. nourishment of the periodontal ligament

D. repair of damaged enamel

61. As the dental pulp ages, the

A. pulp acquires denticles and the odontoblastic cells tend to regress

B. pulp chamber becomes smaller and the cells increase in number

C. fiber content decreases and the amount of secondary dentin increases

D. defense mechanisms are increased and the innervation is reduced

62. The narrow cell-free layer between the odontoblasts and the cellular part of the pulp is designated as the
    A. zone of Weil
    B. granular layer
    C. peridenture
    D. interglobular dentin

63. Cementum arises from the
    A. dentinal papilla
    B. dental sac
    C. epithelial root sheath
    D. dental follicle

64. Afferent nerves from the dental pulp conduct which of the following sensations to the central nervous system?
    A. pain
    B. heat
    C. cold
    D. pressure

65. Which of the following cellular elements are considered defense cells in the pulp?
    A. fibroblasts
    B. histiocytes
    C. lymphoid cells
    D. A and B
    E. B and C

66. Of the three major salivary glands, which is a pure serous-producing gland?
    A. submandibular
    B. parotid
    C. sublingual

67. At the cementoenamel junction, which of the following occurs?
    A. Cementum meets enamel.
    B. Cementum overlaps enamel.
    C. Cementum does not meet enamel.
    D. Any of the above.

68. Acellular cementum is sometimes missing along the root surface. The area where this MOST FREQUENTLY occurs (and where cellular cementum is found instead) is the
    A. coronal third
    B. middle third
    C. apical third

69. Cellular cementum (contrasted with acellular cementum) is
    A. newly formed from cementoid
    B. cementum that is resorbing
    C. cementum that contains cementocytes
    D. the part of the cementum that is adjacent to the dentin

70. Which of the following statements describes cementum?
    A. It is lighter in color than dentin, contains 40 to 50 percent inorganic substance, and is permeable.
    B. It is yellowish in color, has more luster than enamel, and contains 50 to 55 percent organic material and water.
    C. It is penetrated by Sharpey's fibers, derived from endoderm, and contains some elastic fibers—hence its yellowish color.
    D. It is developed under the influence of odontoblasts and contains collagen fiber bundles.

71. The embryonic structures that form the palate (roof of the mouth) are the
    A. premaxilla and frontal processes
    B. median nasal process and the frontal process
    C. lateral nasal process and the median palatine process
    D. right and left maxillary processes and the globular process

72. When a cementoblast is embedded in the cementum matrix, it is called
   A. a cementocyte
   B. an epithelial rest
   C. a cementicle
   D. coronal cementum

73. Cementum differs from dentin in that cementum
   A. contains more organic material than dentin
   B. may contain cells, whereas dentin contains cells as well as cell processes
   C. contains some elastic fibers, whereas dentin contains only collagenous fibers
   D. is produced by cells of the periodontal ligament, but dentin is produced by pulp cells

74. In cementum, an oval space from which canaliculi radiate is a
   A. lacuna
   B. cementoblast
   C. cementocyte
   D. cementoid

75. The connective tissue between the cementum and the alveolar bone is called
   A. periosteum
   B. precementum
   C. periodontal ligament
   D. elastic connective tissue

76. The periodontal ligament consists predominantly of
   A. bundles of collagenous and elastic fibers
   B. regularly arranged bundles of collagenous fibers
   C. fibrous elements that are formed by the cementoblasts
   D. large bundles of oxytalan fibers

77. If a normal tooth loses its antagonist, its periodontal ligament

A. becomes more vascular
B. becomes more cellular
C. becomes more sensitive
D. becomes more collagenous
E. does not show evidence of change

78. Bone consists of approximately how much inorganic matter?
   A. 25%
   B. 35%
   C. 50%
   D. 65%
   E. 75%

79. The principal fibers of the periodontal ligament are
   A. collagenous
   B. reticular
   C. ostocollagenous
   D. elastic

80. The periodontal ligament serves the function of
   A. maintaining the relation of the tooth to the surrounding hard and soft tissue
   B. maintaining the functional capacity of ligament
   C. providing osteoplastic and cementoblastic activity
   D. providing sensation of touch, pressure, and pain
   E. regulating blood through the apical foramen

81. Which of the following principal fiber groups has (have) NO attachment into the bone of the alveolar process?
   A. alveolar crest fibers
   B. free gingival fibers
   C. transseptal fibers
   D. A and B
   E. B and C

82. The periodontal ligament does NOT contain
    A. nerves
    B. cartilage
    C. lymphatics
    D. fibroblasts

83. Cleft lip (bilateral or unilateral) results from failure of the maxillary prominences to meet and merge with the
    A. lateral nasal processes
    B. nasal septum
    C. secondary palate
    D. median nasal prominences
    E. premaxilla

84. The upper part of the face, nasal septum, and anterior part of the roof of the mouth are derived from
    A. frontal process
    B. branchial arch I
    C. branchial arch II
    D. branchial arch III

85. Which of the following structures is NOT derived embryonically from the mandibular arch?
    A. lower jaw
    B. pharynx
    C. part of the tongue
    D. lower part of the cheeks

86. The globular process eventually forms the philtrum. During the formation of the interior of the mouth, it gives rise to the anterior part of the palate, the premaxillary area.
    A. Both statements are true.
    B. Both statements are false.
    C. The first statement is true; second statement is false.
    D. The first statement is false; second statement is true.

87. Sebaceous glands that are embryonically trapped in oral mucous membrane are termed
    A. Koplik's spots
    B. embryonic fusions
    C. clefts
    D. globular processes
    E. fordyce granules

88. Sharpey's fibers are
    A. found in dentin
    B. embedded in cementum and serve to attach the surrounding bone
    C. found only in anterior teeth
    D. formed in immature elastic fibers and run in an axial direction to the periodontal ligament
    E. found only around the periodontal ligament

89. Bone and cementum have many common characteristics. One of the characteristics shared by bone and cementum is that their cells lie in a space known as
    A. an incremental space
    B. tubules
    C. lacunae
    D. canaliculi
    E. odontoid

90. Which of the following types of cells predominate in the presence of periodontitis?
    A. macrophages
    B. polymorphonuclear leukocytes
    C. lymphocytes
    D. plasma cells
    E. osteoclasts

91. Which of the following are microscopic characteristics of gingiva in the presence of gingivitis?
    A. exudate of inflammatory cells in the gingival lamina propria
    B. junctional and sulcular epithelia proliferate into inflamed gingival lamina propria
    C. leukocytes migrate through the junctional epithelium into the gingival sulcus
    D. blood vessels surrounded by perivascular inflammatory infiltrate
    E. all of the above

92. Embryonically, which organ develops from Rathke's pouch?
    A. thyroid gland
    B. pituitary gland
    C. posterior lobe of the hypophysis
    D. anterior lobe of the hypophysis

93. A tough connective tissue membrane that covers the outside surface of bone is the
    A. endosteum
    B. perimysium
    C. periosteum
    D. periochondrium

94. Skeletal muscle is
    A. striated voluntary muscle
    B. striated involuntary muscle
    C. smooth
    D. intercalated

95. Neurons are unique in that
    A. they do not possess a nucleus
    B. they do not possess cytoplasm
    C. they do not multiply
    D. they cannot repair
    E. all of the above

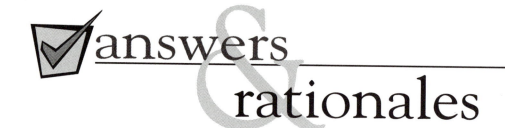

answers & rationales

1.

D. The epithelium of the oral mucous membrane may be keratinized, parakeratinized, or nonkeratinized, depending on its location in the oral cavity. Keratinized tissue is composed of cells that form scales of keratin on the superficial layers, and the cells lose their nuclei. A stratum granulosum is present. The superficial layers of parakeratinized tissue have cells that retain pyknotic nuclei and show some signs of being keratinized. The stratum granulosum is usually absent. Nonkeratinized cells are nucleated and show no signs of keratinization. (1:352–362; 2:83, 104; 5:101; 6:221–223)

2.

A. Normal keratinized areas of the oral mucosa include the vermillion border of the lips, the hard palate, and the gingiva. The buccal mucosa, floor of the mouth, inferior surface of the tongue, and soft palate are nonkeratinized oral mucosa under normal conditions. All oral mucosa, whether keratinized, parakeratinized, or nonkeratinized, is of the stratified squamous type of epithelium. (1:345–362; 2:83–104; 5:101; 6:222)

3.

D. The right and left medial nasal folds and the intervening tissue are termed the frontonasal (frontal) process. The right and left medial nasal folds are derived from the olfactory placodes. The mesenchyme of the right and left nasal folds becomes continuous during the fifth week in utero. (1:30–31; 4:236–237, 239; 5:43; 6:27–28, 33)

4.

D. The anterior two-thirds of the tongue develop from the tuberculum impar and adjacent tissue. The first indication of tongue development appears around the fourth week in utero. Two fused distal tongue buds also help develop into the anterior two-thirds of the tongue. (1:37–39; 4:233–235; 5:57–60; 6:38–40; 7:215–218)

5.

B. The cheeks are formed by fusion of the maxillary and mandibular processes. The maxillary and mandibular processes are derived from the first branchial (visceral) arch. These processes are innervated by the fifth cranial nerve. (1:29–32; 4:227–238; 5:42–45; 6:23–42; 7:219–225)

6.

B. Embryonically, the deep cleft between the growing maxillary and mandibular processes is the primitive mouth, or stomodeum. This stomodeum is lined with ectoderm. At 24 to 27 days in utero, the buccopharyngeal membrane ruptures and establishes a connection with the foregut. (1:26–28; 4:216, 219, 222; 5:42; 6:25–30; 7:83–84, 198–201, 220, 256)

7.

E. In the development of the face, the following play a major role: two mandibular processes, two maxillary processes, two lateral nasal processes, and one medial nasal process. The last three processes are collectively called the frontonasal (frontal) process. All of these processes are derived from branchial arches. (1:30–33; 4:227–238; 5:42–45; 6:28–33)

8.

C. The premaxilla contains the tooth buds of incisors. It forms the anterior portion of the hard palate and the rim of the piriform aperture. The maxilla is the other bone that forms the premaxilla. (1:45–46; 5:55; 6:35–36)

9.

A. The premaxilla has a single center of ossification which is in the anterior part of the palate (primary palate). The premaxilla may never be independent from the maxilla. Nevertheless, the premaxilla and maxilla are separate and distinct structures. (1:45–46; 5:55; 6:35–36)

10.

D. The salivary glands arise from oral mesenchyme. During fetal life, each salivary gland is formed in a specific location in the oral cavity. The primordia of the parotid and submandibular salivary glands appear 7 to 8 weeks in utero. (1:319; 4:223, 235–236; 6:255–257; 7:218–219)

11.

C. The two mineralized connective tissues of the periodontium are cementum and alveolar bone; the two fibrous connective tissues are the periodontal ligament and the lamina propria of the gingiva. The periodontium is a connective tissue organ, covered by epithelium that attaches teeth to the jaw bones and functions to support the teeth. (1:253–287; 6:173–217, 155–169, 237–250)

12.

C. The nasal passageway connecting the olfactory pit with the roof of the primitive oral cavity develops and fuses, forming the primary palate. The primary palate forms the roof of the anterior portion of the primitive oral cavity. It also forms the initial separation between the oral and nasal cavities. (1:33–37; 6:23–40; 7:227–230)

13.

A. The orthodontic movement of the teeth is enhanced because cementum does not resorb. When teeth are orthodontically moved, bone is resorbed on the side of the pressure. New bone is formed on the side of tension. It is bone resorption that leads to orthodontic tooth migration. (1:310–311; 6:169–171)

14.

E. The stomodeum is separated from the foregut (primitive pharynx) by the buccopharyngeal membrane. This membrane ruptures at about 24 days in utero. When this membrane ruptures, it brings the digestive tract in communication with the amniotic cavity. (1:26–28; 4:216, 219, 222; 5:42; 6:23–40; 7:83–84, 198–201, 220, 256)

15.

D. Osteoclasts are cells that resorb bone and tend to be large and multinucleated. The osteoclast accomplishes both demineralization and disaggregation of the organic matrix. (1:76–77, 105, 111–112, 122–126; 2:63, 76; 3:237; 6:190, 192, 211)

16.

B. Cells found in the periodontal ligament that can undergo proliferation under certain pathologic conditions to produce cysts and tumors of jaws are the epithelial rests. These epithelial rests are remnants of Hertwig's epithelial root sheath. Epithelial rests are found in normal periodontal ligaments. (1:98–99, 244, 262; 5:204; 6:37)

17.

E. The lamina propria that supports the oral epithelium does so by interlocking with epithelium through epithelial rests. Epithelial pegs, rete pegs, and rete ridges are names for the same structure. The lamina propria is the connective tissue component of oral mucosa. (1:348; 2:66; 3:188; 5:106; 6:219–235)

18.

B. Keratinized oral epithelium has four layers: the basal layer, the spinous layer, the granular layer, and the cornified layer. These layers are named due to their microscopic structure. The basal layer is the deepest layer and the cornified layer is the outermost layer. (1:352; 6:220)

19.

C. The major part of the alveolar ridge of the upper jaw develops from the maxillary part of the first branchial arch. This alveolar ridge is innervated by the trigeminal or fifth cranial nerve. (1:24–29; 6:23–40)

20.

A. The buccopharyngeal membrane is formed when the stomodeum ectoderm grows toward the foregut until it touches the endoderm and forms the double-layered membrane. The formation of the buccopharyngeal membrane establishes the primitive oral cavity, the stomodeum. This primitive oral cavity is lined with stratified squamous epithelium. (1:26–28; 5:42; 6:23–40; 7:83–84, 198–201)

21.

A. The first indication of tongue development is seen as a median elevation, the tuberculum impar (median tongue bud). This elevation is first seen at approximately 4 weeks in utero. This median elevation is located in the floor of the pharynx, rostral to the foramen cecum. (1:37–38; 4:233–235; 5:57–60; 6:38–40; 7:215–218)

22.

D. The developmental stages of the teeth include the bud stage, the cap stage, and the bell stage. While the shapes and sizes of individual teeth vary, all teeth pass through similar stages of development. (1:82–89; 2:1–12; 3:186–187; 4:523–526; 6:43–72; 7:489–493)

23.

B. The area of the foramen cecum of the tongue is produced embryonically because the thyroglossal duct invaginates from this region to allow the thyroid follicle to migrate toward the future site. The foramen cecum marks the junction between the anterior two-thirds and posterior one-third of the tongue. (1:28; 5:57–60; 6:39; 7:215–218)

24.

C. Von Ebner's glands, located behind the circumvallate papilla of the tongue, are the source of salivary lipase. These serous glands also serve to wash out the soluble elements of food from the circumvallate papilla. (1:376–379; 6:232, 258)

25.

D. Bitter and sour taste sensations of the tongue are mediated by the glossopharyngeal nerve. Sweet and salty tastes of the tongue are mediated by the intermediofacial nerve. Taste occurs when a chemical substance contacts a receptor cell in the taste bud. (1:376–382; 3:180; 6:232, 234–235)

26.

D. The first evidence of tooth development occurs when an epithelial thickening (the dental lamina) occurs over each developing arch, with the thickening having continuity around the arch. (1:78–89; 4:523–526; 5:64; 6:43–72; 7:489–493)

27.

D. The remnants of Hertwig's epithelial root sheath are called the epithelial rests of Malassez. These epithelial rests may become calcified and form cementicles in the periodontal ligament. Under pathologic conditions, these rests may initiate the development of cysts or tumors of the jaws. (6:37)

28.

E. Hertwig's epithelial root sheath is derived from the union of inner dental epithelium and outer dental epithelium. It does not contain a stratum intermedium or stellate reticulum. Hertwig's epithelial root sheath therefore develops from two layers of the enamel epithelium. (1:95, 128, 143, 145–146, 169, 236–239, 244, 262; 6:70, 75, 189–190, 270–271)

29.

C. After the tooth is formed, the dental papilla becomes confined within the dentin walls forming the primordium of the dental pulp. The dental papilla is derived from the inner enamel epithelium. (1:84, 86; 4:523–526; 6:43–72, 137)

30.

C. Hunter-Schreger bands are best demonstrated by oblique reflected light as alternating dark and light strips of varying width. Hunter-Schreger bands are established by the change in direction of enamel rods. These bands originate at the dentinoenamel junction and pass outward, ending some distance from the outer enamel surface. (1:229–230; 6:86)

31.

B. The rhythmical formation of enamel matrix is called apposition. Appositional growth of enamel is a layer-like deposition of the extracellular matrix. This is an additive type of growth. Periods of activity and rest alternate at different intervals during tooth formation. (1:89, 95–96, 197–216; 5:166; 6:62–66)

32.

B. The incremental lines of Retzius illustrate the successive apposition of layers of enamel during formation of the crown. These incremental lines represent variations in structure and mineralization that occur during the growth of enamel. The presence of incremental lines of Retzius is considered normal. (1:224–233; 2:18; 6:92–93, 95, 104)

33.

B. The hardest tissue in the human body is enamel. It is composed of 96 to 98 percent inorganic matter in the form of hydroxyapatite. The structure and hardness of enamel render it brittle. (1:72, 199, 201–203; 3:184; 6:31)

34.

B. The primary enamel cuticle is formed by the ameloblasts just prior to tooth eruption. At this point the enamel matrix is formed. The remnant of the primary enamel cuticle after eruption is referred to as Nasmyth's membrane. (6:65, 85–86)

35.

E. Enamel lamellae can be differentiated into three types: those composed of poorly calcified rod segments, those consisting of degenerated cells, and those that arise in erupted teeth where the cracks are filled with organic material, such as saliva. Enamel lamellae may arise in planes of tension. (1:230–231; 2:20; 6:92–94, 96–97, 104)

36.

A. An age change that takes place in the enamel is that enamel becomes harder, therefore more caries-resistant. Localized increases of certain elements such as nitrogen and fluoride have been found in superficial enamel layers of older teeth. (6:111)

37.

C. On the normal human enamel, incremental lines are termed lines of Retzius. They were named so in 1837 after Retzius, who described the rods as having a clear crystalline appearance and a hexagonal round to oval arrangement resembling fish scales in cross section. (1:224, 226–228, 232–233; 2:18; 6:92–93, 95, 104)

38.

D. Intercalated ducts of salivary glands collect secretions of terminal secretory units of salivary glands. Also, they empty salivary secretions into striated ducts. Intercalated ducts are thin branching tubes of variable length that connect terminal secretory units to the next larger ducts. (1:332–334; 6:262)

39.

C. The region where gnarled enamel is found to the greatest extent is under the tips of cusps or incisal edges. This gnarled enamel is so named due to the irregular intertwining of the bundles of enamel rods in cusp tips or incisal edges. (1:229; 2:20)

40.

B. The ameloblasts enter their formative stage after the first layer of dentin has been formed. The presence of dentin seems to be necessary for the beginning of enamel matrix formation, just as it is necessary for epithelial cells to come into close contact with the connective tissue of the pulp during differentiation of the odontoblasts and the beginning of dentin formation. (1:197–216; 6:51, 64)

41.

B. Structures confined to the enamel rod are cross-striations. (6:81–112)

42.

C. Enamel tufts are narrow ribbon-like structures that consist of hypocalcified enamel rods and interprismatic substance. Enamel tufts arise at the dentinoenamel junction and reach into one-fifth to one-third of the enamel thickness. Enamel tufts extend in the direction of the long axis of the crown. (1:230–231; 2:21; 5:173; 6:92, 95, 99, 104)

43.

C. The tooth pulp is initially called the dental papilla. The dental papilla controls early tooth formation. It also controls whether the forming enamel organ is an incisor or molar. (1:84–93; 6:47, 137)

44.

D. Mineral-poor ectodermal structures in enamel include tufts and lamellae, both of which are defined as hypomineralized structures. Enamel lamellae are thin leaf-like structures that extend from the enamel surface toward the dentinoenamel junction and reach into the enamel to about one-fifth to one-third of its thickness. (1:230–231; 2:20–21; 5:173; 6:92–98, 101, 104)

45.

E. The secondary cuticle is secreted by the reduced enamel epithelium which consists of remaining parts of outer and inner enamel epithelium, stratum intermedium, and stellate reticula. The secondary enamel cuticle is not a mineralized structure. (1:100, 247, 295; 6:66, 86)

46.

C. As a general rule, enamel rods in the middle one-third of the enamel run at 90 degrees to a line drawn tangent to the external surface of the tooth. In the cervical and central parts of the crown of a deciduous tooth, they are approximately horizontal. (6:85)

47.

C. Interglobular dentin is hypocalcified. Mineralization of the dentin sometimes begins in small globular areas that normally fuse to form a uniformly calcified dentin layer. If fusion does not take place, hypomineralized regions remain between the globules. These are termed interglobular dentin. (1:160–161; 2:28–29; 6:124–126)

48.

C. Comparing the dentinal tubules near the pulp with those near the dentinoenamel junction in a newly erupted tooth, those near the pulp are closer together and of larger caliber. Because the outer surface of dentin is larger than the inner surface by about five to one, this will mean that the tubules are farther apart on the outside than the inside. (1:165; 6:113, 116, 118–121)

49.

C. Dentin is a type of connective tissue that is softer than enamel but harder than bone. It contains 90 percent inorganic matter; bone contains 50 percent inorganic matter. (1:287; 3:183; 6:113)

50.

C. The most highly mineralized region of the dentinal matrix has been demonstrated to be the peritubular dentin. Peritubular dentin is more highly mineralized than intertubular dentin. (1:143–144, 155, 158, 179; 3:183; 5:180; 6:117)

51.

A. Deposition of calcium salts into dentinal tubules produces transparent dentin or sclerotic dentin. This is due to obliteration of the tubules and equalization of the refractive indices between the odontoblastic process and tubule. (1:158–161; 6:129–131)

52.

E. All of the structures may be found in dentin except striae of Retzius because they exist in enamel, appearing as incremental lines representing stages of appositional formation of enamel. (1:224–233; 6:113–132)

53.

A. The external resorption of dentin is repaired by dentin apposition. Extensive wear, erosion, caries, or operative procedures lead to damage of the odontoblasts. These damaged odontoblasts are replaced by migration of the dentinal surface of undifferentiated cells from the deeper layers of the pulp. (1:152–153; 6:62–63, 124–152)

54.

D. The narrow layer of minute areas of interglobular dentin near the dentinocementum junction is known as Tomes's granular layer. Tomes's granular layer is only found in the root. It does not follow an incremental pattern. (1:152, 162–163; 5:182; 6:134–135)

55.

A. Terminal branches of dentinal tubules are found somewhat adjacent to the dentinoenamel junction. Dentinal tubules end perpendicular to the dentinoenamel junction and the dentinocementum junction. (1:150, 163–165; 6:113, 116, 118–121)

56.

E. A histologic feature that readily distinguishes dentin of the root from coronal dentin is the presence of Tomes's granular layer. This layer is a hypomineralized structure representing a lack of uniformity in mineralization. (1:124, 135, 152, 162–163)

57.

A. Primary dentin is considered to be vital because it contains Tomes's processes and tissue fluid. However, primary dentin may become sclerotic when dentin is exposed to irritants, necessitating deposition of reparative dentin. (1:138–140, 150–151; 6:124, 135)

58.

B. Sclerotic dentin differs from primary dentin in having relatively less organic material than primary dentin. Primary dentin (or original dentin) undergoes changes by depositing calcium salts and obliterating the tubules, equalizing the refractive index between the process and tubule. (1:158–161; 2:35; 6:129–131)

59.

D. Nerve fibers of the central part of the dental pulp are myelinated with short internodes. The nerves of the pulp mediate the sensation of pain. The nerve supply of the pulp follows the distribution of the blood vessels. (1:184–190; 6:173, 176)

60.

B. One of the functions of the tooth pulp is the production of reparative dentin. This is one of the attempts the pulp can make to wall off the pulp from its source of irritation. The pulp responds to chemical, thermal, mechanical, and bacterial irritations. (1:414–415, 149; 5:181–183; 6:62–63, 124, 152)

61.

A. As the dental pulp ages, the pulp acquires denticles and the odontoblastic cells tend to regress. In general, fibrosis and pulp stone formation are the hallmarks of an aging pulp. Pulp stones (denticles) can appear in either or both the coronal and root portions of the tooth. (1:192–195; 2:43; 6:146–147)

62.

A. The narrow cell-free layer between the odontoblasts and the cellular part of the pulp is designated as the zone of Weil, or subodontoblastic layer. It is believed that the cell-free zone is the area where odontoblasts are mobilized and replaced. The cell-rich layer is composed principally of fibroblasts and undifferentiated mesenchymal cells. (1:86, 185–186)

63.

B. Cementum arises from the dental sac when the dentin of the root has begun to form under the organizing influence of the epithelial root sheath. It is separated by epithelium from the surrounding connective tissue. However, the continuity of the epithelial root sheath is soon broken either by partial degradation of the epithelium or by active proliferation of the connective tissue. Thus, contact of the connective tissue with the surface of the dentin is established. Cells of the periodontal connective tissue, now in contact with the root surface, form cementum. (1:100, 236–242; 5:76–80; 6:155–169)

64.

A. Afferent (sensory) nerves from the dental pulp conduct only pain to the central nervous system. The sensory response in the pulp cannot differentiate between heat, touch, pressure, or chemicals. Most nerves of the pulp are myelinated. (1:184–190)

65.

E. Histiocytes and lymphoid cells are the defense cells of the pulp. Maximov defined histiocytes as resting macrophages which, when they become activated by inflammatory stimuli, will become motile. Lymphoid wandering cells, including lymphocytes and monocytes, perform a phagocytic function. (1:180; 6:137–153)

66.

B. The parotid gland is a pure serous gland. The submandibular gland is a mixed (mixes mucous and serous fluid) gland. The sublingual salivary gland is a mixed type of salivary gland. (1:7, 316, 332–333; 3:188–190; 5:150–153; 6:137–153)

67.

D. At the cementoenamel junction, cementum may meet enamel at a sharp line in 30 percent of cases, while cementum may overlap enamel in 60 percent of cases; both cementum and enamel may not meet but become separated by a gap in 10 percent of cases. (1:256–258; 2:54–55; 6:155–169)

68.

C. Acellular cementum may be missing and instead replaced by cellular cementum most frequently at the apical third of the root. Acellular cementum may extend from the cementoenamel junction to about two-thirds of the root length but may be missing in the apical one-third. Thickness of acellular cementum varies from 20 micra at the cementoenamel junction to 150 micra at the apex. (1:5, 239, 253–256; 2:48; 6:161–163)

69.

C. Cellular cementum (contrasted with acellular cementum) is characterized by the fact that it contains cementocytes. (1:243; 2:49; 6:161–163)

70.

A. Cementum is lighter in color than dentin, contains 40 to 50 percent inorganic substances, and is permeable. (1:243; 2:49; 6:161–163)

71.

D. Embryonically, the palate arises from the right and left maxillary processes and the globular process. The palate shows marked development by the end of the second month in utero. (1:33–37, 440–457; 6:164)

72.

A. A cementoblast embedded in the cementum matrix is called a cementocyte. Cementocytes reside in the lacunae of cementum. Cementocytes are similar to osteocytes found in the lacunae of bone. (2:53; 6:164)

73.

D. Cementum differs from dentin in that cementum is produced by cells of the periodontal ligament (cementoblasts), but dentin is produced by pulp cells (odontoblasts). (1:241–242; 6:161)

74.

A. In cementum, the oval space from which canaliculi radiate is a lacuna. (1:241–242, 254; 6:161)

75.

C. The connective tissue between the cementum and the alveolar bone is called the periodontal ligament. The space the periodontal ligament occupies is the periodontal space. This extends coronally to the most apical part of the lamina propria of the gingiva. (1:253–256; 3:186; 6:173–193)

76.

B. The periodontal ligament consists predominantly of regularly arranged bundles of collagen fibers. These fibers are described as white, collagenous, wavy bundles extending from bone to cementum. (1:253–256; 3:186; 6:173–193)

77.

E. If a normal tooth loses its antagonist, its periodontal ligament would not show evidence of change with regard to vascularity, cellularity, sensitivity, or collagenous content. (6:173–193)

78.

D. Bone consists of approximately 65 percent inorganic material and 35 percent organic material. The inorganic portion is hydroxyapatite. The organic portion is Type 1 collagen. (1:104; 5:108; 6:195–212)

79.

A. The principal fibers of the periodontal ligament are collagenous. There are no elastic fibers in the periodontal ligament. (1:60, 64; 6:183–189)

80.

A. The periodontal ligament serves the function of maintaining a constant relationship between the tooth and the surrounding hard and soft tissue. (1:253–256; 3:186; 6:195–212)

81.

E. The free gingival and transseptal fibers do not attach to the bone of the alveolar process. The free gingival fibers are attached to the lamina propria of the gingiva, while the transseptal fibers attach the cementum of one tooth to another. (1:263–269; 5:206–207; 6:237–250)

82.

B. The periodontal ligament does not contain cartilage. It is made up of collagenous fibers, cells, penetrating blood vessels, lymphatics, and nerves. (1:256, 259–277; 6:173)

83.

D. Cleft lip, either bilateral or unilateral, results from failure of the maxillary prominences to meet and merge with the median nasal prominences. Unilateral cleft lip results from failure of the maxillary prominence on the affected side to merge with the medial nasal prominences. Bilateral cleft lip results from failure of the maxillary prominences to meet and merge with the median nasal prominences. (1:46–49; 4:248–252; 5:47; 6:32)

84.

A. The frontal process will give rise to the development of the upper part of the face, nasal septum, and anterior part of the roof of the mouth. The frontal process is comprised of ectoderm and mesoderm. All branchial arches are located below the frontal process. (1:45; 5:42–45; 7:219–222)

85.

B. The mandibular arch gives rise to the development of the lower jaw, part of the tongue, and lower part of the cheeks. The mandibular arch is derived from the first branchial arch, as are the maxillary processes. (1:24–29; 5:42–45; 6:23–42)

86.

A. The globular process forms the philtrum. During the formation of the interior part of the mouth, the globular process gives rise to the anterior part of the palate and the premaxillary area. The globular process is a single median structure which grows downward below the olfactory pits and lies between the right and left maxillary processes. (1:24–49; 5:42–45; 6:23–42)

87.

E. Sebaceous glands that are embryonically entrapped in oral mucous membrane are termed Fordyce granules. Fordyce granules can appear laterally along the inside of the cheek from either corner of the cheek. Fordyce granules may also appear in the lips. (1:347–348, 384; 6:33)

88.

B. Sharpey's fibers are embedded in cementum and serve to attach the tooth to surrounding bone. Each Sharpey's fiber passes well into the cementum. Sharpey's fibers are composed of collagen. (1:106, 266–267, 277; 5:205; 6:164, 166–169, 173, 180–181)

89.

C. Bone and cementum have many common characteristics. One outstanding feature that they share is that their cells lie in spaces known as lacunae. The cells in bone that lie in these lacunae are osteocytes. The cells in cementum that lie in these spaces are cementocytes. (1:287; 5:108, 196; 6:160)

90.

D. Plasma cells are the predominant type of cell found in the presence of periodontitis. Additional types of cells found in the presence of periodontitis include lymphocytes, polymorphonuclear leukocytes, and macrophages. (3:188)

91.

E. The microscopic characteristics of gingivitis include the presence of inflammatory cells in the gingival lamina propria, lysis of gingival fibers, proliferation of junctional and sulcular epithelium into the inflamed gingival lamina propria, and migration of leukocytes from vessels in the lamina propria through the junctional epithelium into the gingival sulcus. Additionally, blood vessels can be found surrounded by perivascular inflammatory infiltrate. (3:188)

92.

D. Rathke's pouch is the embryonic origin for the anterior lobe of the hypophysis. The posterior lobe of the hypophysis is embryonically derived from the brain. (6:26)

93.

C. The outside surface of bone is covered by a tough connective tissue membrane, the periosteum. The endosteum covers the inner surface of compact bone. The perimysium is a covering of muscle fibers. The perichondrium is a connective tissue membrane that covers cartilage. (1:104–106; 3:236, 246; 5:196; 6:195, 206)

94.

A. Skeletal muscle is striated voluntary muscle. Striated involuntary muscle is known as cardiac muscle. Smooth muscle is found in the walls of blood vessels, in the walls of the intestines, and around hair roots. (1:396; 6:18–19)

95.

C. Neurons, like other cells, do have a nucleus and cytoplasm. However, unlike other body cells, they do not multiply. Some neurons in the peripheral nervous system do have the ability to undergo some repair. (6:15–17)

10 Microbiology

DIRECTIONS Each of the questions below is followed by several suggested answers. Select the best answer in each case.

---

1. Cells that phagocytize microorganisms are which of the following types?
   A. neutrophils
   B. macrophages
   C. lymphocytes
   D. B and C only
   E. A and B only

2. The cell wall of gram-positive microorganisms may include all of the following EXCEPT
   A. lipopolysaccharides
   B. lipoteichoic acids
   C. peptidoglycans
   D. penicillin binding proteins
   E. teichoic acids

3. Serious complications of untreated group A streptococcal pharyngitis are
   A. acute glomerulonephritis
   B. rheumatic fever
   C. moniliasis
   D. B and C only
   E. A and B only

4. Microbiological safety equipment for protection of healthcare workers recommended in OSHA standards includes
   A. gloves
   B. face mask or shield
   C. eye goggles
   D. gowns and aprons
   E. all of the above

5. Prevotella (Bacteroides) melaninogenicus is best characterized as
   A. an aerobic gram-negative rod
   B. an anaerobic gram-positive rod
   C. a virulent oropharyngeal pathogen
   D. a common agent of caseous necrosis
   E. an anaerobe that produces pigmented colonies

6. The only "cold sterilizer" solution capable of destroying bacterial spores, viruses, and vegetative bacteria is
   A. 90% isopropyl alcohol
   B. 2% glutaraldehyde
   C. chlorhexidine
   D. iodophors
   E. quaternary ammonium

7. Autoclave efficiency should be checked regularly by using
   A. heat-activated autoclave tapes that change colors
   B. plastic strips designed to melt at 121° centigrade
   C. culture plates of viable bacteria

D. vials of culture media containing a pH indicator and a thermophilic spore-forming bacteria
E. vials with different acid and base chemical indicators

8. The best method for sterilizing cutting instruments is
   A. autoclave for 15 minutes at 15 pounds of pressure at 121° C
   B. benzalkonium chloride
   C. boiling water
   D. 10% hypochlorite
   E. 70% ethyl alcohol

9. A gram-negative anaerobic organism normally found in the upper respiratory tract and in mixed anaerobic infections is
   A. Clostridium perfringens
   B. Enterococcus faecalis
   C. Prevotella (Bacteroides) melaninogenicus
   D. Streptococcus pneumoniae
   E. Bordetella pertussis

10. Animal experimentation has contributed much to our knowledge of caries, particularly experimentation of the gnotobiotic rat. The BEST definition of this term is
    A. a completely germ-free rat
    B. any rat being fed a cariogenic diet
    C. a previously germ-free rat that has been inoculated by a known organism
    D. a germ-free rat that has been inoculated by an unknown organism

11. Which of the following is a gram-negative anaerobic rod?
    A. Fusobacterium nucleatum
    B. Clostridium prefringens
    C. Peptostreptococcus
    D. Candida albicans
    E. Neisseria meningitidis

12. Microorganisms that may produce alpha or partial hemolysis on blood agar include all of the following EXCEPT
   A. Streptococcus viridans
   B. Streptococcus pneumoniae
   C. Enterococcus faecalis
   D. Streptococcus pyogenes
   E. Streptococcus mutans

13. An opportunistic fungus with a high affinity for afflicting individuals with diabetes mellitus is
   A. Blastomyces dermatiditis
   B. Histoplasma capsulatum
   C. Actinomyces israelii
   D. Mucor
   E. Sporothrix schenckii

14. Herpes zoster is thought to be the adult counterpart of which of the following diseases?
   A. chickenpox
   B. measles
   C. mumps
   D. smallpox
   E. rubeola

15. An anaerobic Streptococcus is classified as a member of genus
   A. Neisseria
   B. Peptostreptococcus
   C. Hemophilus
   D. Lactobacillus
   E. Enterococcus

16. For optimal growth, microaerophilic bacteria grow best with
   A. free access to air
   B. the presence of molecular oxygen only
   C. a complete absence of oxygen
   D. an atmosphere of low oxygen tension

E. a mixture of nitrogen and hydrogen

17. MacConkey's agar is a medium best suited for selective growth of microorganisms such as
   A. Streptococcus pyogenes
   B. Staphylococcus aureus
   C. Lactobacillus species
   D. Escherichia coli
   E. Hemophilus influenzae

18. Lactobacillus acidophilus is a
   A. gram-positive coccus
   B. gram-positive rod
   C. gram-negative coccus
   D. gram-negative rod
   E. gram-variable spiral bacteria

19. Viruses that infect bacteria are known as
   A. saprophytes
   B. commensals
   C. protoplasts
   D. bacteriophages
   E. spheroplasts

20. A substance that helps prepare bacteria for phagocytosis is a (an)
   A. bacteriolysin
   B. interferon
   C. antitoxin
   D. opsonin
   E. hemolysin

21. Which characteristic is the MOST outstanding feature of genus Mycoplasma?
   A. slow-replicating viruses
   B. temperate bacteriophages
   C. extracellular rickettsia
   D. spiral bacteria
   E. cell wall–deficient organisms

22. Chemotaxis is a function of which of the following cells?
    A. erythrocytes
    B. leukocytes
    C. epithelial
    D. endothelial
    E. all of the above

23. Diseases of lower animals that are transmissible to humans are known as
    A. zoonoses
    B. phycomycoses
    C. geophilic
    D. anthrophilic
    E. dermatophytes

24. Ethylene oxide has which of the following action on bacteria?
    A. bacteriostatic
    B. antiseptic
    C. disinfects
    D. sterilizes
    E. sanitizes

25. Immunoglobulins are produced by which of the following cell types?
    A. neutrophils
    B. macrophages
    C. T lymphocytes
    D. B lymphocytes
    E. basophils

26. Active immunity may BEST be described as
    A. the inability of a host to react to a battery of common skin test antigens
    B. an immunity passed from one animal species to another species
    C. an altered state of immune reactivity or hypersensitivity
    D. acquired by deliberate introduction of an antigen into a responsive host
    E. normal species immunity acquired genetically

27. Passive immunity is BEST defined as
    A. protection provided by antigens from nonspecific proteins
    B. protection achieved by the introduction of preformed antibody or immune cells into a nonimmune host
    C. immunity from any source
    D. protection acquired by introduction of hormones into a nonimmune host
    E. acquired by deliberate introduction of an antigen into a responsive host

28. An infection that is not likely to be transmitted by blood transfusion is
    A. hepatitis A
    B. hepatitis B
    C. hepatitis C
    D. human immunodeficiency virus
    E. cytomegalovirus

29. Fusobacterium nucleatum is commonly characterized by the presence of
    A. bacilli with terminal spores
    B. acid-fast spores
    C. bacilli with pointed or tapered ends
    D. gram-positive endospores
    E. gram-positive rods with metachromatic granules

30. The most infectious stage(s) of syphilis is (are) the
    A. primary stage
    B. secondary stage
    C. latent phase
    D. tertiary stage
    E. A and B

31. T lymphocytes are capable of enhancing immune reactivity by liberation of a collection of soluble materials termed
    A. lymphokines
    B. prostaglandins
    C. immunoglobulins
    D. fibrinolysins

32. Infectious mononucleosis is a disease that occurs mostly in adolescents and is caused by
    A. varicella virus
    B. Hemophilus influenzae
    C. herpes simplex type 2
    D. Epstein-Barr virus
    E. herpes simplex type 1

33. Acquired immunodeficiency syndrome (AIDS) is caused by a single-stranded RNA virus known as a
    A. retrovirus
    B. tumor virus
    C. adenovirus
    D. arbovirus
    E. parvovirus

34. Rubella immunity in healthcare workers is important because
    A. the fetus of a pregnant female is at major risk until the third trimester
    B. of progression of infection to an acute cutaneous illness known as "scabby mouth"
    C. of chronic and persistent gastronephritis
    D. of limited serological tests of diagnosis of rubella
    E. immunity can only be determined by electron microscopy

35. The presence of large amounts of lipid in the cell wall of mycobacteria is primarily responsible for the
    A. characterization as an acid-fast bacilli
    B. rapid growth and ease in treatment and eradication of disease
    C. most common mechanism for resistance to anti-tuberculosis drugs
    D. B and C
    E. A and B

36. Significant diagnostic findings in exudates from cases of human actinomycosis include
    A. strongly acid-fast slender beading rods
    B. black granules
    C. large encapsulated gram-negative rods
    D. sulfur granules
    E. ascospores

37. The presence of capsules may be helpful in protecting bacteria by which of the following mechanisms?
    A. interfering with phagocytosis
    B. assisting bacteria in colonization
    C. eliciting production of antibody against bacteria and initiating opsonization
    D. B and C
    E. A and B

38. Virulence mechanisms that aid bacteria in disease are
    A. adhesins such as fimbria
    B. phase and antigenic variation of external proteins
    C. excretion of enzymes and toxins that destroy host tissues
    D. all of the above

39. The term *universal precautions* means that
    A. all procedures are performed as though the patient were known to be infectious
    B. personal protective equipment must be worn
    C. all healthcare workers must use precautions when treating infectious patients
    D. any precautions taken are adequate
    E. only gloves are worn during exposure to infectious agents

40. Many bacteria contain small, circular, covalently closed, double-stranded DNA molecules separate from the bacterial chromosome known as
   A. plasmids
   B. spores
   C. ribosomes
   D. flagella
   E. pili

41. Mutation and selection are important factors in the evolution of bacteria. Among the factors that speed these changes are the processes of genetic transfer which include
   A. transformation
   B. transduction
   C. conjugation
   D. A, B, and C
   E. A and B only

42. Which of the following are normal host barriers or defenses against infection?
   A. intact skin or tissue
   B. saliva secretion and mechanical actions
   C. antagonism by normal microbial flora
   D. bactericidal components of body fluids
   E. all of the above

43. Capnocytophaga species are thin rods with tapered ends that are motile on agar surfaces by which of the following mechanisms?
   A. phagocytosis
   B. pili
   C. gliding
   D. endocytosis
   E. pincytosis

44. Hypochlorite (10%) has been found to be MOST effective against
   A. mycoplasma and rickettsia
   B. pathogenic respiratory fungi

C. all groups of mycobacteria
   D. most viruses including HIV and hepatitis
   E. only non-spore-forming bacteria

45. Recent concern for the emergence of multiple drug resistant (MDR) strains of Mycobacterium tuberculosis has probably been due to which of the following factors?
   A. increased numbers of TB-infected homeless and HIV patients
   B. noncompliance of patients in treatment protocols
   C. potential transmission of MDR strains of Mycobacterium tuberculosis to healthcare workers
   D. all of the above

46. A common opportunistic agent that causes pneumonia in AIDS patients is
   A. Leishmania
   B. Plasmodium
   C. Pneumocystis
   D. Bahesia
   E. Cryptosporidium

47. Patients with HIV infection often acquire a species of Mycobacterium that is intrinsically resistant to a wide range of antimycobacterial agents. This mycobacterium is
   A. Mycobacterium tuberculosis
   B. Mycobacterium bovis
   C. Mycobacterium leprae
   D. Mycobacterium chelonae
   E. Mycobacterium avium-intracellulare

48. Lyme disease owes its etiology to
   A. Rickettsia rickettsii
   B. Borrelia burgdorferi
   C. Rickettsia quintana
   D. Rickettsia prowazekii

49. Treponema pallidum is responsible for which of the following diseases?
    A. gonorrhea
    B. pneumonia
    C. measles
    D. chickenpox
    E. syphilis

50. In bronchopneumonia, the inflammatory consolidation is regular in distribution. The most common microorganisms are influenza rickettsia, staphylococcus, pneumococcus, and streptococcus.
    A. The first statement is true; second statement is false.
    B. The first statement is false; second statement is true.
    C. Both statements are true.
    D. Both statements are false.

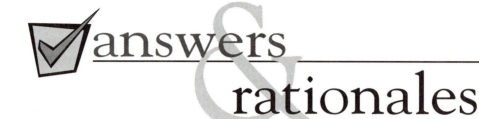

answers & rationales

1.

E. Two cell types are involved in phagocytosis: the polymorphonuclear neutrophil and macrophage. Neutrophils are present in the bloodstream and are short-lived cells. Macrophages, on the other hand, are long-lived cells present throughout the connective tissue and around the basement membrane of small blood vessels. Both cell types migrate to sites of inflammation to engulf bacteria and discharge granules consisting of microbicidal substances. (1:4)

2.

A. Lipopolysaccharide (or endotoxin) is the most significant structure in the cell wall of gram-negative bacteria. It accounts for a variety of immunologic reactions. (2:128)

3.

E. Rheumatic fever and acute glomerulonephritis are non-suppurative complications of group A streptococcal disease. In rheumatic fever, inflammatory changes in the heart, joints, blood vessels, and subcutaneous tissue are evident. Acute inflammation of the glomerulus with edema, hypertension, hematuria, and proteinuria are seen in glomerulonephritis caused by nephrogenetic strains of group A streptococci. (2:186)

4.

E. All body fluids from patients should be considered potentially infectious. The health care worker should exercise precautions as mandated by OSHA by using personal protective equipment which includes gloves, goggles, face shields, gowns or lab coats, and aprons. (3:52)

5.

E. Prevotella (Bacteroides) melaninogenicus is one of the members of anaerobic gram-negative bacteria that produces a dark pigment after several days' growth in blood agar plates. (3:544)

6.

B. A solution of 2% glutaraldehyde is an alkalyzing agent highly lethal to essentially all microorganisms if sufficient contact time is provided and there is absence of extraneous organic material. It is effective for sterilizing apparatuses that cannot be heated. Other products such as alcohols, iodophors, chlorhexidine, and quaternary ammonium compounds are disinfectants. (4:191, 198)

7.

D. Autoclaves should be quality controlled to ensure that the appropriate temperature, pressure, packing, and timing are correct. A thermophilic microorganism, usually Bacillus stearothermophilus, is used as a biological indicator. These organisms are supplied with vials of culture medium containing a pH indicator. The vial is placed in the autoclave with the load and the autoclave is run under normal conditions. The vial is removed and the culture medium is released to mix with the thermophilic microorganisms. The vial is placed in an incubator for a specified period of time and then checked for growth of the organism. If no organisms grow, the autoclave was effective. If the organisms grow in the culture media, the autoclave did not render the contents of that load sterile. (4:191, 198)

8.

A. Autoclaves are usually operated at 121°C which is achieved at a pressure of 15 psi for 15 minutes. Under these conditions, spores are killed. The velocity of the killing increases logarithmically with a steam temperature of 121°C and is more effective than 100°C or boiling. (4:173)

9.

C. Prevotella (Bacteroides) melaninogenicus is normal flora of the mouth and oropharynx. It may be found in anaerobic infections which are frequently polymicrobic. (4:326)

10.

C. The term *gnotobiotic* has been used to designate an animal bearing a known microbial flora. Gnotobiotic may also be used to include the germ-free animal, but common usage has restricted this term to animals bearing one or more known and no unknown microorganisms. For animals born and reared in the usual animal quarters, the term *conventional* has been used. (5:384–385)

11.

A. Fusobacterium nucleatum is a gram-negative non-spore-forming anaerobic rod. Clostridium prefringens is a gram-positive spore-forming rod. Candida albicans is a yeast. Neisseria meningitidis is a member of the aerobic gram-negative cocci. Peptostreptococcus is a gram-positive cocci. (4:339)

12.

D. Streptococcus pyogenes produce a 2–3 mm zone of beta hemolysis on sheep blood agar plates. All of the other organisms listed produce alpha hemolysis, including Enterococcus which may sometimes produce no hemolysis but is only rarely found to be beta hemolytic. (4:293)

13.

D. Zygomycosis (Mucormycosis) is a term applied to infection with any of a group of zygommycetes, the most common of which are Absidia, Rhizopus, and Mucor. Diabetic acidosis has particularly strong association with mucormycosis. (4:659)

14.

A. Reactivation of the varicella-zoster virus, the agent of chickenpox seen most commonly in children, is associated with herpes zoster. It increases in frequency with age and is seen most commonly in adults. (4:566)

15.

B. An anaerobic Streptococcus is classified as a member of genus Peptostreptococcus. (4:326)

16.

D. Microaerophilic bacteria grow best at low oxygen concentration and cannot grow without oxygen. (4:33)

17.

D. MacConkey's agar is a differential and selective medium that supports the growth of organisms such as E. coli and other members of the enteric bacilli. Gram-positive organisms like Streptococci do not grow. Hemophilus influenzae is fastidious and requires a heme-containing medium for growth. (3:360)

18.

B. Lactobacillus acidophilus is a gram-positive rod commonly found in the oropharyngeal flora. It has been believed to play some role in the pathogenesis of dental caries. (4:319)

19.

D. Viruses are capable of reproduction only inside living cells. Those that grow inside bacteria are known as bacteriophages. (4:56)

20.

D. Substances that prepare bacteria for phagocytosis are known as opsonins. They attach to the surface of the microbe and activate the complement pathway. The complement fragment C3b and a calcium-dependent mannose-binding protein are examples of opsonins. (1:14)

21.

E. Mycoplasma are the smallest known free-living microorganisms, intermediate in size between bacteria and viruses. Although they evolved from gram-positive ancestors, they lack a cell wall which is their most distinguishing feature. (6:491)

22.

B. Some bacteria produce chemical substances known as chemotaxins which directionally attract leukocytes. The adherence of bacteria to the leukocyte activates the membrane and initiates engulfment. (1:6)

23.

A. Many bacterial, rickettsial, and viral diseases are classified as zoonoses because they are acquired by humans either directly or indirectly from animals. (4:489, 498)

24.

D. Ethylene oxide is an alkylating agent which is an effective sterilizing agent for heat-liable devices that cannot be treated at the temperatures achieved in the autoclave. (4:175)

25.

D. The role of lymphocytes in the production of antibody was established many years ago. It is now known that lymphocytes of a subset known as B lymphocytes are programmed to make a single, specific antibody which can be found on the outer surface of the cell to act as a receptor. (1:22–23)

26.

D. Primary active immunity is induced prior to exposure to the biological agent. Active immunity or immunization may be acquired with living or dead microorganisms or recombinant proteins. (7:673)

27.

B. Immunity may be acquired by passively administering either preformed immunoreactive serum or cells or by actively presenting a suitable antigenic stimulus to the host's immune system. The most common form of passive immunity is the introduction of whole serum or fractionated concentrated immune gamma globulin that is predominantly IgG obtained from a host who has recovered from the infectious disease or has been immunized. (7:669)

28.

A. Approximately 40 percent of acute hepatitis cases result from hepatitis A, which is spread by person-to-person contact, usually via fecal–oral route or by exposure to contaminated food or water. Sexual or close personal contact may facilitate spread. The virus is present in blood only transiently but present in feces in high concentration for several weeks. (2:702–703)

29.

C. Fusobacterium nucleatum is a thin, gram-negative rod characterized by tapered or pointed ends. It is found in the mouth, genital, gastrointestinal, and upper respiratory tracts of humans and is commonly encountered in clinical infections. (3:539–540)

30.

E. The most infectious stages of syphilis are the primary stage, when a syphilitic chancre has numerous spirochetes present, and the secondary stage, when mucocutaneous lesions with spirochetes are distributed over various areas of the body. (4:898–899)

31.

A. A subpopulation of T lymphocytes called T helper cells, if primed to a specific antigen, will recognize and bind to the combination of antigen with class II MHC molecules on the macrophage surface and produce a variety of soluble factors called lymphokines. (1:28)

32.

D. Epstein-Barr virus has been established as the major cause of infectious mononucleosis worldwide. The virus infects and is shed by epithelial cells in the oropharynx into blood and saliva. (2:586)

33.

A. The most important human retrovirus infection, the acquired immunodeficiency syndrome (AIDS) is caused by one of two groups of retroviruses termed human immunodeficiency virus (HIV-1 and HIV-2). Retroviruses are enveloped, single-stranded RNA viruses. They encode reverse transferase (an RNA-dependent DNA polymerase) that copies their genome into proviral double-stranded DNA. (4:603)

34.

A. Humans are the only host for rubella. The virus is spread by respiratory secretions and is generally acquired in childhood. Congenital disease is the most serious outcome of rubella infection. The fetus is at major risk until the 20th week of pregnancy. A major objective of the vaccination program is development of "herd immunity" in the population which will significantly reduce the chance of exposure to the virus. (2:662)

35.

A. Mycobacteria are rod-shaped organisms that have an unusual cell wall structure that contains a very high lipid content (up to 60%) which renders the surface hydrophobic and makes the bacilli difficult to stain with commonly used basic aniline dyes at room temperature. The bacilli can be stained by prolonged application of heat, and once stained, they resist decolorization with acid alcohol; thus they are described as acid-fast bacilli. (4:443)

36.

D. Actinomycosis exists in several forms. Infection of the cervicofacial area, the most common site of actinomycosis, is usually related to poor dental hygiene, tooth extraction, or some trauma to the mouth or jaw. Once the organism transgresses the epithelial cell barrier under conditions that produce sufficiently low oxygen tension for their multiplication, lesions filled with keratocytes surrounded by an indurated fibrous tissue reaction discharge sulfur granules which are masses or clumps of bacilli. (4:464)

37.

E. Capsules can protect bacteria because copious amounts of polysaccharide capsules may interfere with phagocytosis as in the case with Streptococcus pneumoniae and Hemophilus influenzae type b. Capsules also may aid in colonization and assist bacteria to attach to surfaces; for example, Streptococcus mutans and Streptococcus salivaris cells adhere to the surface of teeth because of the polysaccharide capsules of these bacteria. However, if the capsule elicits the production of antibodies which attach to the bacteria, opsonization and phagocytosis may occur. (4:15–16)

38.

D. Organisms that cause disease have specific determinants of virulence that allow them to avoid eradication by the body's defenses. Among these are adhesins such as fimbria which are responsible for the ability of bacteria to colonize surfaces and cells and excretion of enzymes and toxins that destroy host tissues. Fimbrial adhesins and other proteins may change their antigenic nature due to regulatory proteins that genetically alter their expression on the bacteria and allow a population of the bacteria to escape attachment and colonization, which protects them from eradication by host defenses. (4:6, 23)

39.

A. There has been a dramatic increase in the number of regulations, guidelines, and recommendations and standards affecting the practices of health care workers. Among these, several are well-defined approaches to control occupational health hazards. The practice of "universal precautions" means that health care workers should treat all patients as though they were known to be infectious. (6:38–39)

40.

A. In addition to the large, circular chromosome of supercoiled, double-stranded DNA, many bacteria may contain small, circular, covalently closed, double-stranded DNA molecules separated from the chromosome known as plasmids. (4:25)

41.

D. It is well recognized that the sharing of genetic information within and between related species is quite common and occurs in at least three fundamentally different ways. Transformation involves the release of DNA into the environment by lysis of the bacteria cells followed by direct uptake of that DNA by the recipient cells. Another means of transfer is called transduction, whereby DNA is introduced into the recipient's cell by a nonlethal donor cell. The third process of transfer by conjugation involves actual contact between donor and recipient cell by a plasmid, which is an autonomously replicating extrachromosomal molecule of circular double-stranded DNA. In conjugation, donor and recipient bacterial cells are referred to as male and female respectively. (4:53–54)

42.

E. The major line of defense for the body against infection is intact skin or tissue. The mechanical action of mucous on membranes and the bactericidal contents serve as a protective barrier to infection. The presence of normal bacteria flora in an area of the body suppresses growth of potentially pathogenic bacteria by competition for nutrients and production of inhibiting substances that are bactericidal. (1:2)

43.

C. Strains of Capnocytophaga demonstrate gliding motility on the surface of agar plates. These bacteria have a natural habitat in periodontal pockets of humans and are a cause of a number of infectious processes under certain conditions, including periodontal disease in juveniles. (8:225)

44.

D. Chlorine is a highly effective oxidizing agent which accounts for its lethality against microbes. In concentrations of less than 1 part per million, chlorine is lethal within seconds to most negative bacteria and inactivates most viruses. However, chlorine reacts rapidly with protein and many other organic materials which may render it ineffective. For this reason, it is normally applied as a 5 to 10 percent solution of sodium hypochlorite. (4:177)

45.

D. A national action plan to combat the spread of multiple-drug-resistant Mycobacterium tuberculosis has been implemented by the Centers for Disease Control (CDC) and the Department of Health and Human Services. The number of MDR strains of tuberculosis has increased among HIV patients, the homeless, and other patients who fail to complete or comply with prescribed therapeutic regimens. Some patients have been found to have strains of Mycobacterium tuberculosis that are resistant to as many as six to eight drugs, leaving no alternative treatment for such cases. There is national concern to prevent transmission to health care workers and other workers who are at risk because of close contact with patients and/or their respiratory secretions. (9:No.RR-11)

46.

C. As many as 85 percent of individuals with AIDS will develop pneumonia caused by Pneumocystis carinii. This extracellular opportunistic organism is toxonomically related to fungi, although in most cases, it is classified as a parasitic organism. (2:471–472)

47.

E. Mycobacterium avium-intracellulare is actually two species of mycobacteria, Mycobacterium avium and Mycobacterium intracellulare. However, they are very difficult to distinguish clinically and taxonomically, thus they are known as Mycobacterium avium-intracellulare. Many AIDS-infected patients usually acquire this organism along with other opportunistic infections. Mycobacterium avium-intracellulare is resistant to most common antimycobacterial agents. The mechanism of resistance is not clearly understood but is not related to patient compliance with treatment regimens. (2:336)

48.

B. Human Lyme disease, named after the Connecticut town where it was first reported, is caused by the spirochete Borrelia burgdorferi which is transmitted mainly by a tick. (11:413)

49.

E. The organism Treponema pallidum is responsible for syphilis. Syphilis causes disability and death mainly when the heart, blood vessels, and nervous system become affected. Any organ, however, can become affected. (10:181–189; 11:118, 130, 548; 12:29–245)

50.

D. The inflammatory consolidation found in bronchopneumonia is irregular in distribution. The most common microorganisms involved are influenza bacillus, staphylococcus, streptococcus, and pneumococcus. Tuberculosis, tularemia, and plague are specific types of bronchopneumonia. (10:409–411; 11:239, 241)

11 Oral Microbiology

DIRECTIONS Each of the questions below is followed by several suggested answers. Select the best answer in each case.

1. Necrotizing ulcerative gingivitis (NUG) is associated with an increase in the proportion of which microorganisms in the oral flora?

    A. fusiform bacilli

    B. spirochetes

    C. Streptococcus sp.

    D. A and B

    E. A, B, and C

2. Saliva plays a role in determining susceptibility or resistance to caries by

    A. physically flushing away food particles and bacteria from the teeth

    B. antibacterial substances it contains such as secretory IgA

    C. reducing enamel solubility via the common ion effect of its soluble minerals

    D. all of the above

3. Cellulitis differs from a soft-tissue abscess in that cellulitis
   A. rarely arises as a complication of untreated caries
   B. is invariably of viral etiology
   C. is not well-circumscribed
   D. is synonymous with Ludwig's angina

4. Oral manifestations of AIDS include
   A. hairy leukoplakia
   B. candidiasis
   C. aphthous ulcers
   D. Kaposi's sarcoma
   E. all of the above

5. A type of caries most often noted in the elderly is
   A. acute root caries
   B. smooth surface caries
   C. pit and fissure caries
   D. chronic caries

6. A common occurrence during scaling and curettage is
   A. a bacteremia which is handled successfully by the reticuloendothelial system
   B. a septicemia which generally causes asymptomatic abscesses in organs
   C. a local infection which repairs by morbid granulation tissue
   D. a toxemia which produces manifestations of infectious disease

7. Extrinsic dental stains include
   A. gray or brownish stains caused by tetracycline
   B. red to brown stain caused by congenital porphyria
   C. brown, black, green, or orange stains caused by chromogenic bacteria in plaque
   D. green to brown stain caused by erythroblastosis fetalis

8. Which of the following microorganisms would be LEAST dominant in nine-day-old plaque?
   A. Actinomyces sp.
   B. Neisseria sp.
   C. Veillonella sp.
   D. Streptococcus viridans
   E. Fusobacterium sp.

9. The principal oral site for the growth of spirochetes, fusobacteria, and other anaerobes is
   A. dental plaque
   B. the gingival margin
   C. the gingival sulcus
   D. saliva
   E. calculus

10. The predominant microorganisms of saliva are members of which of the following species?
    A. Streptococcus
    B. Staphylococcus
    C. Bacteroides
    D. Fusobacterium

11. Dextrans and levans are synthesized from sucrose by plaque bacteria primarily as extracellular polymers. Dextrans are polymers of what sugar?
    A. fructose
    B. lactose
    C. glucose
    D. galactose

12. Bacteria isolated from human oral flora that cause caries when introduced into gnotobiotic rats include
    A. Streptococcus mutans
    B. Actinobacillus actinomycetemcomitans
    C. Actinomyces viscosus
    D. Streptococcus fecalis
    E. A, C, and D
    F. A, B, C, and D

13. A fungal infection indigenous to the Mississippi Valley and often manifesting in the oral cavity is
    A. tuberculosis
    B. tetanus
    C. histoplasmosis
    D. pharyngitis

14. Denture-sore mouth is often related to an overgrowth of
    A. herpes simplex
    B. Candida albicans
    C. lactobacilli
    D. Streptococcus viridans

15. Soft-tissue emphysema following overzealous use of compressed air is a complication because of
    A. infection
    B. edema
    C. hemorrhage
    D. atrophy

16. A nonvital pulp that maintains its general histologic characteristic is known as
    A. pulpal abscess
    B. dry gangrene
    C. suppuration
    D. pseudomembranous necrosis

17. The dominant white cell noted in the inflammatory infiltrate of necrotizing ulcerative gingivitis is
    A. eosinophil
    B. basophil
    C. macrophage
    D. neutrophil

18. Hairy leukoplakia represents an opportunistic infection related to the presence of
    A. Candida albicans
    B. Epstein-Barr virus

C. cytomegalovirus
D. human papillomavirus

19. Affinity for the tooth surface is characteristic of
    A. Streptococcus mitis and S. pyogenes
    B. Streptococcus mutans and S. salivarius
    C. group D streptococci and Streptococcus mitis
    D. Streptococcus sanguis and S. mutans

20. The primary acidogenic microorganisms in the oral cavity are
    A. Fusobacterium
    B. Streptococci
    C. yeasts
    D. Lactobacilli

21. Bacteroides sp. produce an enzyme known as
    A. mucinase
    B. coagulase
    C. collagenase

22. Secondary oral herpes simplex virus infections differ from minor oral aphthous ulcers in which of the following parameters?
    A. number of ulcers
    B. duration
    C. location
    D. pain
    E. A, B, C, and D
    F. A and C only

23. The principal oral site for the growth of spirochetes, fusobacteria, and other anaerobes is
    A. dental plaque
    B. the gingival margin
    C. the gingival sulcus
    D. saliva

24. Which of the following is formed in large quantities following the degradation of sucrose by Streptococcus mutans?
    A. lactic acid
    B. acetic acid
    C. butyric acid
    D. propionic acid

25. A 7-year-old girl has a temperature of 102°F. Her mother states that the child has had an upper respiratory infection for several days. Examination reveals a few small white dots surrounded by a reddish halo on the buccal mucosa. The oral lesions most probably are indicative of
    A. rubeola
    B. herpangina
    C. varicella
    D. herpes zoster
    E. hand-, foot-, and mouth-disease

26. The tooth-plaque interface layer is derived from
    A. salivary glycoprotein
    B. bacterial glycoprotein
    C. salivary and bacterial glycoprotein

27. The bacteria that initiate caries on smooth enamel must have the ability to
    A. produce mucin
    B. produce proteolytic enzymes
    C. produce extracellular insoluble dextran
    D. survive in a high pH environment

28. Putative periodontopathic organisms for adult periodontitis include
    A. Actinobacillus actinomycetemcomitans
    B. Porphyromonas gingivalis
    C. Bacteroides intermedius
    D. A and C only
    E. A, B, and C

29. Most of the current efforts in controlling preventable oral disease (caries, periodontal disease) are directed toward the pathogenic potential of
    A. sulcular fluid flow
    B. fluoride
    C. diet
    D. supragingival dental plaque

30. Which of the following types of bacteria compose the predominant bacterial population in dental plaque in all stages of its maturation?
    A. Bacteroides
    B. Veillonella
    C. Fusobacterium
    D. Streptococci
    E. Staphylococci

31. Which of the following microorganisms has been implicated in the dental caries process?
    A. Streptococcus salivarius
    B. Streptococcus mitis
    C. Streptococcus mutans
    D. Veillonella sp.

32. Oral bacterial infections associated with HIV infection include
    A. HIV-associated gingivitis
    B. HIV-associated periodontitis
    C. Klebsiella stomatitis
    D. A and B only
    E. A, B, and C

33. The most common neoplasm seen in AIDS patients is
    A. squamous cell carcinoma
    B. basal cell carcinoma
    C. Kaposi's sarcoma
    D. non-Hodgkin's lymphoma

34. Caries immunization studies with rodents and primates have clearly suggested a role for which class of immunoglobulin (Ig) in protection against caries?
    A. IgM
    B. IgE
    C. IgA
    D. IgG

35. Which of the following types of cells is the predominant inflammatory cell found in the chronic stages of gingivitis?
    A. mast cells
    B. lymphocytes
    C. plasma cells
    D. erythrocytes
    E. macrophages

36. Which of the following microorganisms is most commonly implicated with the etiology of juvenile periodontitis (JP)?
    A. Wolinella recta
    B. Actinomyces israelii
    C. Streptococcus sanguis
    D. Veillonella parvula
    E. Actinobacillus actinomycetemcomitans

37. Which of the following microorganisms has been associated with advanced and/or highly inflamed destructive lesions in adult forms of periodontal disease?
    A. Porphyromonas gingivalis
    B. Actinomyces naeslundii
    C. Rothia dentocariosa
    D. Streptococcus mitis
    E. Streptococcus sanguis

38. Which of the following organisms is commonly implicated with the etiology of necrotizing ulcerative gingivitis (NUG)?
    A. Prevotella intermedia
    B. Streptococcus sanguis

C. Actinomyces israelii
D. Streptococcus uberis

39. Prepubertal periodontitis (PPP) occurs in localized and generalized forms. Organisms most frequently associated with this form of periodontitis include
    A. Selenomonas sputigena
    B. Porphyromonas gingivalis
    C. Prevotella intermedius
    D. Capnocytophaga sputigena
    E. A, C, and D

40. In rapidly progressive periodontitis (RPP), there is a more complex picture of bacterial types than that seen in juvenile periodontitis. These bacteria include
    A. a zone of primarily gram-positive organisms
    B. a zone of gram-negative bacteria with many spirochetes and flagellated bacteria
    C. A and B

answers & rationales

1.

D. Spirochetes with a characteristic ultrastructural morphology invade the epithelium and connective tissue in NUG. Fusiform bacilli can also be seen in necrotic zones superficial to the zone of spirochete infiltration. (1:171; 2:545)

2.

D. Saliva can have a major role in host resistance to caries ranging from nonspecific mechanisms such as reducing plaque accumulation by mechanical cleansing of the teeth to specific aggregation of bacteria and the resultant reduction in their adherence to tooth surfaces. The importance of saliva in defense against caries is illustrated by the marked increase in caries incidence that usually occurs when salivary flow is reduced or eliminated, as in xerostomia. (1:143; 2:533)

3.

C. Cellulitis is a diffuse inflammation of soft tissue that is not circumscribed or confined to one area and is due to infection by organisms (facultative and strict anaerobes) that produce significant amounts of hyaluronidase. Cellulitis of the face and neck most commonly results from dental infection. Cellulitis may cause the patient to be moderately ill with elevated temperature and leukocytes. (1:511–516; 2:223–228)

4.

E. These and several other conditions, including lymphoma, gingivitis/periodontal disease, and xerostomia, have a greater than expected frequency in AIDS patients. These oral manifestations are sometimes the first clinical signs of HIV infection and AIDS. (1:419; 2:109)

5.

A. Acute root caries or senile caries is initiated at the cementoenamel junction. Root caries is found in 60 percent to 70 percent of individuals between 60 and 70 years old. Strains of Streptococcus mutans, S. sanguis, Arthobacter sp., Veillonella sp., Rothia dentocariosa, Actinomyces viscosus, and A. naeslundii have been isolated from human root caries. The etiology and pathogenesis of the lesions are related to gingival recession and often to xerostomia. The xerostomia may be due to Sjogren's syndrome, radiation therapy, or malfunction of the salivary glands. (1:419–459; 2:348)

6.

A. Transient bacteremias are known to follow almost all surgical procedures and are cleared by cells of the reticuloendothelial system. Transient bacteremias usually do not lead to a distant injury or to a new focus of infection. However, they may lead to isolated infections such as osteomyelitis or bacterial endocarditis. (3:176–177)

7.

C. Other examples of extrinsic stains, or those on the tooth surface that can be removed with abrasives, are those caused by pigments in dietary substances such as tea and coffee, or by tobacco tar. Tetracycline ingestion, congenital porphyria, and erythroblastosis fetalis result in intrinsic staining or discoloration. (1:157; 2:517–520)

8.

B. Neisseria sp. would be least dominant of those listed in a nine-day old plaque. Streptococcus sp., Bacteroides sp., Veillonella sp., and fusiform bacteria make up mature plaque. Streptococcal organisms basically compose immature plaque. (4:273–274; 5:476–477, 778)

9.

C. The gingival sulcus is the principal oral site for the growth of spirochetes, fusobacteria, and other anaerobes. At the orifice to the gingival sulcus, a dense mixed population of organisms exists. Within the pocket, spirochetes and other gram-negative organisms are present. (4:294)

10.

A. Streptococcus salivarius, S. mitis, and S. sanguis, members of the "viridans" group of streptococci, are predominant in saliva. Gram-positive filaments such as Actinomyces, Nocardia, and Rothia species are also found in saliva, as well as gram-negative Veillonella species. (2:322; 5:777–778)

11.

C. Dextrans are a type of glucan, a homopolymer of glucose. Mutans are the other type of glucan. These are produced by Streptococcus sanguis, S. mutans, S. salivarius, and Lactobacillus species. Levans are polymers of fructose and are made by S. salivarius and S. mutans. S. mutans, however, is unique in using these polysaccharides to aggregate into large masses in the accumulation of dental plaque. (2:334–335)

12.

E. Streptococcus mutans, S. fecalis, and Actinomyces viscosus may be etiologically related to dental caries as well as S. salivarius, S. sanguis, A. naeslundii, A. israelii, and Lactobacillus casei. Actinobacillus actinomycetemcomitans (Aa) is a putative periodontopathic organism for adult periodontitis. (1:541; 2:528)

13.

C. The fungus (Histoplasma capsulatum) causing histoplasmosis is apparently spread by the excreta of birds, and the Mississippi Valley is a major migratory route. It is also seen in the Ohio Valley. Humans

are infected by inhaling the spores into the lungs. Eighty to 100 percent of the population in endemic areas have experienced primary acute histoplasmosis by age 18. Oral lesions occur in at least 30 percent of patients, usually as multiple ulcerations of the gingiva, tongue, and palate. Oral lesions may be the first clinical manifestation of the disease. (1:390; 5:973; 6:28–29, 746)

14.

B. The most common cause of denture-sore mouth (or denture stomatitis) is poor oral hygiene and unclean dentures. Denture-sore mouth may also be due to salivary duct obstruction, with reduced flow of saliva into tissues and subsequent inflammation, and, in very rare cases, by contact allergy to the denture material. In denture-sore mouth caused by Candida albicans (chronic atrophic candidiasis), there is actual (although superficial) invasion of tissue. However, the typical white patches of thrush may not be seen; the clinical appearance is that of a bright red, somewhat velvety to pebbly surface. This form of candidiasis occurs in up to 65 percent of geriatric individuals who wear complete maxillary dentures. It usually occurs on the palatal mucosa and most often occurs in women. (1:396, 551; 6:482–483; 7:122)

15.

A. Fatal air embolism may occur following overzealous use of compressed air in treating soft-tissue emphysema. A more likely complication is infection due to the microorganisms carried by the air into the soft tissues. Thus, antibiotic therapy is recommended for soft-tissue emphysema. (1:570)

16.

B. Dry gangrene (or mummification) sometimes occurs when the pulp dies for some unexplained reason; it may result from ischemic necrosis or infarction. Being nonpurulent, the pulp maintains its general histologic characteristics. (1:486; 3:60–61)

17.

D. Neutrophils are the dominant cells of most acute inflammations. Their chief function is phagocytosis of bacteria and tissue fragments. They migrate through the vessel walls and proceed by their ameboid activity, influenced by chemotaxis, to the site of injury. (3:82–83)

18.

B. Hairy leukoplakia represents an opportunistic infection caused by the Epstein-Barr virus (EBV) and is associated with subsequent or concomitant development of AIDS in up to 80 percent of the cases. The virus is present in the lesion as well as in the normal oral epithelium of AIDS patients. The human papilloma virus may facilitate the entry, replication, and persistence of EBV in epithelial cells. There can also be a suprainfection with Candida albicans. (2:109)

19.

D. Streptococcus sanguis (as well as Neisseria) appear to dominate in the early plaque, whereas S. mutans colonizes later; streptococcal organisms compose immature plaque. In mature plaque, after a week or so, cocci are reduced to about 50 percent of the plaque flora, with other bacteria such as Fusobacterium, Veillonella, Nocardia, Neisseria, vibrios, and spirochetes being present. (4:284–294; 8:487–490)

20.

B. Streptococci are the dominant acidogenic microorganisms. Of the organic acids formed in dental plaque, lactic acid is the main cause of enamel decalcification. The ratio of streptococci to lactobacilli is approximately 100,000:1. Lactobacilli represent approximately 1 percent of the oral flora. (2:349–351; 4:360–363)

21.

C. Bacteroides sp. (including Porphyromonas gingivalis, formerly Bacteroides gingivalis), Clostridium sp., Bacillus sp., and Actinobacillus actinomycetemcomitans (Aa) produce collagenase. The enzyme may assist in destruction of collagen fibers and thus in the initiation and progression of periodontal disease. (2:362; 4:440)

22.

F. Herpes usually manifests as multiple confluent ulcers on the border, hard palate, and gingiva, while minor aphthae usually appear as a single oral ulcer and can occur on all mucosal sites other than the border, hard palate, and gingiva. Both types of ulcers are painful, are recurrent, and usually resolve in 1 to 2 weeks. Other differences between herpes and minor oral aphthae include cause (herpes simplex virus type I versus focal immunodysregulation), occurrence of a vesicular stage (yes versus no), and method of treatment (antiviral drugs versus steroids). (7:4–9)

23.

C. The environmental nutrients of the gingival sulcus, such as gingival fluid, desquamated epithelial cells, blood cells, and nonviable neutrophils, apparently favor the growth of anaerobic microorganisms. Subgingival plaque associated with cementum is dominated by gram-negative rods, cocci, and spirochetes, including the anaerobic bacteria Veillonella and Fusobacterium nucleatum. (2:361)

24.

A. Large quantities of lactic acid are formed from the fermentation of sugars by Streptococcus mutans. S. mutans is a homofermentable lactic acid former. S. mutans and certain lactobacilli (i.e. Lactobacillus casei) are active acid producers, even at pH 5. (2:347)

25.

A. These oral manifestations of rubeola are pathognomonic of the disease and appear 2 to 3 days before the skin eruptions appear. They are called Koplik's spots. (1:378)

26.

C. Initially, the acquired pellicle is formed on teeth from glycoproteins in saliva. Subsequently, there is deposition of bacterial extracellular polysaccharides and glycoprotein by the initially adherent plaque bacteria. It has been demonstrated that the pellicle or absorbed glycoproteins on the tooth surface can be utilized for bacterial metabolism. (2:326–328)

27.

C. Dextran protects the bacteria from being removed from the teeth by saliva, foods, liquids, and masticatory forces. Glucans occur as dextran or mutans. Dextran is a homologous polymer of glucose. (2:334)

28.

E. Actinobacillus actinomycetemcomitans, Porphyromonas gingivalis and Bacteroides intermedius are all periodontopathic organisms. Porphyromonas gingivalis was formerly known as Bacteroides gingivalis. Other bacteria associated with adult periodontitis include Fusobacterium nucleatum, Wolinella recta, and Selenomonas sputagena. (1:147–197; 2:538–542)

29.

D. Most of the current efforts in controlling oral disease are directed toward the pathogenic potential of supragingival dental plaque because 1) a great deal is now known about the mechanisms responsible for the formation of supragingival plaque; 2) much is known concerning the pathogenic potential of plaque with respect to its microbiologic content and metabolism; and 3) plaque is readily accessible for sampling and study and for the application of preventive and control procedures. (9:476)

30.

D. Streptococcal bacteria compose the predominant bacterial population of dental plaque at all stages of plaque maturation. Dental plaque contains very few species of Bacteroides, Veillonella, and fusiform bacteria in early stages of development, whereas more mature dental plaque contains significant numbers of these bacteria. Because the microbial composition of supragingival plaque is mixed and in a dynamic state of change and succession, it is not surprising that the bacterial composition of plaque samples varies from tooth surface to tooth surface and even from site to site on the same tooth surface. (9:477)

31.

C. Streptococcus mutans has been implicated in dental caries formation. Evidence to support its role in dental caries formation includes: 1) human isolates of S. mutans have been shown to cause multisurface dental caries when administered as monoinfectants into a variety of animal models; 2) there are up to 10 times as many S. mutans organisms present in pooled plaque samples obtained from caries-active individuals as compared to similar plaque samples from caries-inactive patients; 3) S. mutans is present at extremely high concentrations over small localized surfaces of the teeth on which demineralization occurs; 4) tooth surfaces infected with S. mutans develop carious lesions, and surfaces uninfected with the organism generally remain sound; and 5) S. mutans can be isolated from almost all human coronal carious lesions. This organism may serve as a "target organism" in the development of methods to control this plaque-related oral disease. (9:479)

32.

E. Other oral bacterial lesions associated with HIV infection include infections of Mycobacterium avium/intracellulare complex. HIV-associated gingivitis may involve the attached gingiva and alveolar mucosa in addition to the free gingival margin; is often seen in clean mouths; and does not respond to conventional periodontal therapy. In HIV-associated periodontitis, there is extensive soft-tissue necrosis, severe loss of periodontal attachment, and spontaneous bleeding, often with severe, deep-seated pain. (8:417–422)

33.

C. Kaposi's sarcoma (KS) in the past was a relatively rare tumor, occurring most frequently in elderly men of Mediterranean heritage. Oral lesions of KS are now seen in 50 percent of AIDS patients. Its etiology has not been established but may be viral. Oral KS is most often seen on the hard palate. The lesions are red, blue, or purple and may be flat, raised, solitary, or multiple. (6:625; 8:417–422)

34.

C. Secretory IgA (sIgA) is the predominant Ig in external secretions of the body including saliva. sIgA is involved in first-line defenses such as trapping microorganisms at mucous surfaces, inhibiting bacterial adherence, and bacterial lysis. In monkeys, local injection and instillation of Streptococcus mutans antigen into the parotid duct induced production of sIgA and resulted in reduced levels of S. mutans on the animals' teeth. (8:507–508)

35.

C. Plasma cells are the predominant inflammatory cell in chronic gingivitis. In early stages of gingivitis, lymphocytes are the predominant inflammatory cell. (10:331)

36.

E. The microorganism most commonly implicated with the etiology of juvenile periodontitis (JP) is Actinobacillus actinomycetemcomitans (Aa). JP is a relatively rare form of periodontitis, characterized by rapid vertical loss of alveolar bone around permanent first molars and incisors. The rapidity and severity of the bone loss in JP are out of proportion to the intensity of local factors. The prevalence of Actinobacillus actinomycetemcomitans, as well as serum antibody levels to Aa, is greater in JP than in other periodontal conditions. Aa has several means of evading host defense mechanisms including inhibiting neutrophil chemotaxis and the killing of neutrophils and monocytes by the secretion of leukotoxin. (10:173–175; 376–392)

37.

A. Porphyromonas gingivalis has been associated with advanced and/or highly inflamed destructive lesions in adult forms of periodontal disease. Actinomyces naeslundii, Rothia dentocariosa, Streptococcus mitis, and Streptococcus sanguis are all associated with healthy gingiva. (10:173)

38.

A. Prevotella intermedia is associated with the etiology of necrotizing ulcerative gingivitis. (10:173)

39.

E. Selenomonas sputigena and Prevotella intermedius are frequently recovered in oral cultures taken from PPP patients. Increased serum antibody titers to Capnocytophaga sputigena are also associated with PPP. (10:392–393)

40.

C. Based on structural studies of in situ plaque associated with RPP, the zone of primarily gram-positive organisms is attached to the tooth surface. Between this zone and the epithelium, there is a zone of gram-negative bacteria and spirochetes, extending to the apical portion of the pocket. RPP is most commonly seen in young adults in their twenties and thirties, and is characterized by marked inflammation, rapid bone loss, and periods of spontaneous remission. (10:175–177; 393)

12 Nutrition

DIRECTIONS Each of the questions below is followed by several suggested answers. Select the best answer in each case.

---

1. Of the following substances, the ones that are generally MOST readily usable as a source of energy for heterotrophic bacteria are
   A. proteins
   B. vitamins
   C. carbohydrates
   D. ammonium salts

2. Formation of glucose from noncarbohydrate substances is called
   A. gluconeogenesis
   B. glycogenesis
   C. glucogenesis
   D. glycolysis

3. Pernicious anemia is associated with
   A. iron deficiency
   B. aminopyrine therapy
   C. vitamin K deficiency
   D. vitamin B12 deficiency

4. An adequate intake of vitamin C is necessary for good repair of a wound because it promotes
   A. growth of epithelium
   B. production of collagens
   C. budding of capillaries
   D. phagocytosis of cell fragments

5. The pH of foodstuffs is a very important consideration in predicting the cariogenicity of food. The safe pH area is considered to be
   A. 5.5 to 6.0
   B. above 6
   C. above 6.5
   D. about 7

6. The average American diet is lower in calcium than the recommended dietary allowance because calcium readily forms insoluble compounds.
   A. Both statement and reason are correct and related.
   B. Both statement and reason are correct but not related.
   C. The statement is correct but the reason is not.
   D. The statement is not correct but the reason is an accurate statement.
   E. Neither statement nor reason is correct.

7. Certain polyunsaturated fatty acids are essential in the human diet because human tissues are not capable of producing polyunsaturation in fatty acids.
   A. Both statement and reason are correct and related.
   B. Both statement and reason are correct but not related.
   C. The statement is correct but the reason is not.
   D. The statement is not correct but the reason is an accurate statement.
   E. Neither statement nor reason is correct.

8. Iodine is useful in colloid goiter therapy because iodine stimulates the production of thyroxine.
   A. Both statement and reason are correct and related.
   B. Both statement and reason are correct but not related.
   C. The statement is correct but the reason is not.
   D. The statement is not correct but the reason is an accurate statement.
   E. Neither statement nor reason is correct.

9. Certain amino acids are termed essential because they
   A. are components of protein essential for life
   B. are required for the clotting of blood
   C. can be converted into essential hormonal substances
   D. cannot be synthesized within the body at a sufficient rate to meet body requirements
   E. are essential for the formation of high-energy complexes

10. Certain amino acids need NOT be present in the diet of an animal because of its ability to synthesize them. An important source of the carbon of these amino acids is
    A. the metabolism of carbohydrates
    B. the metabolism of fatty acids
    C. carbon dioxide
    D. nucleic acid

11. The effect of vitamin C deficiency is primarily on
    A. epithelial tissues
    B. connective tissues
    C. nervous tissues
    D. muscular tissues
    E. hematopoietic tissues

12. Nutrition is of special importance to the oral tissues
    A. directly, when food is masticated in the oral cavity
    B. systemically, when nutrients are returned through the circulatory system to nourish and maintain the oral tissues
    C. neither A nor B
    D. both A and B

13. The bulk of iron stored in the intestinal wall is
    A. ferritin
    B. apoferritin
    C. $FeSO_4$
    D. hemoglobin
    E. cytochrome C

14. The prime food factor responsible for dental caries is
    A. the sugar content of a particular food
    B. frequent between-meal eating of sweets
    C. firm, detersive foods
    D. drinking fluoridated water
    E. ingestion of a balanced, adequate diet

15. Which of the following is formed in the animal from dietary tryptophan?
    A. niacin
    B. thiamin
    C. folic acid
    D. riboflavin
    E. pyridoxine

16. Which of the following elements is essential for plant growth but not for animal growth?
    A. boron
    B. copper
    C. iodine
    D. magnesium
    E. sulfur

17. Several investigators have demonstrated that neonatal protein deficiency in laboratory rats can increase the susceptibility of the teeth in adulthood to
    A. staining
    B. caries
    C. abrasion
    D. periodontal disease
    E. ridge resorption

18. The electrolyte potassium
    A. is the principal cation in intracellular fluid
    B. is derived solely from dietary intake including meat, milk, and many fruits
    C. is widely distributed in the health-promoting foods
    D. is present in very small amounts in the extracellular fluid
    E. all of the above

19. In reviewing the diet report, special attention should be paid to
    A. frequency of carbohydrate ingestion
    B. presence of retentive fermentable carbohydrates
    C. presence and position of detergent foods in the diet
    D. A and B only
    E. A, B, and C

20. In the dental office, the dental health education program should include material regarding
    A. diet and the caries process
    B. toothbrushing technique
    C. toothbrushing application of fluoride
    D. benefits of toothbrushing habits
    E. all of the above

21. Hypochromic anemia is associated with
    A. iron deficiency
    B. vitamin K deficiency
    C. aminopyrine therapy
    D. vitamin B12 deficiency

22. A disease caused by interference with the intrinsic-extrinsic factor mechanism is called
    A. aplastic anemia
    B. sickle-cell anemia
    C. iron-deficiency anemia
    D. pernicious anemia

23. Beriberi is prevalent in the Orient because a diet made up primarily of polished rice is deficient in
    A. thiamin
    B. vitamin A
    C. vitamin C
    D. riboflavin

24. The daily NRC/RDA (1989) requirement for iron by a normal adult female during childbearing years approximates
    A. 15 mg
    B. 18 mg
    C. 100 mg
    D. 1 g
    E. 10 g

25. The dominant factor in controlling the absorption of iron from the gastrointestinal tract is the

A. excretion of iron in the urine
B. excretion of iron in the stools
C. presence of reducing substances in the gut
D. physiologic saturation of the mucosal cells with iron
E. concentration of the ferrous iron in bone marrow, spleen, and liver

26. Although rare, toxicity to vitamin excess by eating naturally occurring foodstuffs has been reported for vitamins
    A. A and D
    B. D and K
    C. B1 and C
    D. B2 and K
    E. B2 and B6

27. Which of the following nutrient deficiencies is frequently found in the diet of children in developed countries and has been associated with increased caries susceptibility in laboratory animals?
    A. iron
    B. zinc
    C. vitamin E
    D. protein
    E. calcium

28. Amino acids are building blocks for
    A. vitamins
    B. minerals
    C. proteins
    D. all of the above

29. Taking mineral oil at mealtime is inadvisable because it
    A. interferes with vitamin absorption
    B. interferes with fat-soluble vitamin absorption
    C. causes food to be digested more slowly
    D. causes indigestion

30. Carbohydrates primarily responsible for causing dental caries are the
    A. polysaccharides
    B. monosaccharides
    C. disaccharides
    D. both B and C

31. Skimmed milk is preferred to whole milk in adults because
    A. it has more vitamins
    B. it has less lipids
    C. it is easier to digest

32. Calcium metabolism is dependent on and controlled by
    A. diet
    B. parathyroids
    C. the kidneys
    D. the liver
    E. muscle tissue

33. An excessive accumulation of a vitamin in the body leading to toxic symptoms is the definition of
    A. hyperantivitamins
    B. hypervitaminosis
    C. avitaminosis
    D. provitaminemisis

34. Which of the following groups includes only amino acids essential for humans?
    A. valine, serine, leucine
    B. leucine, lysine, glycine
    C. tyrosine, threonine, tryptophan
    D. phenylalanine, methionine, proline
    E. tryptophan, methionine, isoleucine

35. Gingival lesions occur in scurvy, which is caused by a dietary deficiency of
    A. citric acid
    B. pyruvic acid
    C. ascorbic acid
    D. acetoacetic acid

    E. pantothenic acid

36. A trace mineral not essential for humans, but which promotes mineralization of teeth (may exchange with phosphorus in apatite tooth substances), and which may inhibit cholesterol synthesis, is
    A. tin
    B. molybdenum
    C. nickel
    D. silicon
    E. vanadium

37. Proteins that contain all the essential amino acids in sufficient quantity and in the right ratio to maintain nitrogen equilibrium and permit growth of the young are
    A. essential proteins
    B. complete proteins
    C. incomplete proteins
    D. nonessential proteins
    E. limiting amino acids

38. The amino acid(s) most likely to be found in low amounts or missing in foods is (are) which of the following?
    A. tryptophan
    B. lysine, methionine
    C. phenylalanine, leucine, lysine
    D. A and B
    E. tryptophan, leucine, isoleucine

39. The average amount of heme iron in the American diet is
    A. 2–10%
    B. 10%
    C. 10–15%
    D. 25%–35%
    E. 100%

40. The two types of essential iron are
    A. storage and myoglobin

B. heme and nonheme

C. storage and heme

D. ferritin and hemosiderin

41. Vital minerals associated with physiologic fluid balance are

    A. sodium and potassium

    B. iron and iodine

    C. chlorine and sulfur

    D. calcium and phosphorus

    E. iron and ascorbic acid

42. In broad terms, a precursor of a vitamin or provitamin is a substance that

    A. reactivates a vitamin

    B. is a biologically inactive form of a vitamin

    C. prolongs the action of a vitamin

    D. acts as an enzyme in promoting vitamin metabolism

    E. all of the above

43. An experimental dietary magnesium deficiency can adversely affect the periodontal structures because it could produce a reduction in the rate of alveolar bone formation, widening of the periodontal ligament, and gingival hyperplasia.

    A. Both statement and reason are correct and related.

    B. Both statement and reason are correct but not related.

    C. The statement is correct but the reason is not.

    D. The statement is not correct but the reason is an accurate statement.

    E. Neither statement nor reason is correct.

44. The most active and potent metabolite of vitamin D3 (cholecalciferol) is believed to be

    A. 25-OH-D3

    B. 1, 25-(OH)2-D3

C. 24, 25-(OH)2-D3

D. 7-dehydrocholesterol

E. cholecalciferol

45. In order to have carbohydrate on hand when needed, the body stores some of it in the liver and muscles. Glycogen is

    A. the body's reserve supply of carbohydrates

    B. a polysaccharide

    C. both A and B

46. One important function of fat is to

    A. provide nitrogen for cellular metabolism

    B. serve as a catalyst in the breakdown of proteins

    C. assist in the absorption of iron

    D. act as a carrier of fat-soluble vitamins

47. Fat is primarily considered as

    A. a concentrated source of energy

    B. the cheapest source of energy

    C. a tissue-building substance

    D. a food substance to be avoided

48. The most important carbohydrate available to the body, whether it be by absorption from the diet or by synthesis within the body, is

    A. galactose

    B. starch

    C. sucrose

    D. glucose

49. When the intake amount of nitrogen is equal to the amount excreted, a person is said to be in a state of

    A. positive nitrogen balance

    B. negative nitrogen balance

    C. nitrogen equilibrium

    D. shock

50. In summary, the Food and Nutrition Board's DRIs and RDAs are
    A. acceptable levels of intake for population groups
    B. allowances and estimates of nutrients that should meet the needs of nearly all healthy individuals within a group
    C. generally in excess of nutrient requirements except for energy and the mineral iron
    D. insurance for normal growth and maintenance of the health of most people
    E. all of the above

51. The relationship between protein nutrition and oral health and disease might be discussed in all EXCEPT which of the following ways?
    A. There is no relation between protein nutrition and oral health and disease.
    B. Protein substances make up the majority of the organic portions of enamel and dentin.
    C. Protein deficiency may be one reason for delayed eruption and hypoplasia of deciduous teeth.
    D. Protein malnutrition (even the subclinical type) can and very likely will enhance oral infection.
    E. On the basis of our present biochemical knowledge concerning the periodontal tissues and periodontal disease, it appears that dietary protein is a very important consideration in maintaining the health of this tooth-supporting structure.

52. An assay of serum that shows a low level of vitamin A may reflect
    A. a reduced store of the vitamin
    B. a deficient intake of the vitamin
    C. an increased intake of carotene
    D. an increased prothrombin time
    E. both A and B

53. The active form of vitamin D is calcitriol; therefore, a prolonged deficiency may result in
    A. rickets
    B. osteomalacia in adults and rickets in children
    C. faulty tooth formation
    D. B and C only
    E. A, B, and C

54. In relation to dental health, two important functions of the trace mineral zinc are
    A. maintaining normal blood calcium levels and regulating phosphorus concentrations in the body
    B. healing wounds and manufacturing red blood cells
    C. being an essential constituent of carbonic anhydrase and combining with insulin for storage of the hormone

55. An essential macromineral closely associated with calcium and phosphorus in the structure of bones and teeth is
    A. copper
    B. fluoride
    C. magnesium
    D. selenium
    E. zinc

56. Which of the following diet and dental health studies have NEVER been done?
    A. in vivo plaque pH changes in human beings consuming different foods
    B. large-scale, long-term prospective studies on food intake and dental health in noninstitutionalized populations
    C. animal studies in which human foods rather than laboratory chows were used to feed the animals
    D. large-scale, cross-sectional studies on food intake patterns in children and caries prevalence

57. A diet that will cause a severe alteration in bone because of a low calcium or phosphorus intake will
    A. not affect the formative tooth
    B. cause resorption of the formed tooth
    C. halve the growth and calcification of the teeth
    D. cause only slight changes in the formative tooth
    E. form defective areas in the tooth that may be repaired by the body when an adequate intake is again provided

58. The coenzyme systems involved in biochemical reactions concerned with the transfer of CCH_3, $HCOOC$, or CCH_2OH groups from one compound to another contain a derivative of
    A. folic acid
    B. vitamin B1
    C. vitamin B2
    D. d-ascorbic acid
    E. pantothenic acid

59. Intake of which of the following amino acids will lead to increased sulfur excretion?
    A. glycine
    B. arginine
    C. methionine
    D. tryptophan
    E. phenylalanine

60. Vitamin A functions to
    A. prevent pellagra
    B. promote the absorption of calcium
    C. promote differentiation of epithelial cells
    D. maintain the integrity of connective tissue
    E. prevent rickets

61. Pantothenic acid is an integral part of
    A. NAD (nicotinamide adenine dinucleotide)
    B. cobalamin
    C. folic acid
    D. coenzyme A
    E. pyridoxine phosphate

62. Normal production of sound dentin and enamel requires adequate amounts of which of the following vitamins?
    A. vitamin A
    B. vitamin C
    C. vitamin D
    D. all of the above

63. The role of this substance in human nutrition may include helping to prevent diabetes. It is essential to the body's use of sugars and fats. A long-term deficiency has been associated with cardiovascular disease in adults.
    A. zinc
    B. chromium
    C. molybdenum
    D. selenium
    E. fluoride

64. The possible mechanisms of periodontal host defense that are modified by nutrition include
    A. gingival fluid: flow rate, composition
    B. saliva: developmental effects, flow rate, composition
    C. microflora community and mucoepithelial barrier
    D. responsiveness of the repair process
    E. all of the above

65. An increased mucosal permeability has been shown to occur in experimental animals that are deficient in which of the following?
    A. ascorbate
    B. folate
    C. zinc
    D. all of the above

66. Published reports and studies have demonstrated that humans and experimental animals who suffered from this type of malnutrition had reduced mitotic activity in epithelial tissue including that of the oral cavity.

    A. zinc

    B. folate

    C. calorie and/or protein

    D. vitamin A

    E. ascorbate

67. Which of the following ingredients listed on a product label indicates that it contains sugar?

    A. high fructose corn syrup

    B. dextrose

    C. levulose

    D. glucose

    E. all of the above

68. A number of animal feeding experiments have shown that a deficiency of this substance can cause changes in the gingival epithelium and bone of the periodontium.

    A. vitamin A

    B. protein

    C. vitamin C

    D. iron

    E. zinc

69. According to scientific information available at this time, the true essential fatty acids necessary in human nutrition are

    A. linoleic acid and alpha linolenic acid

    B. arachidonic acid and alpha linolenic acid

    C. eicosapentaenoic acid (EPA) and linoleic acid

    D. docosahexaenoic acid (DHA) and arachidonic acid

70. Perifollicular hemorrhages are associated with a dietary deficiency of

    A. ascorbic acid

    B. choline

    C. vitamin B complex

    D. vitamin K

    E. vitamin E

71. In experimental animals deficient in this substance, there is microscopic evidence of destruction of the periodontal fibers, disturbance in the alveolar bone formation, increased osteoclastic resorption, and engorged capillaries.

    A. vitamin A

    B. vitamin C

    C. B6

    D. iron

    E. B12

72. An important nutrient present in low concentration in milk is

    A. carbohydrate

    B. calcium

    C. protein

    D. iron

    E. riboflavin

73. Dyssebacea is the clinical term used to designate a series of disturbances of the sebaceous glands characterized by increased oiliness and dermatitis, fissuring, and exfoliation. These disturbances can be caused by

    A. vitamin A deficiency

    B. ascorbic acid deficiency

    C. riboflavin, niacin, and pyridoxine (B6) deficiency

    D. vitamin K deficiency

74. Follicular hyperkeratosis, generally seen on the extremities, is caused by a deficiency of

    A. vitamin D

    B. vitamin B complex

    C. vitamin A and unsaturated fatty acids

    D. multiple nutrients

    E. vitamin K

75. Filiform papillary atrophy is a nutritional deficiency caused by a lack of
    A. vitamin B complex and iron
    B. niacin and B12
    C. iron and folic acid
    D. vitamins C, B12, folic acid, and iron
    E. both B and C

76. A patient has cheilosis, angular stomatitis, glossitis, and red, itching eyes. The periodontal surgery that was performed one week ago has not healed properly. A deficiency of which of the following vitamins is most likely?
    A. thiamin
    B. riboflavin
    C. tocopherol
    D. calciferol
    E. pantothenic acid

77. The interrelationship among which vitamins is so close that a deficient intake of one will impair the utilization of the others?
    A. fat-soluble
    B. all
    C. water-soluble
    D. vitamin B complex

78. The oral symptoms associated with the anatomic signs of a B-complex vitamin deficiency are
    A. sore lips and pain on opening the mouth
    B. persistent burning and tingling of the tongue
    C. difficulty in swallowing caused by tenderness of the tongue
    D. excessive salivation
    E. all of the above

79. On a functional basis, the B-complex vitamins that are primarily involved in the release of energy from carbohydrates and fats are
    A. biotin, thiamin, riboflavin, niacin, pantothenic acid
    B. B6, B12, folic acid
    C. choline, lipoic acid, inositol
    D. bioflavonoids and para-aminobenzoic acid
    E. all of the above

80. Which of the following conclusions can be drawn from the current available evidence about the local effect of the physical consistency of food on periodontal health?
    A. Fibrous foods do not remove plaque at the gingival half of the tooth.
    B. Fibrous or firm foods stimulate salivary flow and therefore can aid in the oral clearance of food debris.
    C. Selecting fibrous foods rather than soft, retentive sweet foods may indirectly reduce plaque formation because there will be less dietary sucrose available for conversion to glucans.
    D. Chewing fibrous or firm foods does not increase gingival keratinization, but it can have a beneficial stimulatory effect on strengthening the periodontal ligament and increasing the density of the alveolar bone.
    E. All of the above.

81. Even though many assume that this substance is not toxic because of its water-soluble properties, massive (mega-) doses of this vitamin can cause liver toxicity and peptic ulcer.
    A. thiamin
    B. pyridoxine
    C. riboflavin
    D. niacin
    E. pantothenic acid

82. A deficiency of which substance is probably the most common hypovitaminosis in the human race?
    A. vitamin A
    B. folic acid
    C. cobalamin
    D. pyridoxine
    E. ascorbate

83. Many nutrients are involved in the formation and structure of blood. However, the major nutrients that deal with blood formation (hematopoiesis) are
    A. iron and copper
    B. vitamin E and folic acid
    C. vitamin B12 and folic acid
    D. iron and vitamin C
    E. vitamin B6 and vitamin B12

84. The MOST cariogenic carbohydrate, under some but not all conditions, and the LEAST cariogenic are
    A. sucrose, starch
    B. fructose, starch
    C. fructose, dextrose
    D. glucose, levulose
    E. sucrose, dextrose

85. The MOST common source of fructose in our diet is from
    A. fructose sources
    B. galactose sources
    C. maltose sources
    D. lactose sources
    E. sucrose sources

86. There is growing concern among health professionals that the average U.S. diet may be deficient in
    A. iron
    B. vitamin B6
    C. vanadium
    D. zinc
    E. magnesium

87. Which of the following principles should be applied to dietary intervention in the prevention and control of periodontal diseases?
    A. Diet is nutritionally optimal over the long term, meeting or exceeding the Food and Nutrition Board's Dietary Reference Intakes.
    B. Provides variety and is in accordance with the U.S. Dietary Goals.
    C. Diet should contain a variety of firm, fibrous foods with optimal intakes of the B-complex vitamins and vitamin C.
    D. Calcium–phosphorus balance should be ensured by ingestion of low-fat dairy products.
    E. All of the above.

88. There are several guides available that deal with desirable amounts of food and/or nutrients that should be eaten. Each is characterized by a different approach and/or serves a special purpose. Appropriate guides include
    A. the USDA Food Guide and U.S. Dietary Goals
    B. the Food and Nutrition Board's DRIs
    C. the U.S. Recommended Daily Allowances (U.S. RDA)
    D. all of the above

89. Which is the MOST toxic of the vitamins when ingested in excessive amounts?
    A. vitamin C
    B. vitamin A
    C. vitamin K
    D. vitamin D
    E. vitamin E

90. Which has a role in the formation of collagen, particularly in the process of wound healing?
   A. vitamin A
   B. thiamin
   C. vitamin C
   D. vitamin D
   E. vitamin E

91. Combining foods that contain incomplete proteins is a concept known as
   A. complete protein feeding
   B. complementary protein feeding
   C. incomplete protein feeding
   D. nitrogen balance feeding
   E. protein excess feeding

92. Inflamed gingiva, erosion and ulceration of buccal mucosa, and a pale mucosa with anemia are suggestive of a deficiency of which substance?
   A. vitamin B12
   B. vitamin B6
   C. folic acid
   D. zinc

93. A thickening of the epithelium in the oral cavity suggests a deficiency of
   A. folic acid
   B. iron
   C. vitamin C
   D. zinc
   E. calcium

94. A deep red to purple inflamed gingiva with edema, hyperplasia, spontaneous hemorrhaging, ulceration, and necrosis is strongly suggestive of a deficiency of
   A. zinc
   B. vitamin B12
   C. vitamin C
   D. pyridoxine

E. folic acid

95. Hypersensitivity and burning sensation in the oral cavity (particularly the tongue) is strongly suggestive of a deficiency of
   A. riboflavin
   B. pyridoxine
   C. vitamin B12
   D. thiamin and/or niacin
   E. folic acid

96. Which mineral aids in the metabolism of glucose, and therefore may act to lower elevated blood sugar in diabetics?
   A. zinc
   B. chromium
   C. copper
   D. chloride
   E. molybdenum

97. This mineral protects the body from rapid aging and the effects of pollutants. Children who ingest foods grown in soils that are high in this mineral experience a higher than usual dental caries occurrence.
   A. maganium
   B. selenium
   C. vanadium
   D. fluoride
   E. manganese

98. This mineral is essential for bone formation because it aids in the creation of a protein structure into which calcium is deposited.
   A. manganese
   B. magnesium
   C. vanadium
   D. selenium
   E. chromium

99. The rare metallic element that is believed to play a role in lipid metabolism and mineralization of teeth, and that may mimic the role of insulin in the body is
    A. selenium
    B. manganese
    C. vanadium
    D. sulfur
    E. chromium

100. Scurvy, characterized by gingivitis, petechiae, follicular hyperkeratosis, fatigue, depression, and cessation of bone growth, is caused by a deficiency of which vitamin?
    A. vitamin A
    B. vitamin C
    C. vitamin D
    D. vitamin K

101. Following periodontal surgery, dietary intake can be influenced by complications of anorexia, nausea, dysphagia, and oral discomfort. A liquid diet may be required for the first
    A. 1 to 2 hours
    B. 1 to 2 days
    C. 1 to 2 weeks
    D. 1 to 2 months

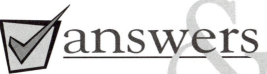
answers & rationales

1.

C. A low-carbohydrate diet will reduce the number of lactobacilli, Streptococcus salivaris, iodophilic polysaccharide-storing streptococci, and Streptococcus mutans. (1:47; 3:65)

2.

A. When the body metabolism requires glucose which is not available from recently digested carbohydrates, it calls on the liver to convert its stored glycogen into glucose through the process of glycolysis. When the store is depleted, the liver begins to make new glycogen from amino acids. This partial conversion of protein to glycogen in the liver is known as gluconeogenesis. (1:17; 2:217)

3.

D. Pernicious anemia is usually due to a lack of intrinsic factor which prevents the absorption of physiologic amounts of vitamin B12. (1:109; 2:400–401)

4.

B. Ascorbic acid is absolutely essential for the fibroblast to produce its fibrous protein, collagen. An ascorbic acid deficiency will bring about a reversal of the differentiated cells to the more immature cell types. However, if ascorbic acid is administered, the defect is promptly corrected. (1:116–117; 2:402–407)

5.

B. One must consider the pH of food as well as the sugar content; one cannot predict the cariogenicity of food by the sugar content alone. A pH above 6 is the safe area; 6.0-5.5 is doubtful; below 5.5 is a danger area for solubility of the tooth. (1:32; 2:84)

6.

B. The Adequate Intake (AI) of calcium for adults 19 to 50 in the United States is 1 gram per day. Under ordinary conditions, about 20 to 30 percent of the calcium is absorbed; the remaining amount is excreted in the feces, urine, and perspiration. (1:149; 2:437–438)

7.

A. Polyunsaturated fatty acids have two, three, or four double bonds per molecule. An example is the essential fatty acid, linoleic acid, found in soybean, cotton, cottonseed, and other vegetable oils. (1:53; 2:103)

8.

B. The classic experiment of Marine and Kimball demonstrated that potassium iodide in small doses could completely eliminate the incidence of goiter in children. Twenty-six percent of 1800 untreated girls (controls) developed goiter, whereas no goiter developed in any of the 800 girls given small doses of potassium iodide during two 10-day periods. In the epithelial cells of the thyroid gland, the iodotyrosine compounds are converted to thyroxine, which, in turn, combines with globulin to form thyroglobulin, the form in which it is stored in the thyroid gland. On demand, iodine is mobilized from thyroglobulin and passed into the circulation as inorganic iodide and as protein-bound iodine. (1:207, 265; 2:610)

9.

D. The body cannot synthesize adequate amounts of some amino acids; therefore, they must be provided every day from the diet. There are nine amino acids that must be included in the diet: lysine, tryptophan, phenylalanine, leucine, isoleucine, histidine, threonine, methionine, and valine. (1:69–70; 2:139–146)

10.

A. Carbohydrates contain carbon, hydrogen, and oxygen, with hydrogen and oxygen occurring in a 2:1 ratio as in water. We now know that carbohydrates are not hydrates of carbon but are polyhydroxy-aldehydes, ketones, and their condensation products (these being combinations between aldehyde and ketone polyhydric alcohols with the elimination of water). (1:13; 2:67–100)

11.

B. Without ascorbic acid for collagen biosynthesis, connective tissue formation would be impaired, and so would healing and scar tissue formation and maintenance. This means that ascorbic acid is essential for the formation and maintenance of intercellular substances in connective tissue. (1:114; 2:402–407, 625)

12.

D. A carbohydrate food must come in local contact with the tooth surface for the decay process to take place. After digestion, nutrients return via the circulatory system to nourish and maintain the oral tissues. (1:34–44, 309–311; 2:84; 3:365)

13.

A. Iron is stored as soluble ferritin within most body tissues, but especially within the reticuloendothelial system and the liver parenchyma. Some iron is held in less mobile masses of aggregate ferritin, called hemosiderin. (1:198–199; 2:461–469, 480)

14.

B. The Vipeholm study proved several points regarding the dental caries-refined carbohydrate relationship. One point is that the frequency of using sugar is the prime factor in caries activity. (1:36–41; 2:84; 3:370–371)

15.

A. Foods that are a good source of tryptophan, such as animal protein (with the exception of gelatin) and vegetable protein, are good sources of niacin because the body has the capacity to convert tryptophan into niacin. (1:95; 2:238, 388)

16.

A. Boron is essential for plant growth but not for animal growth. Boron could possibly be a caries inhibitor. (1:211; 2:482)

17.

B. A protein-deficient diet fed to experimental animals during the period of preeruptive tooth development increases their susceptibility to caries. This may be caused by a quality defect in the matrix of the tooth enamel or by alterations in salivary gland morphology and function. (1:75; 2:160–164; 3:85–86)

18.

E. Potassium is the principal cation in intracellular fluid, and it is present in very small amounts in the extracellular fluid. The potassium content of the body is derived solely from dietary intake—the health-promoting foods: meat, milk, vegetables, and many fruits. (1:83–85; 2:424, 435–436, 451)

19.

E. In reviewing the diet report, frequency of eating sweets, physical nature of the sweets, permeability of the dental plaque, and detersive foods should all receive special attention. (1:290–291; 2:84; 3:370–371)

20.

E. Procedures necessary to the prevention and control of dental caries include: 1) decreasing sucrose intake (diet); 2) decreasing plaque formation (caries process); 3) increasing oral clearance (toothbrushing technique); 4) increasing resistance of enamel surface (application of fluoride); and 5) interfering with bacterial enzyme activity (benefits of toothbrushing habits). (1: Chapter 17; 2:84; 3:365–367, 372–375)

21.

A. Iron deficiency is the most common type of nutritional anemia. A deficiency of iron prevents the synthesis of adequate amounts of hemoglobin. In anemia, the pigmented red cells are classically designated as hypochromic and microcytic. (1:200; 2:464–466, 474)

22.

D. Pernicious anemia is usually due to a lack of intrinsic factor which prevents the absorption of physiologic amounts of vitamin B12. (1:109; 2:400–401)

23.

A. Beriberi is the thiamin deficiency disease. It is commonly found among those populations for whom polished rice is a dietary staple. Thiamin is found in the bran and germ layer of brown rice, but polished white rice has had the bran and germ layer removed, thus removing the source of thiamin. In the United States, thiamin is replaced during enriching processes for rice and other grains. (1:92; 2:382–383)

24.

A. The recommended daily allowance of iron for a woman of childbearing age is 15 mg per day which will allow for accumulation of iron stores and will help take care of the increased needs for iron during menstruation and pregnancy. Previous editions of the Food and Nutrition Board's Dietary Reference Intakes have recommended 18 mg per day for a woman of childbearing age. (1:72, 447; 2:40, 467–468)

25.

D. Humans have difficulty in absorbing iron efficiently. Absorption is improved in the presence of amino acids and ascorbic acid. The theory is not well understood but, according to the explanation of Granick's "mucosal block theory," iron absorption is dependent upon the availability of apoferritin, a protein found in the intestinal mucosa, in order to complex the iron and form ferritin. When apoferritin becomes completely saturated with iron, no further absorption can take place. (1:151; 2:461–464)

26.

A. Toxicity can develop if 20 to 30 times the recommended allowance of vitamin A or carotene is ingested for long periods of time. It is best to avoid vitamin D intake in excess of 400 units per day. Huge amounts of vitamin D will induce a very intense calcification of the bone and even calcification of the arteries, as well as the formation of renal calculi. (1:131–132; 2:11, 356–357)

27.

A. The mineral iron is often found to be deficient in the diet of children in both developed and developing countries. There is suggestive animal experimental evidence of a relationship between an iron-deficient diet and increased caries susceptibility. The caries occur primarily on the smooth buccal surface because of reduced salivary volume and interference with the biosynthesis of salivary proteins, which are dependent on iron. (1:200; 2:353; 3:237)

28.

C. Amino acids are ordinarily required for synthesis of tissue proteins, and the absence of any one of them could prevent the formation of proteins in the body. (1:66–67; 2:139–144)

29.

B. Mineral oil is a lubricant-type laxative that solubilizes the fat-soluble vitamins A, D, E, K, and beta-carotene and thus causes malabsorption of these nutrients. (1:350; 2:350)

30.

D. Monosaccharides, such as glucose, fructose, galactose, sorbitol, and mannitol, are carbohydrates that are cariogenic. Disaccharides (sucrose, lactose, maltose, and raffinose) are also considered to be cariogenic. (1:14–15, 49; 2:84; 3:54–56)

31.

B. Excessive amounts of foods rich in saturated fats should be eliminated from the diet. A suitable diet for the elderly should contain enough fat to provide about 25 percent of the calorie intake. Skimmed milk and powdered dry milk are excellent sources because they have a low fat content and are a source of low-cost protein. (1:238, 354–355; 2:104, 134)

32.

B. The maintenance of the normal level of serum calcium is regulated by parathyroid hormone. When the serum calcium falls below 7 mg per 100 mL, the parathyroid hormone will promote release of calcium from the hydroxyapatite crystals and form intercrystalline materials. On the other hand, when the calcium rises to about 10 mg per 100 mL, the parathyroid action will be inhibited. (1:147–148; 2:437–447, 451)

33.

B. Hypervitaminosis is the excessive accumulation of any of the vitamins that leads to toxic conditions in the body which can include birth defects, bone pain, loss of appetite, dry skin, and vomiting. (1:131; 2:356–357)

34.

E. Tryptophan, methionine, histidine, lysine, phenylalanine, threonine, valine, leucine, and isoleucine are considered essential amino acids for humans. (1:69–70; 2:140–144)

35.

C. The characteristic oral manifestation of scurvy (vitamin C deficiency) in humans is an enlargement of the marginal gingiva or bleeding gingiva. Additional symptoms can include poor wound healing and bleeding skin. (1:118–120; 2:625)

36.

E. Vanadium resembles phosphorus in chemical behavior. There appears to be an inverse correlation between the vanadium content of water supplies and dental caries, i.e., with increased amounts of vanadium, there is decreased caries. There have been no firm conclusions regarding the significance of vanadium as a cariostatic trace mineral. (1:212; 2:482–483)

37.

B. When a food protein consists of all light essential amino acids in significant amounts and in proportions fairly similar to those found in body protein, it is called a complete protein. (1:71; 2:139–171)

38.

E. The amount of tissue protein that is produced is limited by the essential amino acid which is present in the smallest amount in relation to the need of the organism. This is called the most limiting amino acid which can be either tryptophan, leucine, or isoleucine. (1:69–70, 72; 2:143–144)

39.

C. Iron absorption from foods varies from 3 to 40 percent. About 10 to 15 percent of iron in the American diet is heme iron and usually 25 to 35 percent is absorbed. Nonheme iron makes up the rest and usually is absorbed at rates of 2 to 20 percent. (1:197; 2:461)

40.

B. The two types of essential iron are heme and nonheme iron. Heme iron is provided from animal tissues in the diet as hemoglobin and myoglobin and it is readily absorbed. Nonheme iron is provided from plant sources and animal tissues other than myoglobin and hemoglobin. (1:199; 2:461)

41.

A. Maintenance of a high concentration of sodium ions in the extracellular fluid and a correspondingly high concentration of potassium ions in the intracellular fluid depends on the energy derived from adenosine triphosphate (ATP) which promotes active transport. It is by this means that the sodium and potassium ions are maintained in a steady state away from equilibrium. (1:81–85; 2:431–432)

42.

B. Ergosterol (the plant form of vitamin D) is an example of a substance from which the animal organism can form a vitamin. (1:132; 2:360)

43.

A. A magnesium deficiency can produce a reduction in the rate of alveolar bone formation, widening of the periodontal ligament, and gingival hyperplasia. (1:164; 2:449–450, 452; 3:174–175)

44.

B. The family of D vitamins are sterols, but only two are of nutritional importance—vitamins D2 and D3. Vitamin D2 is calciferol (or orgocalciferol) derived from provitamin ergosterol. One milligram of vitamin D2 contains 40,000 IU. Vitamin D3 is the natural form of vitamin D. Its precursor is 7-dehydrocholesterol, which is converted into vitamin D3 when irradiated. Vitamin D3 is found in fish liver oils and foods of animal origin such as eggs, butter, milk, and cheese. (1:132; 2:358–363)

45.

C. Glycogen is the animal equivalent of starch and provides a food-storage system for all forms of animal life. The term *glycogen* connotes the capacity for regenerating sugars. It is found in highest concentration in liver and is also stored in muscle. During active muscular work, glycogen is available for energy purposes. (1:16; 2:69, 74, 217, 304)

46.

D. Lipid nutrients are carriers and facilitate absorption of the fat-soluble vitamins A, D, E, and K. (1:56; 2:6–7, 101–137)

47.

A. Fats are an excellent source of energy. They provide 9 calories per gram of substance compared to 4 calories per gram provided by carbohydrate and protein. In short, they are twice as efficient as a source of energy. (1:56; 2:46, 48, 126, 247–249)

48.

D. Glucose is the form of carbohydrate that the body tissues can best use. (1:14; 2:80–83, 97–100, 189–192)

49.

C. A patient is said to be in nitrogen equilibrium or nitrogen balance if the nitrogen furnished by the food he or she ingests is equal to the nitrogen excreted in the urine, the feces, and the skin. (1:69; 2:153–154)

50.

E. The Recommended Dietary Allowances (RDAs) are acceptable levels of intake for population groups, goals at which to aim when providing for the nutritional needs or assessing the nutritional status of groups, and allowances and estimates of nutrients that should meet the needs of nearly all healthy individuals within a group. The RDAs are in excess of nutrient requirements except for iron and energy needs and ensure the growth and maintenance of health of most people. (1:234; 2:36–44)

51.

A. Protein substances make up the majority of the organic portions of enamel and dentin. Protein deficiency may be one reason for delayed eruption and hypoplasia of deciduous teeth. Children who suffer from protein-calorie malnutrition have crowded and rotated teeth. Protein malnutrition can and very likely will enhance oral infection. Dietary protein is a very important consideration in maintaining the health of the periodontal tissues and tends to ward off periodontal disease. (1:73–77)

52.

E. Vitamin A deficiency usually occurs as a conditioned deficiency from disorders affecting fat absorption. Patients with severe liver disease may show a deficiency. A plasma vitamin A level below 10 μg per 100 mL is one indicator of deficiency. The Recommended Dietary Allowance is 5000 IU for adults. About 1000 IU per day additional vitamin A should be provided during the last six months of pregnancy. (1:126; 2:353–356)

53.

D. A prolonged vitamin D deficiency may result in both faulty tooth formation and skin and mucous membrane infections. (1:127–128; 2:353, 487)

54.

B. The trace mineral zinc is very important in the healing of wounds and the manufacture of red blood cells (RBCs). (1:201; 2:469–472, 480)

55.

C. Magnesium is present both in enamel and dentin, but its concentration in dentin is about twice that in enamel. A deficiency will produce a reduction in the rate of alveolar bone formation, widening of the periodontal ligament, and gingival hyperplasia. (1:163)

56.

B. To date, all large-scale, long-term clinical studies of the dental caries-refined carbohydrate/food intake relationship have been done with institutional populations. (1:36–43; 3:65)

57.

D. The diet that causes severe alteration in bone because of low calcium or phosphorus intake will cause only slight changes in tooth formation. (1:153–155; 2:446–447; 3:170, 173)

58.

A. Chemically, folic acid is a compound that results from the linkage of three residues: pterin, p-aminobenzoic acid, and glutamic acid. (1:105; 2:395–398, 405–406)

59.

C. Methionine is the only sulfur-containing essential amino acid. Therefore, increased intake leads to increased sulfur excretion. (1:70; 2:141)

60.

C. One major function of vitamin A is to maintain the integrity of the skin and membranes that line all passages which open to the exterior of the body as well as the glands and their ducts. Vitamin A controls the differentiation of the epithelium in mucus-secreting structures such as the nose, the throat, and the salivary glands. (1:126–127; 2:351–358)

61.

D. One role of pantothenic acid in biologic functions is its incorporation with coenzyme A which assists in the introduction of an acetyl group into an organic molecule (acetylation reactions). (1:99; 2:389–390, 405–406)

62.

D. Enamel begins developing prenatally and continues postnatally. Enamel originates from oral epithelial cells which differentiate into ameloblasts, while dentin originates from the odontoblasts. Differentiation of these two important cells, necessary for enamel and dentin formation, is aided by both vitamins A and C. Prenatally, calcium and phosphorus are essential for calcification of the enamel and dentin. However, this process cannot occur in the absence of vitamin D. Deficiency of this vitamin also causes poor growth of enamel cells (ameloblasts) and dentin cells (odontoblasts). (1:120, 129, 133; 3:147, 151–152, 159)

63.

B. Chromium is another trace element emerging in importance and is probably too low in the average U.S. diet. In addition, studies show that physically stressed and severely traumatized patients exhibit rapid, high urinary loss of chromium. Continued evidence indicates that Americans need to increase their dietary chromium intake. Food sources are whole wheat breads, meat, vegetables, and mushrooms. (1:204; 2:479–481)

64.

E. Many questions regarding the role of nutrition in periodontal health remain to be answered. One question that remains is how metabolic stressors such as nutritional deficiencies act as codestructive factors in periodontal diseases. Investigators have been studying the ways in which malnutrition modifies the innate potential defense mechanisms of the periodontal tissues. For example: How does inadequate or less than optimal nutrient consumption affect the periodontal defense factors—immunity, repair processes, epithelial barrier, gingival fluid, saliva, and microflora? (1:309–311)

65.

D. Oral epithelial tissues play a protective role by their capacity to replace cells rapidly and to act as a functional barrier. It has been stated that these tissues are in a continuous critical period of growth and development. Increased mucosal permeability has been shown to occur in ascorbate-, folate-, and zinc-deficient experimental animals. (1:310; 3:159, 210, 239)

66.

C. Nigerian children suffering from kwashiorkor (protein-calorie malnutrition) had more severe periodontal disease when compared to healthy children. In experimental animals, caloric restriction or protein-calorie malnutrition reduces mitotic activity in epithelial tissues 70 to 80 percent. (1:75; 2:161–162)

67.

E. Corn syrup, dextrose, levulose, and glucose are all sugars. Corn syrup is a viscous liquid and is the product of incomplete hydrolysis of starch. High fructose corn syrup is derived from sucrose or dextrose. Dextrose is another name for glucose and is produced commercially by the hydrolysis of starch. Levulose is an alternate name for fructose or fruit sugar and it is the sweetest-tasting of all the sugars. Glucose is the carbohydrate that body tissues use most efficiently. (1:14–15, 20–22; 2:16, 28–31, 68, 70–71, 87, 91)

68.

A. Vitamin A deficiency can cause changes in the gingival epithelium and bone of the periodontium. Vitamin A deficiency usually produces atrophy of the alveolar bone. However, some investigators have shown that vitamin A–deficient rats developed epithelial hyperkeratosis and deeper periodontal pockets only when local irritating factors were present. (1:129; 2:353–356)

69.

A. Linoleic acid (an omega-6 fatty acid) and alpha linolenic acid (an omega-3 fatty acid) are necessary for the formation of fatty acids which have double bonds before the ninth carbon numbered from the methyl end. These omega-3 and omega-6 fatty acids form parts of body structures, perform important roles in vision and immune function, and help form cell membranes. (1:53; 2:103–104)

70.

A. The hemorrhagic tendency, resulting in abnormal gingival bleeding, may be due to vascular abnormalities associated with vitamin C (ascorbic acid) deficiency. Even though there is no universally accepted agreement as to the mechanism for the weakness of connective tissue, there is evidence of blood vessel fragility with consequent diffuse tissue bleeding. This results in easy bruising, friable bleeding gums, and pinpoint skin and joint hemorrhage. Infection is a consequence of capillary fragility and permeability. (1:114, 265)

71.

B. Vitamin C has a role in the formation of collagen. Vitamin C also contributes to the integrity of odontoblasts, osteoblasts, and fibroblasts. The chemical name for vitamin C is ascorbic acid. (1:114, 118–120; 2:402–407)

72.

D. Milk is nature's most perfect food but it is severely deficient in iron and ascorbic acid. Milk is not perfect because it does not contain all the essential nutrients. Therefore, diets of infants must be supplemented with these nutrients unless a commercially prepared formula is used. (1:238; 2:34, 444–445, 510–511, 527–528, 533)

73.

C. In riboflavin deficiency, a seborrheic dermatitis characterized by a scaly, greasy erythematous lesion develops in the skin around the nasolabial folds. The clinical manifestations of a riboflavin deficiency are difficult to depict because a deficiency of riboflavin is almost always accompanied by deficiencies of other vitamins in the B-complex group. Clinically, glossitis and angular cheilosis are also characteristic of a riboflavin deficiency. (1:98, 257; 2:385)

74.

C. Rough, dry, scaly skin with follicular hyperkeratosis, due to keratotic plugs protruding from hair follicles, can be associated with a lack of vitamin A or insufficient unsaturated fatty acids. (1:128–129, 265; 2:487)

75.

E. In a severe niacin, vitamin B12, folic acid, and iron deficiency, the filiform papillae of the tongue are atrophied, therefore giving the tongue a smooth, shiny red appearance. The tongue may also be swollen. (1:268; 2:353, 474)

76.

B. A severe riboflavin deficiency is characterized by angular cheilosis, glossitis, dyssebacea of the nasolabial fold, and circumcorneal infection. The diagnosis of a riboflavin deficiency depends not only on chemical changes in the mouth, eyes, and skin, but also on laboratory tests and nutritional history. (1:98; 2:385)

77.

D. No single vitamin of the eight B-complex vitamins is more important than the other because the normal chain of metabolism can be broken by the lack of any one of the complex. The same type of close interrelationship between the B-complex that contributes to the metabolism of carbohydrates, proteins, and fats also exists in the deficiency diseases that they create. (1:103; 2:392–406)

78.

E. In the oral cavity (lips, tongue, buccal mucosa), the signs and symptoms of one B-complex vitamin deficiency can very easily simulate and/or overlap the signs of another B-complex deficiency. For example, in cheilosis (inflammation of the lips at the corners of the mouth), glossitis (inflammation of the tongue in which the tongue is magenta or in some cases, fiery red), hypertrophied papillae (pebbly textured), or atrophied papillae (smooth, dry, and glazed appearance), the oral mucosal membrane may become inflamed and swollen, and there may be a degeneration of the epithelial lining of the buccal mucosa. (1:104; 2:400–401, 474; 3:203)

79.

A. The complete metabolism of carbohydrates depends on the presence of adequate amounts of each of the five energy-releasing B-complex vitamins (biotin, thiamin, riboflavin, niacin, and pan-

tothenic acid). The B-complex vitamins also play a role in the metabolism of protein and fats. (1:103; 2:211–217, 302–303)

80.

E. The possible effects of the physical consistency of food on periodontal health are listed in this question. It has been assumed for many years that the mastication of firm fibrous foods might have a positive effect on periodontal health and that the ingestion of sticky, soft foods might have a negative effect. (1:311; 3:381)

81.

D. Megadoses of nicotinic acid can cause transitory vasodilation resulting in a tingling and flushing of the skin. Also, niacin in 3 grams or more may cause errhythmias, GI problems, abnormal chemistry, liver toxicity, and peptic ulcers. (1:97; 2:386–388)

82.

A. Vitamin A deficiency constitutes one of the major public health problems in developing countries. Worldwide, vitamin A deficiency is the leading cause of nonaccidental blindness. Among the world's most destitute nations, hundreds of thousands of children become blind each year because they lack vitamin A; approximately 500,000 die shortly thereafter because of infections. (1:106; 2:395–398, 405–406)

83.

C. Vitamin B12 affects cells that are dividing rapidly such as those involved with the formation of blood. In the absence of vitamin B12, there is a block of DNA synthesis that results in megaloblastic hematopoiesis. Because folic acid is so closely related to the formation of purines and pyrimidines, it is essential for the manufacture and maturation of blood cells. (1:106, 108; 2:398–400)

84.

A. In animal models, all simple sugars (mono- and disaccharides) are highly cariogenic, but sucrose is even more cariogenic. It appears that flour and starches are not nearly as cariogenic as are sugars. As stated in the Vipeholm study, in the Turku clinical trial, and in hereditary fructose intolerance studies, sugars are highly cariogenic and starches are not. (1:48; 2:84; 3:54–56)

85.

E. Sucrose is broken down, absorbed, and utilized as both fructose and glucose. Therefore, fructose is provided in the diet mostly from sucrose sources. (1:43–44; 2:71, 125)

86.

D. Zinc is widely distributed in the protective or health-promoting foods. The best source is red meat and other good sources are seafoods, especially oysters. However, as the quality of the average diet deteriorates, and because foods are not routinely "enriched" with zinc, the population as a whole may not be receiving adequate amounts of this nutrient. (1:202; 2:469–480)

87.

E. The dietary treatment to aid in the prevention and control of periodontal diseases consists of ingesting a very optimal diet over the lifespan. It should meet or exceed the Food and Nutrition Board's DRIs, be in accordance with the U.S. Dietary Goals, and sugar and sugar-containing products should be eaten only sparingly. Optimal amounts of calcium, phosphorus, B-complex vitamins, and ascorbic acid must be consumed. (1:309–337; 2:562; 3:157, 380–381)

88.

D. The four types of guides available that state the desirable amounts of foods and/or nutrients that should be consumed are: the USDA Food Guides, the Food and Nutrition Board's DRIs, the U.S. Recommended Daily Allowances (U.S. RDA), and the U.S. Dietary Goals. When the recommendations of these guides are considered together, they have one objective—to aid the consumer in selecting a protective optimal diet to meet his or her individual dietary needs. (1:231–244; 2:36–44, 558)

89.

D. Research by Dr. Hector DeLuca revealed that vitamin D must be converted to two biologically active metabolites before it can induce physiological changes. Vitamin D is initially hydroxylated in the liver and intestines to 25-hydroxycholecalciferol and is then carried to the kidneys for further hydroxylation to form 1-25-dihydroxycholecalciferol which is the most potent biologically active form, vitamin D3. Large doses are retained for long periods of time, and if excess doses continue, very toxic effects can be produced. (1:131–133; 2:358–363)

90.

C. Vitamin C contributes to the integrity of cells associated with fibroblasts, osteoblasts, and odontoblasts, which are cells involved in the development of connective tissue, bones, and teeth. (1:114; 2:402–406)

91.

B. When two or more proteins combine to compensate for deficiencies in essential amino acid content in each individual protein, the proteins are called complementary. Mixed diets generally provide high-quality proteins. Plant-based diets would rely on complementary proteins to provide all essential amino acids. (1:71; 2:139–144)

92.

C. The junctional epithelium in the gingiva is made up of rapidly multiplying cells, and a deficient intake of folic acid may impair this type of cellular metabolism. Clinically, the patient has tissue anemia characterized by weakness, paleness of the skin and gingiva, and a burning sensation in the tongue and oral mucosa. (1:105)

93.

D. Zinc is an integral of at least 70 enzymes (and maybe as many as 200 in all) that are known as metallo-enzyme, i.e., carbonic anhydrase. Zinc also activates enzymes that function in the digestion of protein. An essential role is also played in the synthesis of DNA and RNA and thus the synthesis of proteins. (1:201–202; 2:469–480)

94.

C. Oral symptoms of vitamin C deficiency are characterized by gingivae that are swollen, bluish red, and soft, and that hemorrhage easily. The inflamed gums can become secondarily infected by organisms that will result in acute necrotizing ulcerative gingivitis. (1:93–99; 2:28, 403–406; 3:387)

95.

D. The oral manifestations of a thiamin and/or niacin deficiency are increased sensitivity of the oral mucosa, burning tongue, and possible loss or decrease in taste acuity. The close metabolic relationship of the B-complex vitamins makes the above oral manifestations possible in many of the B-complex vitamins, i.e., riboflavin, vitamin B6, thiamin, and niacin. (1:93–99; 2:383–384; 3:202, 206)

96.

B. The biologically active form, trivalent chromium, is required for the maintenance of normal glucose levels and energy metabolism. It may act as a cofactor in insulin utilization. Chromium is not toxic in levels and forms found in our food sources. (1:204; 2:479–481)

97.

B. Selenium is an essential component of the enzyme that catalyzes the oxidation of glutathione. Glutathione protects RBCs from oxidative damage. Children who ingest foods grown in soils that are very high in selenium have a higher than usual incidence of decay and sometimes GI disturbances and abnormal fingernails. (1:203, 211; 2:474–480)

98.

A. Even though the clinical signs and symptoms of a manganese deficiency have not been clearly defined, manganese is an essential nutrient for humans. It is needed for normal bone structure because manganese creates a protein structure into which calcium is deposited. (1:206; 2:479–482)

99.

C. The data regarding the role of vanadium in human nutrition are not sufficient to draw firm conclusions. However, with increased amounts of vanadium in the diet, there is usually a decreased number of dental caries. Scientists at the University of British Columbia report that vanadium enhances the effectiveness of the hormone insulin in diabetics and plays a positive role in lipid metabolism. (1:212; 2:483–484)

100.

B. Scurvy is caused by vitamin C deficiency, and is characterized by gingivitis, petechiae, follicular hyperkeratosis, fatigue, depression, and cessation of bone growth. (3:159)

101.

B. Consistency of the diet following periodontal surgery will depend upon the extent of surgery and symptoms of the patient. A liquid diet may be required for the first 1 to 2 days. (3:389)

CHAPTER

13 General Pathology

DIRECTIONS Each of the questions below is followed by several suggested answers. Select the best answer in each case.

1. Which of the following is the term for cell or tissue death?

   A. lysis

   B. phagocytosis

   C. pyknosis

   D. necrosis

   E. karyolysis

2. Caseous necrosis is most commonly seen in which of the following disease processes?

   A. tuberculosis

   B. pneumonia

   C. syphilis

   D. scarlet fever

   E. chickenpox

3. The difference between a benign and a malignant tumor is
   A. the speed with which a patient dies from the tumor
   B. the response to chemotherapy or radiation therapy
   C. the rate of growth
   D. the ability of the tumor to metastasize

4. Addison's disease is characterized by which of the following?
   A. stomach ulcers
   B. decreased adrenal function
   C. increased skin pigmentation
   D. decreased pituitary function
   E. polyps of the gastrointestinal tract

5. Vitiligo describes which of the following conditions?
   A. acquired depigmentation of areas of the skin
   B. benign pigmented nevi
   C. albinism
   D. ochronosis

6. The normal continuous breakdown of red blood cells in the reticuloendothelial system results in deposition of what in the liver and spleen?
   A. white blood cells
   B. hematoidin
   C. hematin
   D. porphyrins
   E. hemosiderin

7. Icterus is a result of
   A. hemorrhage
   B. cirrhosis of the liver
   C. pancreas dysfunction
   D. excessive bilirubin

8. An inflammatory reaction characterized by an outpouring of abundant fluids is known as which type of inflammation?
   A. catarrhal
   B. hemorrhagic
   C. serous
   D. fibrinous

9. Small abscesses of the skin are known as
   A. furuncles
   B. carbuncles
   C. ulcers
   D. fistulas

10. Langerhans' giant cells are characteristically found in
    A. the pancreas
    B. the liver
    C. the kidney
    D. pneumonic lung tissue
    E. tubercle lesions

11. Which of the following types of immunity does an individual exhibit when his or her body has produced its own antibodies through activation of the immune system as a result of antigenic stimulation?
    A. active immunity
    B. passive immunity

12. Highly specialized tissue has what capacity for regeneration?
    A. greater
    B. lesser

13. Which of the following is a septicemia characterized by the specific presence of pyogenic microorganisms?
    A. pyemia
    B. bacteremia
    C. toxemia
    D. sapremia

14. Which of the following tissues do not regenerate?
    A. bone
    B. intestinal mucosa
    C. striated muscle
    D. liver
    E. cartilage

15. An abnormal decrease in white blood cells is
    A. leukoplakia
    B. leukocythemia
    C. leukocytosis
    D. leukopenia

16. Cellulitis is
    A. usually a limited lesion
    B. characterized by the formation of pus
    C. an inflammation characterized by a diffuse spread through tissue spaces
    D. a form of chronic inflammation

17. Which of the following genetic disorders is characterized by microcephaly, mental retardation, hypertelorism, prominent epicanthal folds, low-set ears, and an infantile cry sounding like that of an animal?
    A. Milroy's disease
    B. Huntington's chorea
    C. galactosemia
    D. cri du chat syndrome
    E. phenylketonuria

18. The first step in the sequence of steps in the vascular reaction associated with the inflammatory process is
    A. increased vascular permeability
    B. vasodilation
    C. transient vasoconstriction
    D. margination of leukocytes
    E. slowing of blood flow and stagnation

19. Chemical products released into the blood during the inflammatory process can produce which of the following?
    A. lymphadenopathy
    B. fever
    C. bacteremia
    D. pyemia
    E. leukopenia

20. Inflammation is a nonlocal reactive change in tissues that is both protective and healing. The development of this inflammatory process is dependent upon the initiating irritant, whether chemical, traumatic, physical, or microbiologic.
    A. The first statement is true; second statement is false.
    B. The first statement is false; second statement is true.
    C. Both statements are true.
    D. Both statements are false.

21. AIDS is characterized by a depletion of which type of cells?
    A. polymorphonuclear leukocytes
    B. B lymphocytes
    C. helper T lymphocytes
    D. suppressor T lymphocytes

22. A purulent inflammation is characterized by the production of mucin. It is a creamy opaque substance containing liquefied necrotic material and many red blood cells.
    A. The first statement is true; second statement is false.
    B. The first statement is false; second statement is true.
    C. Both statements are true.
    D. Both statements are false.

23. Granulomatous inflammation is present in which of the following diseases?
    A. tuberculosis
    B. fungal infections
    C. sarcoidosis
    D. all of the above

24. What are the chief cells in granulomatous inflammation?
    A. macrophages
    B. leukocytes
    C. epithelial cells
    D. basophils

25. What kind of healing occurs when the injury is slight and there is a degeneration of parenchymal cells without necrosis?
    A. scar formation
    B. regeneration
    C. resolution
    D. organization
    E. granulation

26. The MOST common presenting feature of AIDS is
    A. oral candidiasis
    B. Kaposi's sarcoma
    C. Pneumocystis carinii pneumonia
    D. cryptosporidium diarrhea

27. A large wound with much tissue loss, rapid healing, and no infection would heal by
    A. primary union
    B. secondary union
    C. tertiary union
    D. quaternary union

28. Which of the following bacteria is (are) most commonly associated with pseudomembranous inflammation?
    A. typhoid
    B. diphtheria
    C. smallpox
    D. encephalitis

29. Which of the following bacteria is (are) most commonly associated with cellulitis?
    A. pyogenic organisms
    B. beta-hemolytic streptococci
    C. staphylococci
    D. all of the above

30. Pedal edema is most likely a result of
    A. hepatic cirrhosis
    B. angineurotic edema
    C. nephrotic syndrome
    D. right-sided heart failure
    E. hypersensitivity reactions

31. When the amounts of sodium and water retained by the body are proportionate, this state is referred to as
    A. hypertonicity
    B. isotonicity
    C. hypotonicity
    D. normonatremic
    E. hyponatremic

32. Electrolytes play a role in which of the following processes?
    A. maintenance of osmotic pressure
    B. distribution of body fluids
    C. normal neuromuscular irritability
    D. preservation of acid-base balance
    E. all of the above

33. The MOST prevalent inherited disease among Caucasian children is
    A. muscular dystrophy
    B. polio
    C. congenital syphilis
    D. cystic fibrosis
    E. sickle-cell anemia

34. An increased volume of blood within dilated blood vessels in an organ or part of the body is referred to as
    A. venous congestion
    B. edema
    C. hemorrhage
    D. hematoma
    E. hyperemia

35. A mass formed from the constituents of the blood within the vessels or the heart (during life) is
    A. an infarct
    B. a capillovenous hyperemia
    C. a thrombus
    D. an embolus

36. Ischemia is a condition in which
    A. there is an increased blood supply to an organ or part of the body
    B. there is an obliteration of the blood supply to a localized part of the body
    C. air is accidentally injected into an artery or vein
    D. all of the above

37. Chills, fever, and petechial hemorrhages of the skin can be clinical manifestations of which of the following?
    A. pneumonia
    B. hypersensitivity
    C. anaphylactic reaction
    D. septicemia

38. One of the MOST common inherited disorders among African Americans is
    A. cystic fibrosis
    B. polio
    C. sickle-cell anemia
    D. muscular dystrophy

39. Whooping cough is associated with
    A. Hemophilus influenzae
    B. Klebsiella rhinoscleromatis
    C. Streptococcus pneumonia
    D. Clostridium welchii
    E. Bordetella pertussis

40. Mycoplasma organisms are MOST commonly involved in infections of the
    A. lung
    B. urinary tract
    C. brain
    D. gastrointestinal tract
    E. A and B

41. Which of the following is the MOST common route of infection of tuberculosis?
    A. inhalation
    B. infection through the alimentary tract
    C. infection through the bloodstream
    D. infection through the skin
    E. congenital infection

42. The primary pulmonary tubercle lesion is referred to as the
    A. Ghon tubercle
    B. tuberculid
    C. atypical tubercle
    D. Group I lesion

43. The MOST common persistent feature of Lyme disease is
    A. erythematous rash
    B. arthritis
    C. heart inflammation
    D. neurological symptoms
    E. swelling at the sight of inoculation

44. A macular or papular skin rash is characteristic of which stage of syphilis?
    A. primary
    B. secondary
    C. tertiary

45. Serum sickness can be classified as a systemic form of the Arthus reaction, which is a local reaction. The MOST common form of inducement is the administration of
    A. antitoxins
    B. antibacterial agents
    C. IgE
    D. IgG
    E. gamma globulins

46. Cervical cancer is associated with
    A. herpes virus type I
    B. herpes virus type II
    C. gonorrhea
    D. human papillomaviruses
    E. syphilis

47. Carcinoma in situ is a condition
    A. in which there is no penetration of subepithelial connective tissue
    B. only seen in the cervical region in females
    C. that can only be treated by chemotherapy
    D. in which invasion and metastasis are inevitable
    E. all of the above

48. Which of the following is NOT a common site for a metastatic tumor?
    A. lymph nodes
    B. lungs
    C. liver
    D. skeletal muscle
    E. bones

49. The common method of spread of sarcomas is through the
    A. bloodstream
    B. lymphatic system
    C. bone marrow
    D. portal system

50. The immediate cause of death in cancer is usually
    A. hemorrhage
    B. pulmonary disorder
    C. cardiac insufficiency
    D. central nervous system (CNS) depression

51. Gonorrhea
    A. is commonly not symptomatic in men
    B. is commonly seen as a testicular infection in men
    C. is controllable by immunization
    D. is commonly asymptomatic in women

52. The presence of Aschoff's cells in the myocardium suggests the presence of which of the following diseases?
    A. tuberculosis
    B. arteriosclerosis
    C. aneurysm
    D. rheumatic fever
    E. hydropericardium

53. A localized, persisting dilation of a vessel is known as
    A. an embolus
    B. a thrombus
    C. an infarct
    D. an aneurysm

54. Heart failure resulting from progressive diseases that weaken the heart directly or cause an increased demand on the heart is known as
    A. congenital heart failure
    B. acute heart failure
    C. left-sided heart failure
    D. right-sided heart failure
    E. congestive heart failure

55. The MOST common tumor affecting the salivary glands is
    A. mucoepidermoid carcinoma
    B. mixed tumor (pleomorphic adenoma)
    C. oncocytoma
    D. basal cell carcinoma

56. The feature of a viral infection called latency is BEST illustrated by
    A. hepatitis A virus
    B. herpes viruses
    C. influenza virus
    D. mumps virus
    E. rhinoviruses

57. Iron-deficiency anemia is caused by all of the following EXCEPT
    A. chronic blood loss
    B. faulty iron absorption
    C. inadequate dietary intake
    D. erythrostasis of red blood cells
    E. increased requirements for iron

58. An abnormal increase in the number of white blood cells in the peripheral bloodstream is known as
    A. leukemia
    B. hemophilia
    C. leukopenia
    D. thrombocytopenia
    E. anemia

59. Rheumatic fever is a systemic, poststreptococcic, nonsuppurative inflammatory disease that seriously affects the heart; however, it never involves any other part of the body.
    A. The first statement is true; second statement is false.
    B. The first statement is false; second statement is true.
    C. Both statements are true.
    D. Both statements are false.

60. Sickle-cell anemia is a hereditary type of chronic hemolytic anemia. All blacks who have the sickle-cell trait exhibit the manifestations of the disease.
    A. The first statement is true; second statement is false.
    B. The first statement is false; second statement is true.
    C. Both statements are true.
    D. Both statements are false.

61. What is the leading cause of death in industrialized Western countries?
    A. cancer
    B. ischemic heart disease
    C. tuberculosis
    D. AIDS
    E. hypertension

62. Early diagnosis of lung cancer is made
    A. rarely because it does not exhibit symptoms
    B. by the presence of blood in the sputum
    C. by persistent cough
    D. when shortness of breath is progressive
    E. during episodes of pneumonia

63. Squamous metaplasia of bronchial mucosa
    A. occurs with many chronic pulmonary irritations
    B. is reversible if smoking is stopped
    C. is not a precursor of bronchogenic carcinoma
    D. all of the above

64. What does a positive PPD test mean?
    A. Live organisms of Mycobacterium tuberculosis are present in the body.
    B. A patient is likely to have syphilis.
    C. A patient has sarcoidosis.
    D. Progressive pelvic inflammatory disease is present.

65. Distention of the air spaces of the lung with destruction of the alveolar septae is called
    A. telangiectasia
    B. atelectasis
    C. empulema
    D. emphysema

66. In the presence of renal disease, loss of plasma albumin and salt retention can lead to
    A. uremia
    B. lipoid nephrosis
    C. edema
    D. renal vein thrombosis
    E. toxemia

67. A well-known cause of focal glomeru-lonephritis is
    A. staphylococcus infection
    B. pneumonococcus infection
    C. toxemia
    D. subacute bacterial endocarditis

68. Renal infarcts are quite commonly a result of
    A. embolism
    B. hyperlastic arteriosclerosis
    C. necrosis of arterial walls
    D. dehydration
    E. edema

69. Tumors of the urinary bladder are more frequent among which sex in the 50- to 70-year age group?
    A. men
    B. women

70. The MOST common cause of agranulocy-tosis is
    A. radiation
    B. excessive blood loss
    C. an allergic phenomenon related to the ingestion of drugs

    D. immature red blood cells

71. Hypertension, albuminuria, edema, and convulsions during the later months of pregnancy can be symptoms of
    A. diabetes
    B. hepatitis
    C. eclampsia
    D. cirrhosis of the liver

72. Toxic hepatitis can be caused by which of the following?
    A. chloroform
    B. carbon tetrachloride
    C. phosphorus
    D. all of the above

73. Which of the following disturbances of the thyroid (specifically, a lack of function) is seen in children and is a congenital metabolic disturbance?
    A. myxedema
    B. acromegaly
    C. gigantism
    D. cretinism
    E. dwarfism

74. Cirrhosis refers to a fibrosis or scarring of the liver. It is a stationary, healed, end stage of injury.
    A. Both statements are true.
    B. Both statements are false.
    C. The first statement is true; second statement is false.
    D. The first statement is false; second statement is true.

75. Portal cirrhosis is often linked with
    A. schistosomiasis
    B. clonorchiasis
    C. syphilis
    D. alcoholism
    E. hemochromatosis

76. The MOST common tumor of the liver is
    A. an amebic abscess
    B. a carcinoma
    C. a cavernous hemangioma
    D. a congenital cyst
    E. a hamartoma

77. Which of the following is an outstanding feature resulting from portal cirrhosis?
    A. atrophy
    B. ascites
    C. fatty liver
    D. ulceration of liver

78. A 34-year-old African American male is admitted for surgery on his left hand to correct a congenital malformation. His left arm up to his shoulder is immobilized for 8 months. After this time, a radiograph of the left hand demonstrates a distinct loss of calcified tissue, as compared with the right arm which appears normal radiographically. A complete body bone scan reveals no other bones with a loss of calcified tissue. This patient probably has
    A. malignant recessive osteopetrosis
    B. generalized osteoporosis
    C. Cushing's disease
    D. benign recessive osteoporosis
    E. local osteoporosis

79. Insulin affects metabolism of which of the following?
    A. carbohydrates
    B. proteins
    C. amino acids
    D. fatty acids
    E. all of the above

80. The body's ability to phagocytize foreign material is provided by the
    A. red blood cells
    B. lymph nodes
    C. reticuloendothelial system
    D. appendix

E. all of the above

81. Which of the following organs plays the largest role in the breakdown of hemoglobin, the filtration of foreign material from the bloodstream, and the formation of antibodies, and also serves as a reservoir for blood?
    A. spleen
    B. liver
    C. kidney
    D. appendix
    E. pancreas

82. An infection of the throat would produce swelling in which of the following lymph nodes?
    A. axillary
    B. inguinal
    C. cervical
    D. all of the above

83. Which of the following has been implicated as a causative factor in infectious mononucleosis?
    A. streptococcus
    B. staphylococcus
    C. herpes simplex virus
    D. Epstein-Barr virus

84. A quantitative deficiency of hemoglobin results in
    A. polycythemia
    B. leukocytosis
    C. agranulocytosis
    D. leukopenia
    E. anemia

85. A severe deficiency of vitamin B12 can result in
    A. angular cheilitis
    B. kwashiorkor
    C. rickets
    D. aplastic anemia
    E. pernicious anemia

86. Considering the etiology of peptic ulcer disease, the MOST recently described factor is
   A. acid secretion
   B. diet
   C. smoking
   D. job stress
   E. bacteria

87. Simmonds' disease, characterized by loss of sexual function, low metabolic rate, weakness, cachexia, and premature senility, is due to
   A. hyperpituitarism
   B. hypopituitarism
   C. hyperthyroidism
   D. hypothyroidism

88. A deficiency of iodine apparently leads to diminished production of thyroid hormone, which in turn causes decreased output of thyroid-stimulating hormone (TSH) from the pituitary gland. This is followed by atrophy of the thyroid gland.
   A. The first statement is true; second statement is false.
   B. The first statement is false; second statement is true.
   C. Both statements are true.
   D. Both statements are false.

89. The MOST acute and severe type of hyperthyroidism is
   A. Cushing's disease
   B. Hashimoto's disease
   C. Graves' disease
   D. myxedema
   E. cretinism

90. Increased serum calcium and phosphatase levels and a decreased serum phosphate level would be expected in which of the following disorders?

   A. hyperthyroidism
   B. hypoparathyroidism
   C. thymus hyperplasia
   D. Wermer's syndrome
   E. hyperparathyroidism

91. Symptoms of low blood pressure, extreme weakness, pigmentation of the skin, and destruction of adrenocortical tissue are characteristic of
   A. Schmidt's disease
   B. vitiligo
   C. anencephaly
   D. Addison's disease
   E. Cushing's disease

92. Sebaceous glands, hair, and teeth can be found in which of the following types of ovarian cysts?
   A. dermoid cyst
   B. epidermoid cyst
   C. cystadenofibroma
   D. Brenner tumor

93. Stevens-Johnson syndrome is a severe form of
   A. lichen planus
   B. erythema multiforme
   C. pemphigus vulgaris
   D. granuloma annulare
   E. erythema nodosum

94. The MOST frequent type of skin cancer is
   A. epidermoid carcinoma
   B. squamous-cell carcinoma
   C. basal-cell carcinoma
   D. leukoplakia
   E. basosquamous carcinoma

95. Osteomalacia is the adult counterpart of
   A. osteoporosis
   B. kwashiorkor

C. rickets

D. scurvy

96. The MOST serious form of skin cancer is

A. basal cell carcinoma

B. squamous cell carcinoma

C. Bowen's disease

D. melanoma

97. Bell's palsy

A. is a unilateral facial paralysis

B. results in an unusual gait

C. is bilateral optical field blindness

D. is the same as tic douloureux

98. Down's syndrome is caused by

A. E-18 trisomy

B. an acrocentric chromosome

C. 49 pairs of chromosomes

D. 40 pairs of chromosomes

99. Marfan's syndrome, Huntington's chorea, Milroy's disease, and von Recklinghausen's neurofibromatosis are all

A. sex-linked dominant diseases

B. autosomal recessive diseases

C. sex-linked recessive diseases

D. autosomal dominant diseases

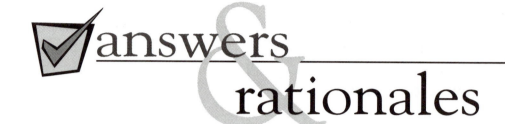

answers & rationales

1.

D. Necrosis refers to cell or tissue death within the living body. The first sign of cell death or necrosis begins with the nucleus. Necrosis may be caused by almost any type of severe injury. (1:40; 4:22–26; 5:11, 23, 113)

2.

A. Caseous necrosis is most commonly seen as necrotic tissue resulting from tuberculosis infection. Caseous necrosis has a cheese-like macroscopic appearance. It is also seen in tularemia and certain fungal infections. (1:43; 4:25; 5:113)

3.

D. The major distinguishing feature between benign and malignant tumors is the ability of the latter to metastasize to distant sites. (4:152, 158)

4.

C. Addison's disease is a clinical condition resulting from chronic adrenocortical insufficiency. It is characterized by skin pigmentation, extreme weakness, and low blood pressure. A hormone is responsible for the increase in skin pigmentation. (1:46, 609–610; 4:435, 439–440; 5:259–260)

5.

A. Acquired depigmentation of areas of the skin is known as vitiligo. The size and distribution of areas of vitiligo can vary. This is not to be confused with partial albinism. (1:46; 4:60)

6.

E. Hemosiderin is deposited in the liver and spleen during the normal continuous breakdown of red blood cells in the reticuloendothelial system. Hemosiderin may be formed locally or systemically where there is an excessive destruction of erythrocytes in the circulation. (1:46–50; 4:82)

7.

D. Icterus is a result of excessive bilirubin in the circulation which produces a yellowish pigmentation. This same condition is also known as jaundice. (1:50, 458; 5:116)

8.

C. Serous inflammation is an inflammatory reaction characterized by an outpouring of abundant fluids. Serous inflammation occurs particularly in acute inflammations of serous cavities. (1:65; 4:85–89; 5:61–71)

9.

A. Furuncles are small abscesses of the skin. Furuncles are also known as boils. A carbuncle is a more extensive spreading abscess of the skin. (1:66; 4:469; 5:28)

10.

E. Langerhans' giant cells are characteristically found in tubercle lesions. Langerhans' giant cells usually have peripheral nuclei. Foreign body giant cells usually have diffuse or central nuclei. (1:61, 138; 4:88–89)

11.

A. An individual will exhibit active immunity when his or her body has produced its own antibodies through activation of the immune system as a result of antigenic stimulation. This differs from passive immunity in which a transient protection is acquired by administration of preformed antibodies. (1:76; 5:77)

12.

B. Highly specialized tissue has a lesser capacity for regeneration. For example, surface epithelium has a marked capacity for regeneration, while neurons of the central nervous system have no power of regeneration. (1:76)

13.

A. A septicemia characterized by the specific presence of pyogenic microorganisms (pus-forming) is a pyemia. Pyemia is spread by the blood and results in multiple abscesses in distant areas. (1:122; 4:146; 5:61)

14.

C. Neurons of the central nervous system and striated voluntary muscles do not regenerate. Myocardium has a very limited capacity for regeneration, probably only in infancy. (1:73–74)

15.

D. An abnormal decrease in white blood cells is leukopenia. Leukocytosis is a term that indicates an increase in the number of white blood cells. (4:284; 5:271)

16.

C. Cellulitis is an acute inflammation characterized by a diffuse spread through tissue spaces. Cellulitis is usually poorly defined and does not necessarily form pus. (1:66–67; 4:87; 5:67, 174)

17.

D. Cri du chat syndrome patients have, as infants, a cry that sounds similar to the meowing of a cat. The cri du chat syndrome is a deletion chromosome disorder. These patients also manifest microcephaly, mental retardation, hypertelorism, prominent epicanthal folds, and low-set ears. (1:14; 4:47)

18.

C. The first step in the vascular reaction associated with the inflammatory process is transient vasoconstriction. This transient vasoconstriction produces a local anemia. It is replaced by hyperemia. (1:53; 4:77–97)

19.

B. Chemical products that are released into the blood during the inflammatory process can produce fever. (1:68–69; 4:77–97; 5:61–71)

20.

B. Inflammation is a local reactive change in tissues that is both protective and healing. The development of the inflammatory process is dependent on the initiating irritant. The irritant may be chemical, traumatic, physical, or microbiologic. (1:53; 5:61–71)

21.

C. AIDS is a disease characterized by a depletion of helper T lymphocytes. (4:102)

22.

D. A purulent inflammation is characterized by the production of pus. It is a creamy opaque substance containing liquefied necrotic material and many white blood cells. A suppurative reaction usually results from a bacterial infection. (1:65-66; 4:85; 5:61–71)

23.

D. Granulomatous inflammation is a form of chronic inflammation. It is characterized by a focal accumulation of mononuclear leukocytes, chiefly macrophages, and is present in important diseases such as TB, fungal infections, and sarcoidosis. (4:89; 5:136)

24.

A. Macrophages are the chief cells in granulomatous inflammation. Other cells present are lymphocytes, histiocytes, plasma cells, and giant cells. Frequently, a proliferation of fibrous tissue is found. (1:67–68; 4:88–89; 5:136)

25.

C. Healing by resolution occurs when the injury is slight and there is a degeneration of parenchymal cells without necrosis. Healing by resolution restores the affected part to a normal state. (1:70–71; 4:91–96; 5:64–73)

26.

C. Pneumocystis carinii pneumonia is caused by a protozoa and is one of the most common presenting features of AIDS. (4:102)

27.

A. A large wound with much tissue loss that heals rapidly with no infection would heal by primary union. Healing by primary union is also known as "healing by first intention." Maximum tensile strength is usually obtained in scar tissue formed in healing by primary union. (1:72–73; 4:91–96; 5:63–64)

28.

B. Diphtheric toxins are most commonly associated with pseudomembranous inflammation. Pseudo-membranous inflammation occurs on mucous surfaces where certain toxins and gases form a false membrane. The surface pseudomembrane is composed of necrotic epithelium, coagulated plasma, and fibrin. (1:67; 4:87; 5:67)

29.

B. Beta-hemolytic streptococci are the bacteria most commonly associated with cellulitis. (1:66–67; 4:87)

30.

D. Pedal edema, involving the ankles where venous return is impaired and easily noted, is caused by right-sided heart failure. (4:212; 5:25, 64)

31.

B. A state in which the amounts of sodium and water retained by the body are proportionate is referred to as isotonicity. Isotonicity is a normal state. Excesses of sodium produce the retention of water. (1:98)

32.

E. Electrolytes function in all of the following processes: maintenance of osmotic pressure, distribution of body fluids, normal neuromuscular irritability, and preservation of acid-base balance. (1:99–101)

33.

D. Cystic fibrosis is the most common inherited disease among Caucasian children, usually of mid-European ancestry. It is a disorder that produces an abnormality of secretion of the exocrine glands. Cystic fibrosis is an autosomal recessive trait. (1:17; 5:57)

34.

E. Hyperemia is an increased volume of blood within dilated blood vessels in an organ or part of the body. It may have an acute onset or occur gradually and be prolonged. Hyperemia may be active or passive. (1:101–102; 4:78; 5:23, 65)

35.

C. A thrombus is defined as a mass formed from the constituents of the blood within the vessels or heart during life. Thrombosis is the process of thrombus formation. Thrombi are sometimes referred to as "antemortem clots." (1:107–111; 4:179–182; 5:23–24)

36.

B. Ischemia is a condition in which there is an obliteration of the blood supply to a localized part of the body. Ischemia may be produced from interference with arterial or venous blood flow. Causes of ischemia can include thrombosis, embolism, vasospasm, and arteriosclerosis, among other conditions. (1:11, 116–117; 4:179; 5:23–24)

37.

D. Clinical manifestations of septicemia are chills, fever, and petechial hemorrhage of the skin. Septicemia is a circulating bacteremia. (1:122; 4:146; 5:61)

38.

C. Sickle-cell anemia is carried as a trait by 10 percent of African Americans and 0.2 percent have sickle cell anemia. (4:277; 5:270)

39.

E. Whooping cough is characterized by a paroxysmal cough and thick sputum. It is most commonly caused by Bordetella pertussis. (4:237)

40.

E. Mycoplasma organisms are most commonly involved in infections of the lung and urinary tract. (4:140)

41.

A. Inhalation is the most common route of infection of tuberculosis. (4:245; 5:28–29)

42.

A. The primary pulmonary tubercle lesion is referred to as the Ghon tubercle. It develops to a size of 1 to 3 cm. Its spread occurs through lymphatics to the mediastinal lymph nodes. (1:140; 4:246–247; 5:28–29)

43.

B. The most common persistent feature of Lyme disease is arthritis, although the first symptoms may include an erythematous rash. (4:413)

44.

B. A macular or papular skin rash is characteristic of the secondary stage of syphilis. However, clinical manifestations can be extremely variable. Latent periods can occur in which there are no clinical signs other than positive serologic reactions. (1:181–189; 4:549–552; 5:29, 245)

45.

A. Serum sickness can be induced by the administration of foreign serum, serum proteins, or antitoxins. Symptoms of the disorder are fever, lymphadenopathy, splenomegaly, urticarial and erythematous skin lesions, and arthralgia. The symptoms may appear days or weeks after exposure to the antigen. (4:106)

46.

D. Human papillomaviruses are associated with cervical cancers and are transmitted sexually. (4:525)

47.

A. Carcinoma in situ is a condition in which there is no penetration of the carcinoma into the epithelial stroma. It is generally believed that carcinoma in situ is a true intraepithelial cancer. If left untreated, it will frequently become an invasive carcinoma. (1:246; 4:160–161)

48.

D. One of the least common sites for a metastatic tumor is in skeletal muscle. Another infrequent site of metastatic tumor is in the spleen. Lymph nodes, lungs, liver, bone, kidneys, and adrenal glands are the most common sites for metastases. (1:247–250; 4:159–163)

49.

A. The most common spread of sarcomas is through the bloodstream. The lung is the most common site for metastatic sarcomatous tumors. Five to 10 percent of metastatic sarcomas occur in the lymph nodes. (1:271; 4:152, 410, 432, 528; 5:122)

50.

B. The immediate cause of death in cancer is usually a pulmonary disorder. The most common fatal infections are pneumonia, septicemia, and peritonitis. Additionally, pyelonephritis is a more common cause of death. (1:252–253)

51.

D. Gonorrhea is commonly asymptomatic in women which is in contrast to symptoms of urethritis in men. There is no protection through immunization. (4:552–553; 5:244–245)

52.

D. The presence of Aschoff's cells in the myocardium suggests the presence of rheumatic fever. An Aschoff's body in the myocardium is an elongated or oval microscopic nodule. It lies interstitially between muscle fibers and often adjacent to a small blood vessel. (4:225)

53.

D. An aneurysm is a localized, persisting dilation of a vessel, usually an artery. The dilation results from a weakness in the vessel wall. In a typical aneurysm, all layers of the blood vessel wall are included. (1:290–293; 4:206–207)

54.

E. Congestive heart failure is the consequence of progressive diseases that directly weaken the heart or cause an increased demand on the heart. Congestive heart failure occurs most commonly in association with atherosclerotic coronary heart disease, valvular deformities, and hypertensive cardiopathy. (1:298–299; 4:35)

55.

B. Benign mixed tumors (pleomorphic adenomas) are the most common tumors found in salivary glands. Ninety percent occur in the parotid gland. Approximately 60 percent occur in females. (1:519; 4:166, 316)

56.

B. Some viruses, like the herpes viruses, can remain dormant in cells for a long period of time, a feature called latency. (4:120)

57.

D. Chronic blood loss, faulty iron absorption, inadequate dietary intake, and increased requirements for iron may cause iron-deficiency anemia. When general anemia results, there is a quantitative deficiency of hemoglobin. It is usually accompanied by a corresponding decrease in the number of red blood cells. (1:497; 4:272–273; 5:136)

58.

A. An abnormal reduction in the number of white blood cells in the peripheral bloodstream is termed leukopenia. Leukemia, however, is an abnormal increase in the number of white blood cells in the peripheral bloodstream. (1:504–508; 4:284–288; 5:271)

59.

A. Rheumatic fever is a systemic, poststreptococcic, nonsuppurative inflammatory disease. It not only affects the heart, but can also affect arteries, joints, tendons, the nervous system, and subcutaneous tissues. (1:90, 305, 310, 416, 722, 752; 4:224–227)

60.

A. Sickle-cell anemia is a hereditary type of chronic hemolytic anemia. However, not all persons who have the sickle-cell trait will exhibit manifestations of the disease. The sickle-cell trait is found in approximately 10 percent of all black persons; sickle cell anemia is seen in 0.2 percent. (4:277; 5:270)

61.

B. Ischemic heart disease is the leading cause of death in Western countries, responsible for over 35 percent of total deaths. (4:216)

62.

A. The diagnosis of lung cancer is rarely made in early stages because of a lack of symptoms. (4:269)

63.

B. Squamous metaplasia of bronchial mucosa is reversible if smoking is stopped. It may lead to bronchogenic carcinoma. (4:149)

64.

A. A positive PPD (purified protein derivative) test, given as a skin test, means that live organisms of

Mycobacterium tuberculosis are present in the body. The larger the reaction, the greater the chances of active disease being present. (4:236)

65.

D. Distention of the air spaces of the lung with destruction of the alveolar septae is called emphysema. It is associated with smoking, pollutants, infection, and genetic factors. (4:260)

66.

C. Loss of plasma albumin and salt retention can lead to edema in the presence of renal disease. Edema is an excess of fluid within tissue spaces or serous cavities. It may be localized or generalized. (1:97–99, 334, 341; 4:376–383)

67.

D. Subacute bacterial endocarditis is a well-known cause of focal glomerulonephritis. The focal glomerular lesion is usually fibroid necrosis. Capillary thrombosis may also occur. (1:341–342; 4:229–233)

68.

A. Renal infarcts are commonly a result of embolism. They may also result from atrial fibrillation and mural thrombosis subsequent to myocardial infarction. (1:349)

69.

A. Males in the 50- to 70-year age group have tumors of the urinary bladder more commonly than females of the same age group. Etiology is usually not apparent. Common types of bladder tumors are papilloma and transitional cell carcinoma. (1:376–377; 4:393)

70.

C. The most common cause of agranulocytosis is an allergic phenomenon related to the ingestion of drugs. Agranulocytosis is a depression of granulocytic leukocyte formation, accompanied by a decrease in the number of white blood cells. (1:504–513; 4:282–283; 5:33)

71.

C. Symptoms of hypertension, albuminuria, edema, and convulsions in the latter months of pregnancy are suggestive of eclampsia. Eclampsia is a toxic complication of pregnancy. (1:442, 663–664; 4:376)

72.

D. Toxic hepatitis can be caused by chloroform, carbon tetrachloride, and phosphorus. These hepatotoxins usually produce zonal necrosis of the liver. Cirrhosis of the liver may even result. (1:442; 4:352–356; 5:30–31)

73.

D. Cretinism is a congenital lack of thyroid function. It may occur due to failure of proper development of the thyroid gland, or the thyroid gland may be aplastic or absent. (1:443–446; 4:443–450; 5:257–258, 265)

74.

C. Cirrhosis of the liver is a progressive disease that refers to a fibrosis or scarring of the liver. It is a chronic condition. All parts of the liver are fibrotically involved. (1:446–453; 4:357–359)

75.

D. Portal cirrhosis of the liver is often linked with alcoholism. It occurs most frequently in the middle decades of life. It is found more frequently in males. (1:447–450; 4:357–359)

76.

C. A cavernous hemangioma is the most common type of tumor found in the liver. Features are dilation of vascular spaces and engorged blood sinuses. (1:295; 4:208; 5:127–128)

77.

B. Ascites is the most outstanding feature resulting from portal cirrhosis. Also, portal circulation is obstructed. Death may occur suddenly from the rupture of varices of the esophagus. (1:447–450; 4:357–359)

78.

E. Local osteoporosis involving individual bones may be seen after single bone immobilization or in an area of bone that is being compressed by a tumor or an aneurysm. Osteoporosis is a reduction in the amount of calcified bone mass per unit volume of the skeletal tissue. (1:703–705; 4:34, 398–399; 5:105, 135–136, 265)

79.

E. Insulin, a protein secreted by the pancreas, stimulates carbohydrate metabolism, glycogen storage, protein synthesis, amino acid uptake, and fatty acid synthesis. (4:454; 5:164, 263)

80.

C. The body's ability to phagocytize foreign material is provided by the reticuloendothelial system. Neutrophilic leukocytes and large mononuclear cells are macrophages which are the most important phagocytic cells. (1:1, 61–63; 4:82; 5:66–68)

81.

A. The spleen functions to break down hemoglobin. It also filters foreign materials from the bloodstream. Additionally, it forms antibodies and serves as a reservoir for blood. (1:447–480)

82.

C. The cervical lymph nodes would be swollen if an infection existed in the throat. Lymph nodes are focal collections of lymphoid and reticuloendothelial cells. (1:480–483; 4:297–298)

83.

D. The Epstein-Barr virus has been implicated in the etiology of infectious mononucleosis. Infectious mononucleosis is a common disease of teenagers and adults. It is sometimes known as the "kissing disease." (1:84, 177, 480, 482; 4:298–299; 5:29, 88)

84.

E. A quantitative deficiency of hemoglobin will result in anemia. Types of anemia include pernicious anemia, aplastic anemia, congenital anemia, and acquired anemia, among others. (1:496–503; 4:270–272, 276; 5:267–271, 276)

85.

E. Pernicious anemia can be the result of a severe vitamin B12 deficiency. This results from a lack of secretion of a gastric intrinsic factor. (1:89, 253, 497–498, 530; 4:274; 5:269)

86.

E. The bacteria Helicobacter pylori is the most recently identified etiological factor in peptic ulcer disease. This suggests that the disease may be treatable with antibiotics. (6:234)

87.

B. Simmonds' disease is due to hypopituitarism. It is characterized by loss of sexual function, weakness, cachexia, premature senility, and low metabolic rate. (1:579–580; 4:436)

88.

D. A deficiency of iodine leads to diminished production of thyroid hormone. This, in turn, causes increased output of TSH from the pituitary gland. This is followed by hyperplasia of the thyroid gland. (1:583–584; 4:71; 5:257–258)

89.

C. Graves' disease is the most acute and severe type of hyperthyroidism. It occurs particularly in young and middle-aged adults. Its incidence is not limited to geographic goiter belts. (1:93, 583, 585–588; 4:447)

90.

E. Hyperparathyroidism produces increased serum calcium and phosphatase levels and a decreased serum phosphate level. The primary form originates in the parathyroid gland. (1:600–601; 4:401, 452–454; 5:100, 258–259)

91.

D. Characteristic symptoms of Addison's disease are low blood pressure, extreme weakness, pigmentation of the skin, and destruction of adrenocortical tissue. Symptoms appear when about 80 percent of adrenal cortical tissue has been destroyed. (1:46, 609–610; 4:435, 439–440; 5:259–260)

92.

A. Dermoid ovarian cysts can contain sebaceous glands, hair, and teeth. These are usually benign cysts. However, approximately 2 percent of dermoid ovarian cysts may become malignant. (1:276, 629–630, 636, 698; 4:492–493)

93.

B. Stevens-Johnson syndrome is a severe form of erythema multiforme. Erythema multiforme is an acute or subacute dermatitis characterized by papules, macules, vesicles, and bullae. Stevens-Johnson syndrome occurs in children and young adults. (1:683; 4:475, 479–481)

94.

C. Basal-cell carcinoma is the most frequent type of skin cancer. It is most commonly found on the upper two-thirds of the face and on the nose and eyelids. This carcinoma is of low-grade malignancy. (1:689–690; 4:486–487)

95.

C. Osteomalacia is the adult counterpart of rickets. It is caused by calcium and vitamin deficiencies. It occurs almost exclusively in women. (1:703; 4:67, 399–401; 5:138)

96.

D. Although representing only 1 percent of all skin cancers, melanoma has a great tendency to metastasize early and does not respond to treatment. (4:488–489)

97.

A. Bell's palsy is a unilateral facial paralysis. It involves the seventh cranial (facial) nerve, unlike tic douloureux or trigeminal neuralgia, which involves the fifth cranial nerve. (4:521)

98.

B. Down's syndrome is caused by an additional acrocentric chromosome. The head is usually small with a prominent tongue. There is an apparent diminished number of cortical neurons. (1:11, 12, 580, 748; 4:47–49, 101, 513; 5:17, 228)

99.

D. Marfan's syndrome, Milroy's disease, Huntington's chorea, and von Recklinghausen's neurofibromatosis are all autosomal dominant diseases. (1:15–16; 4:31, 41, 228, 398)

14 Oral Pathology

DIRECTIONS Each of the questions below is followed by several suggested answers. Select the best answer in each case.

---

1. Radiographically, a periapical cyst and a periapical granuloma

    A. show different peripheral remodeling characteristics

    B. are distinguished by the presence of lamina dura

    C. are indistinguishable

    D. contain foci of calcification

2. A 50-year-old woman is examined in a dental office. She smokes, is sensitive to sunlight, and has had basal cell carcinoma of the lower lip. She has a medical history of intestinal polyps and has had a hysterectomy. Upon dental clinical examination, she is found to have yellow elevated areas on the mucosa of her lower lip and on her buccal mucosa, bilaterally. She is not aware of the presence of these yellow elevated areas. This patient most probably has, from a dental point of view,

    A. stomatitis nicotina

    B. Fordyce granules

C. Peutz-Jeghers syndrome

D. none of the above

3. In the presence of facial hemihypertrophy, the teeth on the affected side are not enlarged. The teeth on the affected side will have the same eruption pattern as the uninvolved side.

A. The first statement is true; second statement is false.

B. The first statement is false; second statement is true.

C. Both statements are true.

D. Both statements are false.

4. Peutz-Jeghers syndrome consists of which of the following symptoms?

A. papules, high fever, Hutchinson's incisors

B. cheilitis, granulomatosa, facial paralysis, scrotal tongue

C. hypertelorism, median cleft of premaxilla

D. macrognathia, cleft of palate

E. intestinal polyposis, oral mucosal pigmentation

5. Which of the following is NOT an oral manifestation of AIDS?

A. Kaposi's sarcoma

B. desquamative gingivitis

C. candidiasis

D. major aphthous ulcers

E. oral hairy leukoplakia

6. A specific presentation of oral candidiasis, sometimes seen in otherwise healthy patients, is

A. fissured tongue

B. geographic tongue

C. benign migratory glossitis

D. hairy tongue

E. median rhomboid glossitis

7. Antibiotics prescribed for a dental infection may cause

A. oral candidiasis

B. oral hairy leukoplakia

C. median rhomboid glossitis

D. geographic tongue

E. desquamative gingivitis

8. Xerostomia is related to which of the following?

A. Peutz-Jeghers syndrome

B. antibiotic therapy

C. Sjögren's syndrome

D. benign tumors of the parotid gland

E. multiple mucoceles

9. The state of teeth joined together only by cementum is diagnosed as

A. fusion

B. concrescence

C. budding

D. gemination

10. Two tooth buds are joined together during development and may appear clinically as a macrodont. The probable diagnosis is

A. budding

B. fusion

C. gemination

D. concrescence

E. dilaceration

11. A radiograph shows that the roots of a lower molar are severely curved to almost 90 degrees. This is diagnosed as

A. Turner's tooth

B. hypoplasia

C. teratology

D. Hutchinson's tooth

E. dilaceration

12. Which of the following is the MOST common site for a supernumerary tooth?
    A. between the mandibular incisors
    B. distal to the maxillary third molar
    C. between the mandibular premolars
    D. between the maxillary central incisors
    E. between the maxillary premolars

13. Which of the following are two types of amelogenesis imperfecta?
    A. formative; mature
    B. autosomal dominant; autosomal recessive
    C. enamel hypoplasia; enamel hypocalcification
    D. yellow; dark brown

14. A patient has lost enamel on the anterior teeth because of a lemon-sucking habit. The diagnosis is
    A. chemico-attrition
    B. attrition
    C. erosion
    D. abrasion

15. A common benign neoplasm originating from surface epithelium is
    A. verruca vulgaris
    B. the fibroma
    C. the teratoma
    D. the papilloma
    E. neurofibromatosis

16. Mottling of enamel due to fluoride can occur at which of the following levels?
    A. 0.2 ppm
    B. 0.6 ppm
    C. 0.8 ppm
    D. 1 ppm
    E. 2 ppm

17. A grayish-white, thickened, multinodular papular appearance of the palate with a small red spot in the center of each nodule, found only in smokers, describes which of the following conditions?
    A. leukoplakia
    B. papillary hyperplasia
    C. candidiasis
    D. galvanism
    E. stomatitis nicotina

18. Carcinoma that does not invade the connective tissue is referred to as
    A. basal cell carcinoma
    B. carcinoma in situ
    C. epidermoid carcinoma
    D. squamous-cell carcinoma

19. A grayish-white area with a coarsely wrinkled appearance, found bilaterally on the buccal mucosa of an African American patient, is probably
    A. leukoedema
    B. leukoplakia
    C. lichen planus
    D. lupus erythematosus

20. Basal cell carcinoma exhibits practically no tendency for metastasis. It is probably the most common type of carcinoma in women.
    A. The first statement is true; second statement is false.
    B. The first statement is false; second statement is true.
    C. Both statements are true.
    D. Both statements are false.

21. Oral squamous cell carcinoma is MOST commonly found at which of the following sites?
    A. lateral tongue and floor of the mouth
    B. lip and soft palate
    C. buccal mucosa and mucobuccal fold
    D. gingiva and alveolar ridge
    E. labial commissure

22. Epidermoid carcinoma of the lower lip is MOST commonly found in
    A. teenage males
    B. menopausal females
    C. children with fair skin
    D. elderly males
    E. elderly females

23. The MOST serious side effect of radiation therapy of the head and neck is
    A. xerostomia
    B. cervical caries
    C. alopecia
    D. candidiasis
    E. osteonecrosis

24. Verrucous carcinoma of the oral cavity is MOST commonly associated with a person who
    A. drinks alcohol
    B. uses an abrasive dentifrice
    C. uses sodium peroxide for mouthwash
    D. chews tobacco
    E. all of the above

25. The MOST serious form of skin cancer is
    A. squamous cell carcinoma
    B. actinic keratosis
    C. basal cell carcinoma
    D. melanoma
    E. merkel cell carcinoma

26. The MOST common benign soft-tissue lesion occurring in the oral cavity is the
    A. papilloma
    B. fibroma
    C. amalgam tattoo
    D. verruca vulgaris
    E. pyogenic granuloma

27. Peripheral giant-cell granulomas always occur
    A. in the mandible
    B. in the maxilla
    C. in edentulous patients
    D. on the gingiva or alveolar process

28. Clinically, the peripheral giant-cell granuloma closely resembles the
    A. pyogenic granuloma
    B. papilloma
    C. cementoma
    D. carcinoma
    E. mucocele

29. The central giant-cell granuloma is not a destructive lesion. Radiographically, it appears radiopaque.
    A. The first statement is true; second statement is false.
    B. The first statement is false; second statement is true.
    C. Both statements are true.
    D. Both statements are false.

30. A congenital tumor characterized by proliferation of blood vessels is
    A. a hematoma
    B. a hemangioma
    C. a telangiectasia
    D. an angiomatosis

31. An outstanding feature of Sturge-Weber disease is
    A. telangiectasia
    B. hematoma
    C. port wine nevi
    D. all of the above

32. The MOST common sites in the oral cavity for lymphoma are the
    A. nasopharynx and maxillary sinus
    B. floor of mouth and tonsils
    C. maxillary sinus and nasal cavity
    D. palate and pharynx
    E. tonsils and nasopharynx

33. A 6-year-old boy has a 1 cm elevated blue lesion on the alveolar ridge in the molar area, distal to the second primary molar. This patient most probably has
    A. a hemangioma
    B. a hematoma
    C. a juvenile nevus
    D. an eruption cyst
    E. a melanoma

34. The MOST outstanding characteristic of von Recklinghausen's disease is
    A. neurofibromatosis
    B. hemorrhage
    C. jaw expansion
    D. vitiligo

35. Which of the following is the MOST common site for a pleomorphic adenoma?
    A. submandibular salivary gland
    B. lip
    C. tongue
    D. parotid gland
    E. buccal mucosa

36. A dentigerous cyst originates through alteration of the reduced enamel epithelium
    A. after the crown and root are completely formed
    B. before the crown is completely formed
    C. after the crown is completely formed
    D. after the crown is formed, but before the root is completely formed

37. A dentigerous cyst is attached to the tooth at
    A. the cementoenamel junction
    B. the apex of the roots
    C. middle third of the roots
    D. the periodontal ligament

38. The ameloblastoma is a neoplasm of a type resembling enamel organ tissue that occurs most frequently in the mandible. It does not cause expansion of the jaw.
    A. The first statement is true; second statement is false.
    B. The first statement is false; second statement is true.
    C. Both statements are true.
    D. Both statements are false.

39. Excess tissue of developmental origin found in a normally occurring area is called
    A. a teratoma
    B. a neoplasm
    C. redundant tissue
    D. a hamartoma

40. The phenomenon of "strawberry tongue" is associated with which of the following diseases?
    A. streptococcal infection
    B. chickenpox
    C. measles
    D. diphtheria
    E. scarlet fever

41. A false membrane consisting of grayish, thick, fibrinous exudate and dead cells is MOST commonly associated with
    A. tuberculosis
    B. measles
    C. diphtheria
    D. scarlet fever
    E. smallpox

42. Tubercle lesions of the oral cavity are relatively uncommon. The possibility that the dentist can contract an infection from a patient with pulmonary or oral tuberculosis is very low.
    A. The first statement is true; second statement is false.
    B. The first statement is false; second statement is true.

C. Both statements are true.

D. Both statements are false.

43. Which of the following are characteristics of congenital syphilis?

A. Turner's tooth

B. gumma

C. mucocutaneous rash

D. eighth nerve deafness

E. chancre

44. The pyogenic granuloma is a true tumor of blood vessels. The pyogenic granuloma is a response of the tissues to a nonspecific irritant.

A. The first statement is true; second statement is false.

B. The first statement is false; second statement is true.

C. Both statements are true.

D. Both statements are false.

45. Upon oral examination, a 4-year-old child is found to have intensely inflamed gingiva, difficulty in swallowing, fever, lymphadenopathy, and small fluid-filled vesicles in the oral cavity. The diagnosis is probably

A. scarlet fever

B. diphtheria

C. Koplik's spots

D. chickenpox

E. primary herpetic gingivostomatitis

46. Recurrent herpes simplex infections should be expected to heal in

A. 2 days

B. 5–7 days

C. 1 week

D. 7–14 days

E. 1 month

47. A 50-year-old man who smokes a pipe is found to have lesions on his palate, underneath his denture. He says he removes the denture only to clean it. The lesions on his palate are erythematous, papillary projections. His chief complaint is an ill-fitting set of dentures that is 10 years old. This patient most probably has

A. stomatitis nicotina

B. traumatic ulcers

C. papillary hyperplasia

D. denture stomatitis

E. epulis

48. A white patch on the oral mucosa that cannot be rubbed off and cannot be ascribed to any other disease is most probably

A. lichen planus

B. leukoplakia

C. erythroplasia

D. squamous-cell carcinoma

E. candidiasis

49. A white plaque which, when scraped or removed from the oral mucosa, leaves a raw, bleeding surface probably is

A. leukoplakia

B. white sponge nevus

C. lichen planus

D. candidiasis

E. hereditary benign intraepithelial dyskeratosis

50. Warts and papillomas are both found on pedunculated bases. Both owe their etiology to viral infections.

A. The first statement is true; second statement is false.

B. The first statement is false; second statement is true.

C. Both statements are true.

D. Both statements are false.

51. Regarding the difference between 1) aphthous ulcers and 2) intraoral herpetic lesions, which statement applies?
    A. Both are viral in origin.
    B. 1) Are recurrent and 2) occur only once.
    C. They cannot be distinguished by clinical exam only.
    D. 1) usually occur on mobile tissue and 2) usually occur on mucosa bound down to periosteum.
    E. Only 1) exist in the oral cavity.

52. Which of the following descriptive words would be MOST appropriately applied to a microorganism that can enter the host's body and cause disease?
    A. emissive
    B. potent
    C. pathogenic
    D. virulent

53. Which drug does NOT cause gingival hyperplasia?
    A. phenytoin
    B. cyclosporine
    C. nifedipine
    D. inderal

54. Recurrent aphthous ulcers
    A. are caused by coxsackievirus
    B. can produce an associated rise in antibody titer against herpes virus
    C. appear to be associated with stress
    D. are caused by herpes simplex virus
    E. are caused by herpes zoster virus

55. A 40-year-old man has routine dental films exposed. Upon examination of the radiographs, an oval radiolucent area is discovered above the maxillary central incisors. The teeth are vital, and the roots are not resorbed. This patient most probably has

A. central giant cell tumor
B. median palatine cyst
C. globulomaxillary cyst
D. nasopalatine duct cyst
E. brachial cleft cyst

56. The MOST common location for a mucocele is the
    A. lower lip
    B. upper lip
    C. palate
    D. retromolar pad
    E. buccal mucosa

57. Herpangina is a virus infection that
    A. produces painful persistent ulcers
    B. produces no lasting immunity
    C. is caused by a coxsackievirus
    D. is identical to the fever blister virus
    E. remains dormant in the trigeminal nerve with numerous recurrences

58. A permanent tooth that displays hypoplasia caused by trauma or infection during development has been termed
    A. Hurst's hypoplasia
    B. "peg" lateral
    C. Hutchinson's incisor
    D. Turner's hypoplasia

59. A 60-year-old man has squamous-cell carcinoma of the floor of the mouth. If it invades other oral structures, it MOST probably will invade the
    A. gingiva
    B. the sublingual and submandibular salivary glands
    C. palate
    D. nasopharynx
    E. parotid salivary gland

60. A cyst that remains after or develops subsequent to extraction of a tooth is a

A. residual cyst

B. primordial cyst

C. dentigerous cyst

D. periapical cyst

61. Salivary gland tumors occur MOST frequently in which salivary gland?

 A. sublingual gland

 B. submandibular gland

 C. parotid gland

 D. minor salivary glands

62. A 50-year-old white man seeks dental attention for a widening of the alveolar ridges of both his maxilla and mandible which has caused his dentures not to fit. Bone scans of his skull and extremities show enlargement and abnormally dense formation of bone. His bones are warm to the touch. He states on his medical history that for the past 18 months he has had frequent headaches, dizziness, and a noticeable loss of hearing. Using the information in the case history, you would conclude that this patient MOST probably has

 A. Paget's disease

 B. osteogenesis imperfecta

 C. craniofacial dysostosis

 D. Treacher Collins syndrome

 E. achondroplasia

63. A ranula is specifically associated with

 A. the parotid gland

 B. the lower lip

 C. the floor of the mouth

 D. the soft palate

 E. the upper lip

64. The condition MOST likely to occur after initiation of therapeutic radiation to the head and neck region is

 A. osteonecrosis

 B. radiation caries

C. candidiasis

D. xerostomia

E. chronic mucosal erythema

65. The MOST common complication in the healing of human tooth-extraction wounds is the condition known as

 A. dry socket

 B. hemorrhage

 C. cellulitis

 D. residual cyst

66. Hand-Schuller-Christian disease is characterized by the class triad of which of the following symptoms?

 A. mucocutaneous pigmentation, pituitary tumor, ectodermal dysplasia

 B. exophthalmos, diabetes insipidus, bone lesions

 C. neurofibromas, intestinal polyps, vitiligo

 D. xerostomia, amelogenesis imperfecta, anhydrosis

 E. Turner's tooth, Hutchinson incisors, mulberry molars

67. Cherubism, hyperparathyroidism, and aneurysmal bone cyst ALL

 A. have etiology in the pituitary

 B. affect soft tissues only

 C. contain multinucleated giant cells histologically

 D. require aggressive therapy

68. A riboflavin deficiency would MOST likely be orally manifested in which of the following structures?

 A. alveolar bone

 B. periodontal membrane

 C. gingiva

 D. floor of the mouth

 E. tongue

69. Pellagra is associated with a deficiency of
    A. folic acid
    B. thiamin
    C. riboflavin
    D. nicotinic acid
    E. pantothenic acid

70. Hyperparathyroidism almost always produces
    A. skeletal lesions
    B. a thickened lamina dura
    C. amelogenesis imperfecta
    D. mucosal pigmentation
    E. diabetes insipidus

71. An outstanding oral manifestation of cleidocranial dysplasia is
    A. elongated roots
    B. oversized crowns
    C. retained primary teeth
    D. enlarged maxilla
    E. enlarged mandible

72. A "cotton-wool" appearance of the skull radiographically is characteristic of
    A. achondroplasia
    B. cleidocranial dysostosis
    C. osteopetrosis
    D. Paget's disease

73. A dentist is often consulted first by a patient with pernicious anemia for relief of
    A. severe gingivitis
    B. edematous buccal mucosa
    C. glossitis
    D. denuded gingiva

74. Which of the following is NOT characteristic of acute necrotizing ulcerative gingivitis?
    A. grayish pseudomembrane
    B. punched-out erosions of interdental papillae
    C. hemorrhage
    D. slow onset
    E. fetid odor

75. Chronic desquamative gingivitis is MOST frequently found in
    A. malnourished children
    B. adult males
    C. adult females
    D. teenage females

76. Which of the following conditions can occur in a mouth in which the hygienic condition is faultless?
    A. gingivitis
    B. Vincent's infection
    C. juvenile periodontitis
    D. periodontitis

77. Cone-shaped teeth are characteristic of
    A. dentinogenesis imperfecta
    B. acromegaly
    C. cleidocranial dysostosis
    D. ectodermal dysplasia
    E. Paget's disease

78. Stevens-Johnson syndrome is a severe form of
    A. herpes simplex
    B. lupus erythematosus
    C. herpes zoster
    D. erosive lichen planus
    E. erythema multiforme

79. White sponge nevus appears to follow a hereditary pattern. However, it is of great clinical significance because of its threat of being malignant and its potential for metastasis.
    A. The first statement is true; second statement is false.

B. The first statement is false; second statement is true.

C. Both statements are true.

D. Both statements are false.

80. Nikolsky's sign is a characteristic feature of
    A. lupus erythematosus
    B. herpes simplex
    C. pemphigus
    D. herpes zoster
    E. eczema

81. Oral radiographs of a patient with scleroderma would show
    A. abnormal trabecular bone formation
    B. a thickened periodontal ligament
    C. absence of lamina dura
    D. horizontal bone loss
    E. vertical bone loss

82. A patient is observed to have a drooping mouth on one side and a watering eye, and complains of having a loss of taste sensation on the anterior portion of the tongue. This patient MOST likely has
    A. Bell's palsy
    B. tic douloureux
    C. Ménière's disease
    D. multiple sclerosis
    E. polio

83. Lace-like white striae present on the buccal mucosa bilaterally may represent
    A. erythema multiforme
    B. pemphigus vulgaris
    C. cicatricial pemphigoid
    D. lichen planus
    E. lupus erythematosus

84. A patient who manifests a peculiar inflammation of the gingiva and demonstrates ulcerated and necrotic epithelium

that sloughs (or peels off) with air blasts probably has
    A. Vincent's infection
    B. redmouth syndrome
    C. periodontosis
    D. desquamative gingivitis
    E. periodontitis

85. Dental caries is an infectious disease. It is the only infectious disease in which tissue is destroyed in the absence of cell injury and inflammation.
    A. The first statement is true; second statement is false.
    B. The first statement is false; second statement is true.
    C. Both statements are true.
    D. Both statements are false.

86. Gingivitis can be accompanied by all of the following EXCEPT
    A. ulceration
    B. hypertrophy
    C. necrosis
    D. serous exudation
    E. purulent exudation

87. Periodontitis is diagnosed when
    A. periods of remissions and exacerbations are demonstrated
    B. proliferation of sulcular epithelium exists
    C. loss of alveolar bone exists
    D. spontaneous hemorrhage exists
    E. pocket depth is over 3 mm

88. Use of aspirin affects which component of the clotting process?
    A. vascular contraction
    B. platelet aggregation
    C. prothrombin time
    D. partial thromboplastin time
    E. fibrin clot stabilization

89. A gingival disease characterized by painful hyperemic gingiva, punched out erosions of the interdental papillae, covered by a gray pseudomembrane, and with an accompanying fetid odor is most probably
    A. acute primary herpetic gingivostomatitis
    B. periodontosis
    C. chronic desquamative gingivitis
    D. necrotizing ulcerative gingivitis
    E. Dilantin hyperplasia

90. Excessive occlusal forces can result in changes in the periodontal ligament and alveolar bone. If these occlusal forces are chronic and repeated over a long time, the periodontal ligament can become more dense, and the periodontal space will widen.
    A. The first statement is true; second statement is false.
    B. The first statement is false; second statement is true.
    C. Both statements are true.
    D. Both statements are false.

91. When the mass of dental tissues in an odontoma radiographically resembles the anatomy of normal teeth, the odontoma is termed
    A. composite odontoma
    B. compound odontoma
    C. complex-compound odontoma
    D. complex odontoma

92. A 26-year-old African American female was examined clinically and radiographically. On a mandibular periapical radiograph that included the central and lateral incisors, radiolucent lesions were found at the apex of each of these four teeth. Six months later, the radiolucent areas were radiopaque. Each of the four teeth

retained its vitality. This patient most likely has
    A. ameloblastomas
    B. teratomas
    C. Gorlin cysts
    D. Pindborg tumors
    E. cementomas

93. A carcinoma categorized as T3 N2 M0 falls into which of the following clinical stage groupings?
    A. Stage I
    B. Stage II
    C. Stage III
    D. Stage IV

94. Which of the following types of the herpes virus is associated with the face and oral cavity, and not necessarily the genitals and skin of the lower body?
    A. herpes simplex, Type I
    B. herpes simplex, Type II
    C. herpes simplex, Type III
    D. herpes simplex, Type IV

95. The nerve ganglia MOST commonly affected by the herpes simplex virus Type I is the
    A. superior posterior alveolar nerve
    B. trigeminal nerve
    C. facial nerve
    D. inferior posterior alveolar nerve
    E. infraorbital nerve

96. Place the following in the correct temporal order with regard to fever blisters: 1) vesicles, 2) erythema, 3) crust.
    A. 1, 2, 3
    B. 2, 1, 3
    C. 3, 1, 2
    D. 1, 3, 2
    E. 3, 2, 1

97. A patient complaining of moderately severe pain, particularly just before, during, and after meals and with evidence of swelling in a salivary gland, would be suspected of having
   A. antrolithiasis
   B. rhinolithiasis
   C. xerostomia
   D. sialolithiasis

98. A herpetic whitlow refers to a herpes infection of the
   A. gingiva
   B. lip
   C. cervix
   D. finger
   E. penis

99. Bottle-baby syndrome is a widespread carious destruction of the primary teeth. Which of the primary teeth are MOST commonly affected?
   A. maxillary central and lateral incisors
   B. mandibular central and lateral incisors
   C. maxillary second molars
   D. mandibular second molars

100. Which of the following groups of permanent teeth has the highest caries susceptibility?
   A. mandibular central and lateral incisors
   B. maxillary canines and premolars
   C. maxillary central and lateral incisors
   D. maxillary second premolars
   E. maxillary and mandibular first molars

101. Bruxism is a pathologic manifestation of which of the following conditions?
   A. abrasion
   B. erosion
   C. attrition
   D. resorption
   E. recession

102. Radiation caries is commonly MOST clinically evident at which area of the tooth?
   A. occlusal
   B. cervical
   C. interproximal

103. Aspirin is not meant for use as an obtundent. If used in this manner, it will produce
   A. erythema
   B. leukoplakia
   C. a burn followed by sloughing
   D. hyperplasia

104. Which of the following medications can produce oral mucosal pigmentation?
   A. anti-inflammatory medications
   B. antimalarial drugs
   C. calcium channel blockers
   D. AZT
   E. more than one of the above

105. A 20-year-old female, upon clinical examination, is found to have a brownish-gray discoloration of her teeth. Her health history reveals that when she was 3 years old, she was quite ill with high fevers. An antibiotic was administered. This brownish-gray discoloration is most likely from
   A. fluorosis
   B. penicillin
   C. erythromycin
   D. aureomycin
   E. tetracycline

106. The MOST common oral reaction to cancer chemotherapeutic agents is
   A. mucosal erosion and ulceration
   B. edema
   C. petechial hemorrhage
   D. rampant cervical caries
   E. osteoradionecrosis

107. Patients with bulimia commonly suffer
from
  A. erosion of the teeth
  B. gastric acid decalcification of the teeth
  C. severe dental caries
  D. all of the above

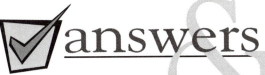

answers & rationales

1.

C. A periapical cyst and a periapical granuloma are indistinguishable radiographically. (2:36–37; 3:173–174; 6:422; 7:118–123)

2.

B. Fordyce granules are ectopic sebaceous glands, entrapped embryonically in oral soft tissues. The most common sites are the buccal mucosa and the lips. They are described clinically as yellow spots, only slightly elevated on oral mucosa. (1:5–7; 2:52–53, 157; 3:39–41; 5:23; 6:26–27; 7:15–16, 24, 43)

3.

D. In the presence of facial hemihypertrophy, the teeth on the affected side are enlarged. The teeth on the affected side erupt sooner than the teeth on the nonaffected side. Although the disproportion will remain throughout life, facial growth ceases by the age of 20 years. (1:34–35; 2:12; 5:199; 6:485–486; 7:255)

4.

E. Familial intestinal polyposis and oromucosal pigmentation are characteristic of Peutz-Jeghers syndrome. The melanin pigmentation of the lips and oral mucosa is usually present from birth and appears as small brown macules measuring from 1 to 5 mm in diameter. Intraorally, the pigmentation occurs most frequently on the buccal mucosa, but also on the gingiva and hard palate. (1:550; 2:70, 74–75, 133; 5:50; 6:38–39, 162–164, 558; 7:394–395)

5.

B. Desquamative gingivitis is an oral manifestation of a number of mucocutaneous diseases such as lichen planus, pemphigus, or pemphigoid. It is not a manifestation of AIDS as are the other choices. (2:64, 92; 3:223; 6:109; 7:162–163, 180–181)

6.

E. Median rhomboid glossitis is a presentation of candidiasis in which a central area on the mid-dorsal surface is devoid of papillae. (2:48–49, 104–105; 3:42; 6:145; 7:8, 18–19, 50, 193–197)

7.

A. Use of antibiotics is one of the many predisposing factors which may lead to the development of oral candidiasis. (2:8, 48, 62, 69, 104, 131; 3:246–247, 252; 4:32, 367, 551; 6:120)

8.

C. Xerostomia (dry mouth) is related to Sjögren's syndrome, an autoimmune process that often includes rheumatoid arthritis and results in the destruction of the salivary glands. (2:18, 46–47; 3:2, 11; 6:261; 7:169–170)

9.

B. The condition of teeth joined together only by cementum is termed concrescence. It is thought to arise as a result of traumatic injury. Concrescence may occur before or after the teeth have erupted. (1:65, 67–68, 3:59–60; 6:497; 7:225, 258–259, 467)

10.

B. Fusion of teeth is a condition produced when two tooth buds are joined together during development and appear as a macrodont. This is not to be confused with true macrodontia in which all teeth are larger than normal. (1:65–67; 2:12–13; 3:60; 6:496; 7:225, 257–258, 468)

11.

E. The condition in which the roots of mandibular molars are severely curved to almost 90 degrees is termed dilaceration. This is thought to be caused by trauma during tooth development. Dilacerated teeth can present problems at the time of extraction. (1:76–78; 3:52–53; 6:497; 7:225, 259–261, 467)

12.

D. The most common site for supernumerary teeth is between maxillary central incisors. Supernumerary teeth have a 2:1 predilection for males. Supernumerary teeth may closely resemble the teeth of the group to which they belong. (1:60–64; 2:12, 14; 3:51–52; 5:311; 6:476–477, 500, 504–506; 7:21, 26, 250–254)

13.

C. Enamel hypoplasia and enamel hypocalcification are two types of amelogenesis imperfecta. Amelogenesis imperfecta represents a group of hereditary defects of enamel unassociated with any other generalized defects. It is entirely an ectodermal disturbance. (1:79–84; 2:16–17; 3:54–57, 271; 6:506; 7:267–269)

14.

C. Erosion is the wearing away of the teeth due to a chemical process. Lemon-sucking is a frequent cause of erosion. Additionally, erosion is a common clinical finding in patients with bulimia. Eroded areas of the teeth occur most frequently on the facial and lingual surfaces. (1:48–50; 2:2–3, 18–19; 3:109; 6:501–502; 7:84–86)

15.

D. A very common benign neoplasm originating from oral epithelium is the papilloma. It is often confused with the fibroma, yet each has definite characteristics. The papilloma is an exophytic growth made up of numerous, small, fingerlike pro-

jections which results in a roughened verrucous or "cauliflower-like" surface. (1:259–262; 2:4, 82, 83, 135; 3:122–123; 5:146, 302; 6:44–45, 179–182; 7:290–291)

16.

E. Mottling of enamel (fluorosis) can occur when the fluoride level in the drinking water is at 2 parts per million. The ingestion of fluoride-containing water during the time of tooth formation may result in mottling. Mottled enamel represents a type of enamel hypoplasia. (1:47; 2:16; 3:56–57; 6:508–509; 7:268)

17.

E. Stomatitis nicotina produces a grayish-white, thickened, multinodular papular appearance of the palate with a small red spot in the center of each nodule. This condition is found exclusively in smokers, and is not a premalignant condition. (1:291–292; 2:56–57; 3:250; 6:20–21, 102; 7:94–98)

18.

B. Carcinoma that does not invade the underlying connective tissue is referred to as carcinoma in situ. Carcinoma in situ clinically may present itself as erythroplakia, not just as a hyperkeratotic lesion. (1:287; 2:62; 4:83, 336; 5:17, 30, 41; 6:105–107, 147)

19.

A. A grayish-white area that presents a coarse wrinkled appearance, found bilaterally on the buccal mucosa of an African American patient, is probably leukoedema. Clinically, leukoedema can resemble leukoplakia. There is no evidence that this is a premalignant lesion. It does appear to have an ethnic association. (1:7–8; 2:52–53, 127; 5:81; 6:21, 93–94; 7:48–49)

20.

A. Basal cell carcinoma does not exhibit a tendency for metastasis. It is probably the most common type of carcinoma in males. Basal cell carcinoma develops most frequently on the exposed surfaces of the skin, face, and scalp. (1:310–312; 3:122–123; 4:378; 6:577–580; 7:299–301)

21.

A. Oral squamous cell carcinoma is most commonly found on the lateral tongue and floor of the mouth. (2:21, 62–63, 98–99, 106, 130, 139; 3:123–124; 4:251; 6:79–81; 7:287, 291–296)

22.

D. Epidermoid carcinoma of the lower lip is most commonly found in elderly males. The greatest incidence occurs between the ages of 50 and 70 years and is commonly related to chronic sun exposure. (6:79; 7:291–296)

23.

E. The most serious side effect of head and neck radiation therapy is osteonecrosis which can result in loss of large segments of bone, especially involving the mandible. (2:14, 18; 4:92, 97, 594; 6:85; 7:454–455)

24.

D. Verrucous carcinoma of the oral cavity is most commonly associated with a person who chews tobacco. Verrucous carcinoma is a form of epidermoid carcinoma. The typical lesion of verrucous carcinoma is usually slow-growing, chiefly exophytic, and superficially invasive. (1:304–306; 2:56–57, 128; 3:250; 5:17–154; 6:46–47, 187–189; 7:299–300)

25.

D. Melanoma is one of the most unpredictable and deadly of all human neoplasms. (2:4; 4:76, 376, 398, 594; 6:167–171; 7:338)

26.

B. The most common benign soft-tissue lesion occurring in the oral cavity is the fibroma which probably represents fibrous hyperplasia. The fibroma appears as an elevated lesion of normal color with a smooth surface and a sessile or pedunculated base. (2:4, 14, 20–21, 80–81, 102, 134; 3:126–127; 6:202; 7:108–112)

27.

D. Peripheral giant-cell granulomas always occur on the gingiva or alveolar process, outside of bone. They occur most frequently anterior to molars. These lesions are most often dark red, vascular or hemorrhagic, and commonly ulcerated. (1:373–374; 2:20–21; 6:30–31, 51, 142–145; 7:106–108)

28.

A. Clinically, not microscopically, the peripheral giant-cell granuloma closely resembles the pyogenic granuloma. It may also resemble a fibroma. The peripheral giant-cell granuloma seems to originate from the periodontal ligament or mucoperiosteum. (1:373–374; 2:20–21; 6:30–31, 51, 142–145; 7:39–42, 104–105, 108)

29.

D. The central giant-cell granuloma is a destructive lesion, appearing radiolucent with a smooth or ragged border in radiographs. The central giant-cell granuloma occurs predominantly in children or young adults. The mandible is more often affected than the maxilla, and it is more commonly found in females than males. (1:453–455; 6:88–89, 409–411; 7:104–105)

30.

B. A hemangioma is a congenital tumor characterized by a proliferation of blood vessels. A hemangioma of the oral soft tissue appears as a flat or raised lesion, usually deep red or bluish red. The most common sites of occurrence are the lips, tongue, buccal mucosa, and palate. (1:390–392; 2:58–59, 129; 3:127–128; 4:148, 359; 6:30–31, 136–142; 7:335–336)

31.

C. Port wine nevi are an outstanding feature of Sturge-Weber disease, as is the presence of typical intercranial convolutional calcification. Port wine nevi (dermal capillary-venous angiomas) are generally present at birth and are almost exclusively confined to the skin supplied by the trigeminal nerve. Ocular involvement occurs in some patients and includes glaucoma, exophthalmus, or angioma of the choroid. (1:392–393; 2:60–61, 129; 3:127; 4:148, 359; 6:139–140)

32.

D. The palate and pharynx are the most common sites in the oral cavity for lymphoma. (2:36, 38–39, 106–107; 4:77, 190, 192; 6:310; 7:345, 450–451)

33.

D. Eruption cysts, a form of a dentigerous cyst, are frequently associated with erupting primary or permanent teeth in children. Blood accumulates in the tissue and a swelling exists over the site of the erupting tooth. The swelling appears purple or blue and is sometimes referred to as an eruption hematoma. (1:496; 2:4; 3:120, 122, 130; 5:105; 6:52–53, 73, 332–333; 7:233)

34.

A. The most outstanding feature of von Recklinghausen's disease is neurofibromatosis, a condition of multiple tumors of nerve tissue origin. Von Recklinghausen's disease is hereditary and affects all races and both sexes. Intraoral neurofibromas may be present. (1:381–383; 2:32, 80; 6:224–227, 558–561; 7:330)

35.

D. The most common site for the pleomorphic adenoma is the parotid gland, but it can occur in any major or minor salivary gland. It occurs in a 6:4 ratio of females to males. This tumor usually does not show fixation to deeper tissues. (1:339–343; 2:32–33, 38–39; 6:265–269; 7:302–306)

36.

C. A dentigerous cyst, which is also an odontogenic cyst, originates through alteration of the reduced enamel epithelium after the crown is completely formed. The dentigerous cyst is always associated with the crown of an unerupted tooth. (1:493–496; 2:14; 6:72–73, 326–332; 7:232–233)

37.

A. A dentigerous cyst is attached to the tooth at the cementoenamel junction. (2:14; 6:326; 7:232–233)

38.

A. The ameloblastoma is a neoplasm of a type resembling enamel organ tissue. It occurs most frequently in the mandible (80 percent of the time) and expands the bone rather than perforating it. (1:512–516; 3:125–126; 6:81, 363–374; 7:311–313)

39.

D. A hamartoma is an abnormal amount of tissue native to that part of the body where the tissue normally is present. (1:555–556)

40.

E. The phenomenon of "strawberry tongue" (the tongue has a white coating and the fungiform papillae are edematous and hyperemic) is associated with scarlet fever. (1:144; 4:528; 6:35,155)

41.

C. A false membrane consisting of a grayish, thick, fibrinous exudate and dead cells is commonly associated with diphtheria. It usually covers the tonsils, larynx, and pharynx. (1:145–146; 3:67; 4:537)

42.

A. Tuberculous lesions of the oral cavity are relatively uncommon. However, the possibility that the dentist or dental hygienist can contract an infection from a patient with pulmonary or oral tuberculosis is very high. (1:150–153; 2:98, 139; 3:28–29; 4:223; 6:10–11, 43–45; 7:185–186)

43.

D. Eighth nerve deafness is a sign of congenital syphilis, one of the triad of Hutchinson including interstitial keratitis and tooth abnormalities. (2:2, 102–103; 3:29, 245; 4:58, 116, 533–555; 6:41; 7:187–189, 269–270)

44.

B. The pyogenic granuloma is not a true tumor. It represents a response of the tissues to a nonspecific irritant. In a pregnancy, the occurrence of the pyogenic granuloma is referred to as a pregnancy tumor. (2:20–21; 3:96–97; 6:142; 7:39–42, 104–105)

45.

E. Upon examination, a 4-year-old child is found to have intensely inflamed gingiva, difficulty in swallowing, fever, lymphadenopathy, and yellowish fluid-filled vesicles. These symptoms are all characteristic of primary herpetic gingivostomatitis. (1:182–183; 2:84–85; 3:236–239; 5:82; 6:5; 7:203)

46.

D. Recurrent herpes simplex infections should be expected to heal in 7 to 14 days. The lesions can occur as often as every month or as infrequently as once a year or less. Recurrent herpes is often associated with trauma, fatigue, menstruation, pregnancy, upper respiratory infection, emotional upset, allergy, gastrointestinal disturbance, or exposure to sunlight. (1:183–184; 2:84–85, 136; 3:236–239; 4:224, 545; 6:4–9; 7:202–208)

47.

C. Papillary hyperplasia is most often associated with ill-fitting dentures. The lesions are red, edematous papillary projections of the palate. (1:367–368; 2:68–69; 6:44–45, 124, 176–177; 7:112–114)

48.

B. Any white patch on the oral mucosa that cannot be rubbed off and cannot be ascribed to any other disease is most probably clinical leukoplakia. Leukoplakia is most often due to tobacco use and chronic irritation. (2:4, 20, 54–55, 102, 127; 3:95, 242, 247; 4:78; 6:98; 7:192–198, 296–297)

49.

D. A white plaque which, when scraped or removed from the oral mucosa, leaves a raw, bleeding surface, probably is candidiasis. Candidiasis is caused by a yeast-like fungus, Candida albicans. Candidiasis may involve the skin, gastrointestinal tract, vaginal tract, urinary tract, and lungs, as well as the oral cavity. (1:163; 2:8, 62, 64, 68–69, 104–105; 3:246–247, 252; 4:332, 367, 551; 7:192–198, 296–297)

50.

C. Warts and papillomas are both found on pedunculated bases. The etiology of both is one of a number of subtypes of human papillomavirus. (2:4, 82–83, 135; 4:361, 546; 6:178; 7:199–200)

51.

D. Recurrent aphthous ulcers and lesions of intraoral herpes are distinguished largely on their location. The former are located primarily on mobile mucosa while the latter are located on tissue bound to periosteum. (2:94–95; 3:1; 4:245; 6:57; 7:148–153, 206)

52.

C. The words *pathogen* and *pathogenic* refer to the ability of a microorganism to enter a host's body and cause disease. (2:156; 3:152)

53.

D. Gingival hyperplasia is caused by phenytoin, cyclosporine, and nifedipine, but not inderal. (2:24–25; 3:219–221; 6:200; 7:112–115)

54.

C. Recurrent aphthous ulcers appear to be associated with stress. The stress factors may include bacterial infection, immunologic abnormalities, iron, vitamin B, or folic acid deficiencies, trauma, endocrine conditions, psychic factors, or allergic factors. Lay persons commonly refer to aphthous ulcers as "canker sores." (1:236–239; 2:94–95; 3:1; 4:245; 6:12–13, 52–60; 7:148–153)

55.

D. Nasopalatine duct cysts are often discovered on routine dental films. They usually manifest as ovoid, round, or heart-shaped radiolucencies above the roots of the maxillary centrals. The lesion is usually bilaterally symmetrical. (1:25–27; 2:36; 3:39–40; 6:74–75, 345–347; 7:240–241)

56.

A. The lower lip, being frequently involved in trauma, is the most common site for a mucocele. (2:32–33, 40–41; 3:41, 112; 6:240; 7:99–101)

57.

C. Herpangina is a viral infection that is caused by a coxsackievirus. The clinical manifestations of herpangina are comparatively mild and of short duration. It begins with a sore throat, low-grade fever, and abdominal pain. Orally, patients will exhibit small gray ulcers with a red periphery. (1:193; 2:84–85, 136; 3:239; 6:5, 14; 7:212–213)

58.

D. A permanent tooth that displays hypoplasia caused by trauma or infection during development is termed Turner's hypoplasia. Usually only a single tooth is involved. The degree of hypoplasia may range from a mild, brownish discoloration of the enamel to severe pitting and irregularity of the tooth crown. (1:45–47; 2:16–17; 3:56–57; 7:371–373)

59.

B. Squamous cell carcinoma of the floor of the mouth may directly invade the sublingual and sub-maxillary glands before it invades any other structures. (1:299–301; 2:21, 62–63, 98–99, 106, 130, 139; 3:119–125; 4:378; 6:505–506; 7:287, 291–296)

60.

A. A residual cyst is one that remains after or develops subsequent to the extraction of a tooth. It results from incomplete removal of an apical periodontal cyst. (1:105–109; 6:73, 326–327; 7:237, 239–240)

61.

C. Salivary gland tumors of all types occur most frequently in the parotid salivary gland. However, any type of salivary gland tumor can occur in any salivary gland, whether it is major or minor. (1:336–339; 2:32–33, 38–39; 3:124–125; 6:55–61; 7:301–310)

62.

A. Paget's disease is often discovered because patients' dentures do not fit due to a widening of the alveolar ridges. Eventually, these patients will complain of some or all of the following symptoms: bone pain, headache, dizziness, deafness, blindness, facial paralysis, and mental disturbance. (1:449–451; 3:264–265; 4:351, 426; 6:102–103, 458–461; 7:36, 422–424)

63.

C. A ranula is specifically associated with the sublingual and submaxillary salivary glands. It develops as a slowly enlarging, painless mass in the floor of the mouth. (2:40–41; 3:41, 113; 6:246; 7:101)

64.

D. Therapeutic radiation in the head and neck region results most commonly in xerostomia. Alterations in the salivary glands may begin within 1 to 2 weeks after the beginning of radiation treatment. With most dose levels, the loss of saliva will be permanent. (2:18, 46–47; 3:1–27; 4:594; 6:85; 7:454–455)

65.

A. The most common complication in the healing of human tooth-extraction wounds is the condition known as dry socket. Dry socket is a term used to describe a focal osteomyelitis in which the blood clot has been lost or undergone disintegration. Symptoms of dry socket include pain and foul odor but no suppuration. (1:119–120)

66.

B. Hand-Schuller-Christian disease is characterized by diabetes insipidus, punched-out bone destruction, and exophthalmos with or without other manifestations of dyspituitarism (such as polyuria, dwarfism, or infantilism). Hand-Schuller-Christian disease occurs early in life, primarily before the age of 5 years. It is more common in boys than girls, with a ratio of 2:1. (1:451–453; 3:276; 6:89, 413; 7:167–168)

67.

C. Cherubism, hyperparathyroidism, and aneurysmal bone cyst all have in common the presence of multinucleated giant cells under histologic examination. (6:347, 461, 469; 7:382–383)

68.

E. A riboflavin deficiency would most likely be manifested orally in the tongue. It begins with a glossitis which begins with soreness of the tip and/or lateral borders of the tongue. In severe cases, all papillae of the tongue may atrophy. (1:601; 6:151)

69.

D. Pellagra is associated with a deficiency of nicotinic acid. Oral characteristics of acute stages of pellagra include fiery red and painful mucosa.

Salivation is profuse and the epithelium of the entire tongue desquamates. Gingiva can be affected by tenderness, pain, redness, and ulceration of the interdental papillae. (1:601; 3:139–140; 4:617; 6:151)

70.

A. Hyperparathyroidism almost always produces skeletal lesions. The bone disturbances found in hyperparathyroidism can be vague to radiographically evident to grossly clinically evident. Orally, the first sign of the disease may be a giant cell tumor or "cyst" of the jaw. (1:612–614; 2:20; 3:100, 258–259; 4:503; 6:102–103, 461–464; 7:108, 413–415)

71.

C. An outstanding oral manifestation of cleidocranial dysplasia is retained primary teeth. Other characteristics include abnormalities of the skull, teeth, jaws, and shoulder girdle, and stunting of the long bones. Cleidocranial dysplasia was referred to as cleidocranial dysostosis prior to 1969. (1:445–446; 2:14–15; 3:52–53; 6:475–476; 7:384)

72.

D. A "cotton-wool" appearance of the skull radiographically is characteristic of Paget's disease. Paget's disease of bone, also known as osteitis deformans, is due to a circulatory disturbance. Paget's disease may consist of any of the following symptoms: bone pain, severe headache, deafness, blindness, facial paralysis, dizziness, and mental disturbance. (1:449–451; 3:264–265; 4:361, 426; 5:276, 279; 6:102–103, 458–461; 7:36, 422–424)

73.

C. A dentist is often consulted first by a patient with pernicious anemia for relief of glossitis. Pernicious anemia has characteristic symptoms that include generalized weakness, a sore, painful tongue, and numbness or tingling of the extremities. (1:604–605; 3:269, 276–277; 4:617; 6:151; 7:427–428)

74.

D. Classic characteristics of necrotizing ulcerative gingivitis include the presence of a grayish pseudomembrane, hemorrhage, fetid odor, and punched-out interdental papillae. (1:124–126; 2:26–27, 104; 3:221–223; 6:545–547; 7:39–41, 189–190)

75.

C. Desquamative gingivitis is most frequently found in adult females. Symptoms of chronic desquamative gingivitis include: red, swollen, glossy gingiva, occasionally with vesicles, and many denuded areas. It represents a gingival manifestation of a mucocutaneous disease such as lichen planus, pemphigoid, or pemphigus. (2:64, 92; 3:223; 6:21; 7:162–163)

76.

C. Juvenile periodontitis can occur in a mouth in which the patient's oral hygiene is faultless. It is most commonly found in females, 18 to 25 years of age, with a higher incidence in blacks. (1:137; 6:551–553)

77.

D. Cone-shaped teeth are a characteristic of ectodermal dysplasia. Patients with cone-shaped teeth may manifest anodontia or oligodontia. The malformation of the teeth can affect the permanent and primary dentitions. (1:541–542; 2:14, 46; 3:51; 4:32; 6:501–503; 7:399–400)

78.

E. Stevens-Johnson syndrome is a severe form of erythema multiforme. It occurs chiefly in young adults. Symptoms include asymptomatic erythematous macules and papules. Oral lesions appear as hyperemic macules, papules, or vesicles which can become eroded and bleed easily. (1:568; 2:90–91, 137; 3:223, 244; 5:93; 6:63; 7:157, 160)

79.

A. White sponge nevus appears to follow a hereditary pattern. It is a perfectly benign condition. The oral mucous lesion appears folded or corrugated with a soft or spongy texture. The lesion has a white opalescent hue. (1:542–543; 2:54–55, 127; 6:21–22, 94–95; 7:394)

80.

C. Nikolsky's sign is a characteristic feature of pemphigus vulgaris. Pemphigus vulgaris is characterized by vesicles and bullae. When the bullae rupture, they leave a raw eroded surface. The loss of epithelium in areas that seem unaffected is termed Nikolsky's sign. (1:559–561; 2:92; 6:16, 23; 7:138, 177, 180, 470)

81.

B. Oral radiographs of a patient with scleroderma would probably show a thickened periodontal ligament. Other oral radiographic features of scleroderma may include bilateral resorption of the angle of the ramus of the mandible or complete resorption of the condyles and/or coronoid processes of the mandible. (1:583–586)

82.

A. When a patient is observed to have a drooping mouth on one side and a watering eye, and complains of having a loss of taste sensation on the anterior portion of the tongue, the patient most likely has Bell's palsy. (1:627–628; 6:581–582)

83.

D. Lace-like white striae, the so-called Wickham's striae, are a classic presentation of lichen planus. (2:2, 4, 64–65, 130; 3:243–244; 6:115; 7:157–164)

84.

D. A patient with desquamative gingivitis will exhibit a peculiar inflammation of the gingiva, with necrotic and ulcerated epithelium that sloughs off with air blasts. (1:128–129; 2:64, 92; 3:223, 244; 6:21; 7:162–163)

85.

C. Dental caries is an infectious disease. It is the only infectious disease in which tissue is destroyed in the absence of cell injury and inflammation. (2:18–19; 3:178–195; 6:521–533; 7:21, 24–25)

86.

B. Gingivitis can be accompanied by ulceration, necrosis, serous exudation, or purulent exudation. It cannot be accompanied by hypertrophy. (1:122–124; 2:26–27, 104–105; 3:219–224; 6:543–547)

87.

C. Periodontitis is diagnosed when a loss of alveolar bone exists. It usually begins as a simple marginal gingivitis. As the marginal gingiva becomes more severely inflamed, there is a tendency for migration (apically) of the epithelial attachment, and a periodontal pocket is formed. (1:133–134; 3:225–229; 6:547–553)

88.

B. Use of aspirin may interfere with the aggregation of platelets, resulting in the increase in clotting time. (6:158)

89.

D. The characteristics given describe those found in necrotizing ulcerative gingivitis. Necrotizing ulcerative gingivitis usually has a rapid onset, and the patient may complain of inability to eat. The patient may also suffer from headache, malaise, and a low-grade fever. (1:124–126; 2:26–27, 104; 3:221-223; 6:545–547; 7:39-41, 189-190)

90.

C. Excessive occlusal forces, when chronic, can cause the periodontal ligament to become more dense, and the periodontal space to widen. The alveolar bone will become denser and the teeth will show wear facets. (2:18)

91.

B. When the calcified dental tissues in an odontoma superficially resemble the anatomy of normal teeth, it is termed a compound odontoma. (3:128–129; 6:390; 7:21, 26, 327, 329)

92.

E. During the early stages, cementomas are characterized by radiolucent lesions at the apex of vital teeth. In later stages, the areas will become radiopaque as the cementoma is completely formed. (1:464–465; 6:388–390; 7:33, 324–326)

93.

D. A carcinoma categorized as T3 N2 M0 falls into Stage IV of clinical stage groupings. Other categories of carcinoma found in Stage IV of clinical stage groupings are: T1 N2 M0, T2 N2 M0, T1 N3 M0, T2 N3 M0, and T3 N3 M0. (1:301–302)

94.

A. Herpes simplex virus, Type I, usually affects the face, lips, oral cavity, and upper body skin. Herpes simplex virus, Type II, usually affects the genitals and skin of the lower body. However, herpes simplex virus, Type II, can be found in the lips or oral mucous membrane, and herpes simplex virus, Type I, can be found on the genitalia. (1:181–182; 2:2, 4, 62, 84, 90, 98, 102, 106–107; 3:237–239; 4:244, 332, 545; 6:4–5)

95.

B. The ganglia most commonly affected by the herpes simplex virus, Type I, is the trigeminal nerve. The lumbosacral ganglia is most commonly affected by the herpes simplex virus, Type II. (1:181; 3:237–239; 4:244, 332, 545; 6:4–9)

96.

B. Recurrent herpetic stomatitis arises as an area of erythema, followed by the appearance of vesicles. These vesicles rupture to form a crust, which ultimately resolves in several more days. (2:84–85, 106–107; 3:237–239; 6:6)

97.

D. Sialolithiasis is the occurrence of calcareous deposits in the salivary ducts or glands. Many patients will complain of pain just before, during, or after meals, owing to the psychic stimulation of salivary flow. The occlusion of the salivary ducts prevents the free flow of saliva, which creates an accumulation of saliva under pressure, which produces pain. (1:326–327; 2:40–41; 3:113; 6:244–245; 7:101–103)

98.

D. Herpetic whitlow represents a herpetic lesion of the finger. Before the routine use of gloves, this was a definite occupational risk of dental professionals. (2:84–85; 6:6; 7:207)

99.

A. Bottle-baby syndrome usually affects the primary maxillary central and lateral incisors, followed by the first molars and cuspids. It is the absence of caries in the mandibular incisors that distinguishes this disease from ordinary rampant caries. (6:521–533)

100.

E. Upper and lower first molars have approximately a 95 percent susceptibility to dental caries attack. Upper and lower second molars have a 75 percent susceptibility to dental caries attack. Lower central and lateral incisors and cuspids have approximately a 3 percent susceptibility to dental caries attack. (6:521–533)

101.

C. Bruxism is a pathologic manifestation of attrition. (1:48; 2:18; 3:108, 282, 287–290; 7:80–83)

102.

B. Radiation caries most often begins and is clinically most evident at the cervical areas of the teeth. The lesion more closely resembles a demineralization than a true caries pattern. Radiation caries can be prevented. (1:219–220; 2:14, 18, 46; 6:85–86; 7:454–455)

103.

C. Aspirin tablets are used mistakenly by patients as an obtundent for relief of toothache. Within a few minutes of placing the tablet next to oral mucosa, a burning sensation will result. The affected tissue will become blanched or whitened, and sloughing and bleeding of the tissue will occur. (1:216; 2:94; 3:249–250; 6:26–27; 7:87–88)

104.

E. Mucosal pigmentation can be induced by antimalarial drugs such as chloroquine, and by AZT, used to treat patients with HIV infection. (3:86–87, 240–242, 251; 6:174)

105.

E. Primary and permanent teeth may be discolored as a result of prophylactic or therapeutic regimens instituted in the pregnant female or postpartum in the infant. The portion of the tooth that is stained by tetracycline is determined by the stage of tooth development and depends on the dosage, length of time over which the administration occurred, and the form of tetracycline. (1:57; 2:68, 102; 3:20, 57; 6:518–520; 7:455, 457)

106.

A. The most common oral reaction to cancer chemotherapeutic agents is mucosal erosion and ulceration. It can occur at any oral site. The lips, tongue, and buccal mucosa are the most common sites. (1:218–222; 2:28, 68; 4:97; 7:455)

107.

D. Patients with bulimia induce vomiting, often after bouts of uncontrolled eating between periods of starvation. Chronic vomiting produces erosion or gastric acid decalcification. These patients may also suffer from severe dental caries due to excessive carbohydrate intake. (1:48; 2:18–19; 3:31; 6:501–502; 7:85–86)

15 Pharmacology

DIRECTIONS
Each of the questions below is followed by several suggested answers. Select the best answer in each case.

---

1. Which of the following drugs does NOT depress the central nervous system?
    A. phenobarbital
    B. Pentothal™
    C. secobarbital
    D. Benzedrine™

2. When considering the prescription and its parts, one thinks of the inscription as being
    A. the information about the patient (name, address, etc.)
    B. directions to the pharmacist
    C. information on patient usage
    D. the drug and the amount prescribed

3. Certain governmental controls are placed on the prescribing of dangerous drugs by the Comprehensive Drug Abuse Prevention and Control Act of 1970. This act is enforced by
   A. the Justice Department
   B. a state-appointed committee
   C. the Department of Commerce
   D. the local sheriffs' department

4. Of the five schedules of controlled drug substances, which schedule has a high potential for abuse, for which no accepted medical use has been shown?
   A. Schedule I
   B. Schedule II
   C. Schedule III
   D. Schedule IV
   E. Schedule V

5. Which of the following formulas may be used in calculating drug dosages when using the weight of a child?
   A. Adam's rule
   B. Young's rule
   C. Beck's rule
   D. Clark's rule

6. Drug allergy may manifest itself in many ways; which of the choices below is a severe life-threatening drug allergy?
   A. anaphylaxis
   B. localized dermatitis
   C. photosensitivity
   D. urticaria

7. If a medication is to be prescribed to be taken at bedtime, the abbreviation used is
   A. p.o.
   B. a.c.
   C. b.i.d.
   D. h.s.

8. In understanding a prescription, the instructions stating "take one tablet every 6 hours" may also be written as
   A. q3h
   B. t.i.d.
   C. q.i.d.
   D. stat

9. A healthcare worker develops a positive reaction to a tuberculin skin test. After proper medical evaluation, the worker may be placed on long-term dosage of
   A. insulin
   B. Rifampin™
   C. Isoniazid (INH)™
   D. Vancomycin™

10. In using nitrous oxide–oxygen analgesia, one must keep in mind that
    A. the patient is put to sleep during the analgesia
    B. local anesthetic is most often used to supplement the analgesia
    C. at most, a concentration of 10% nitrous oxide and 90% oxygen is sufficient for most analgesia
    D. in no way does nitrous oxide analgesia relax the patient

11. In considering the pharmacologic properties of nitrous oxide, one can see that the gas is
    A. an irritant
    B. lighter than air
    C. colorless
    D. an organic solvent

12. Which of the following conditions would NOT require the patient to have antibiotic prophylaxis prior to gingival therapy?
    A. postrheumatic fever
    B. cardiac pacemaker
    C. heart-valve replacement
    D. congenital heart defect

13. A drug that is used for the treatment of epilepsy and that may produce excessive gingival enlargement is
    A. phenobarbital
    B. lincomycin
    C. Dilantin™ (phenytoin)
    D. nystatin

14. A synonym for penicillin V is
    A. phenoxymethyl penicillin
    B. oxacillin
    C. phenoxyethyl penicillin
    D. methicillin

15. The most important advantage of penicillin V over penicillin G is
    A. it costs less per 100 tablets
    B. that V is easier to remember than G
    C. that penicillin V can be given to patients who are allergic to penicillin G
    D. that penicillin V is stable at low gastric pH

16. Codeine, a widely used analgesic in dentistry,
    A. is a natural constituent of opium
    B. may be given only by injection
    C. has a calming effect on gastric mucosa
    D. is contraindicated for use in cough

17. When the following drugs are given parenterally, which is MOST effective for pain?
    A. codeine
    B. oxycodone
    C. meperidine
    D. morphine

18. The Drug Enforcement Administration (DEA) number is required for all of the following drugs EXCEPT
    A. Dolophine™ (methadone)

B. meperidine
C. tetracycline
D. alphaprodine

19. If a patient complained of chest pain and then placed a white tablet beneath his or her tongue, it might be concluded that
    A. it was sugar
    B. it was phenoxypenicillin
    C. it was nitroglycerin for angina pectoris
    D. it was diphenylhydantoin sodium (phenytoin)

20. Dental patients may be seen who are on long-term cortisone therapy and may develop hyperglycemia and glycosuria. Therefore, caution should be used in cortisone therapy for patients with
    A. hypertension
    B. diabetes
    C. peptic ulcer
    D. tuberculosis

21. Another name for mepivicaine hydrochloride is
    A. prilocaine
    B. Carbocaine™
    C. Xylocaine™
    D. procaine

22. Which of the following drugs would be BEST given to a patient with a history of gastric ulcers?
    A. aspirin
    B. acetaminophen
    C. ibuprofen

23. The usual adult dose of aspirin is
    A. 30–60 mg
    B. 650 mg
    C. 1000 mg
    D. 300–600 gr

24. Which of the following drugs may be used as a narcotic antagonist in cases of overdose, etc.?
    A. Dilaudid™ (hydromorphone)
    B. morphine
    C. Nalline™
    D. oxycodone

25. Pharmacologically, the difference between a hypnotic drug and a sedative drug is that the hypnotic will produce
    A. tingling of the extremities
    B. sleep
    C. hunger
    D. nausea

26. Which of these barbiturates can be classed as an ultra-short-acting compound?
    A. amobarbital
    B. thiopental sodium
    C. pentobarbital
    D. phenobarbital

27. When applied topically, the alcohols ethanol and isopropanol are
    A. bactericidal
    B. bacteriostatic

28. If a local bleeding area persists in a prophylaxis patient, topical thrombin may be applied because
    A. it provides vitamin K
    B. it is a vasoconstrictor which is needed now
    C. it clots fibrinogen directly
    D. it really is only salt

29. The topical cortisone MOST commonly used in treating oral ulceration is
    A. triamcinolone acetonide (Kenalog™)
    B. Orabase™
    C. promethazine hydrochloride
    D. oxycodone hydrochloride

30. In prescribing amoxicillin for prevention of bacterial endocarditis, one should give how much amoxicillin 1 hour prior to the oral prophylaxis appointment?
    A. 500 mg
    B. 1000 mg
    C. 3000 mg
    D. 2000 mg

31. Decreased pH in the tissues of an abscess makes complete local anesthesia difficult due to
    A. impairment of the liberation of anesthetic base
    B. neutralization of the anesthetic salt
    C. insolubility of the nerve fiber itself
    D. permeation of the nerve sheath by leukocytes

32. A patient with a mild to moderately severe oral infection who gives a history of allergy to penicillin should be given
    A. cloxacillin
    B. erythromycin
    C. streptomycin
    D. chloramphenicol
    E. cephalexin

33. Pentazocine is sold under the trademark
    A. Ponstel™
    B. Talwin™
    C. Darvon™
    D. Dilaudid™

34. Which of the following is a Schedule II controlled substance?
    A. Demerol™
    B. Phenaphen™
    C. Empirin™ with codeine 1/2 gr
    D. Tylenol™ with codeine

35. In discussing meperidine (Demerol™), one finds that

A. it is commonly used alone as a pre-anesthetic medication for anxiety

B. it has a usual adult dose of 25 mg

C. it is a good substitute drug for morphine

D. its ability to be combined with other drugs (for example, aspirin) is quite limited

36. A good drug to use in preanesthetic sedation in combination with Vistaril™ or Valium™ is

A. aspirin

B. acetaminophen

C. pentobarbital

D. Demerol™

37. In general, barbiturates have the ability to

A. produce long-term cortical depression

B. provide sedation but no analgesia

C. provide sedation and analgesia

D. be sedative but not hypnotic

38. Promethazine (Phenergan™) has all of the following properties EXCEPT

A. anti-inflammatory

B. sedative

C. local anesthetic

D. antihistaminic

39. A patient has just been given a local anesthetic. He suddenly begins to complain of an intense itching of the face and difficulty in breathing. In a matter of seconds, the patient is gasping for breath and losing consciousness. You diagnose this as anaphylaxis and immediately inject

A. Benadryl™ (an antihistamine)

B. epinephrine

C. hydrocortisone

D. aminophylline

40. A primary consideration in the topical use of vasoconstrictors to control severe capillary hemorrhage is

A. the transient effect of their action

B. the difficulty in applying the drug

C. the pain and irritation when they are applied

D. the discoloration of skin where they are applied

41. Methadone hydrochloride is an analgesic drug, well absorbed by the oral route, that may be used in dentistry and is comparable in its potency to

A. morphine

B. codeine

C. pentazocine

D. acetaminophen

42. A drug that may be used in the treatment of epilepsy and that does not produce gingival hyperplasia is

A. atropine

B. tetracycline

C. digoxin

D. phenobarbital

43. The addition of a vasoconstrictor in the anesthetic solution

A. may increase toxicity if the solution is placed close to a vessel

B. will provide a small degree of sedation for the patient

C. makes taking crown impressions easier by prolonging anesthesia

D. aids absorption of the local anesthetic

44. Oxycodone is

A. meperidine

B. Dilaudid™

C. Percodan™

D. Talwin™

45. High doses of aspirin may cause all of the following EXCEPT
    A. increased circulating uric acid
    B. nausea and headache
    C. allergy
    D. alteration of prothrombin production

46. If a patient is allergic to salicylates (aspirin), you may prescribe
    A. Demerol™
    B. Darvon™ compound
    C. Tylenol™
    D. codeine

47. If a patient gives a history of having been on a drug regimen of long-term chlorothiazide, one should be alert to
    A. hypertension and diuresis
    B. diabetes and poor healing
    C. psychosis and mood elevation
    D. heart disease and anticoagulation

48. In the removal of a tooth with a painful periodontal abscess, which sensation is first impeded by the local anesthetic agent?
    A. pressure
    B. proprioception
    C. cold
    D. touch

49. The MOST commonly prescribed antibiotic in healthcare practice is
    A. tetracycline
    B. erythromycin
    C. vancomycin
    D. amoxicillin

50. Which of the following semisynthetic penicillins is NOT effective against penicillinase-producing organisms?
    A. ampicillin (Amcill™)
    B. methicillin (Staphcillin™)
    C. cloxacillin (Tegopen™)
    D. nafcillin (Unipen™)

51. The principal serious toxic effect in patients treated with clindamycin is
    A. skin rash
    B. blood dyscrasia
    C. enterocolitis
    D. dizziness

52. A patient who is a known diabetic on insulin therapy is in your dental chair when he complains of feeling peculiar. You notice that he appears nervous, and his skin is cold and clammy. Examination of the pulse reveals a tachycardia. Suddenly, the patient begins to appear wild-eyed and confused. A probable diagnosis would be
    A. hysterical reaction
    B. epilepsy
    C. hyperglycemia
    D. hypoglycemia

53. Patients with Sjörgen's syndrome commonly have dry mouth and increased susceptibility to caries. The dental hygienist in planning for continued fluoride therapy should advise the patients to
    A. use fluoride mouth rinses only
    B. apply topical fluoride by a cotton tipped applicator daily
    C. mix topical fluoride with an artificial saliva substance for daily rinsing
    D. apply topical fluoride in a custom carrier for five minutes daily

54. Which drug is usually NOT associated with possible tendencies toward prolonged hemorrhage?
    A. aspirin
    B. Demerol™
    C. dicumarol
    D. warfarin

55. Death due to an overdosage of barbiturates would be via which mechanism?
    A. ventricular arrhythmias
    B. shock
    C. pulmonary embolism
    D. respiratory depression

56. Which of the following drugs is used to suppress inflammation and may be taken by dental patients?
    A. thyroid extract
    B. insulin
    C. digitalis
    D. corticosteroid

57. All of the following require a narcotic prescription EXCEPT
    A. codeine
    B. meperidine
    C. oxycodone
    D. acetaminophen

58. The MOST common adverse effect related to penicillin ingestion is
    A. blood dyscrasia
    B. GI disturbance
    C. renal damage
    D. allergic phenomena

59. The lethal adult dose of aspirin is 10 to 30 grams.
    A. true
    B. false

60. Which of the following types of compounds is capable of inhibiting but does not necessarily destroy microorganisms?
    A. disinfectant
    B. germicide
    C. deodorant
    D. antiseptic
    E. bactericide

61. Which of the following agents is capable of killing viruses?
    A. bactericide
    B. virucide
    C. fungicide

62. The only gaseous chemical agent that can be relied on for complete sterilization of instruments is
    A. phenol
    B. isodine
    C. ethylene oxide
    D. hexachlorophene

63. A peculiar bluish translucency of the primary and permanent teeth may develop from ingestion of
    A. pediatric vitamins containing iron
    B. penicillin
    C. tetracyclines
    D. soybean-based infant formulas

64. Which of the following vitamins is NOT correctly matched with the disease produced from its deficiency?
    A. riboflavin—avitaminosis
    B. vitamin C—scurvy
    C. niacin—pellagra
    D. vitamin D—rickets

65. Epinephrine is necessary in an emergency kit for which of the following situations?
    A. syncope
    B. diabetic coma
    C. cardiac arrest
    D. congestive heart failure

66. In addition to epinephrine, which of the following drugs should be administered to a victim of cardiac arrest?
    A. sodium bicarbonate
    B. morphine
    C. Benadryl™
    D. ammonia

67. A patient with syncope should be treated with
   A. nitrous oxide
   B. ethylene oxide
   C. spirits of ammonia
   D. Benadryl™
   E. Valium™

68. Patients with xerostomia are BEST treated with
   A. glycerin
   B. sodium carboxymethyl-cellulose
   C. fluoride
   D. steroids
   E. Orabase™

69. When a patient takes penicillin with salicylates, the resulting effect is
   A. gastric hemorrhage
   B. antagonism
   C. enhanced effect of penicillin
   D. inhibition of penicillin

70. Surgical dental treatment or any procedure involving oral bleeding is not recommended on patients with acute cocaine abuse because of
   A. a tendency toward excess bleeding
   B. rapid hemostasis and clot dissolution
   C. increased incidence of delayed healing
   D. a poor risk for follow-up care by the patient

71. The drug Procardia™ is a commonly prescribed medicine and is frequently part of a patient's medical history. It most often signals the presence of
   A. kidney disease
   B. liver disease
   C. gastrointestinal disease
   D. cardiovascular disease

72. Fexofenadine (Allegra™) is a frequently prescribed antihistamine for use in allergic rhinitis. A major benefit it possesses is
   A. the ability to produce sedation
   B. noninterference of psychomotor functions
   C. significant anticholinergic activity
   D. pronounced beta blocking

73. The goal of antihypertensive therapy, if feasible, is to achieve and maintain a diastolic blood pressure at or below
   A. 80 mm/Hg
   B. 90 mm/Hg
   C. 100 mm/Hg
   D. 110 mm/Hg

74. Systemic treatment for the HIV-infected patient many times consists of therapy with which of the following drugs?
   A. Zidovudine™
   B. Acyclovir™
   C. Dexamethasone™
   D. Mycelex™

75. A single episode of rheumatic fever generally results in residual heart damage (rheumatic heart disease) in about
   A. 50% of all cases
   B. 100% of all cases
   C. 75% of all cases
   D. 65% of all cases

76. If allergy to penicillin is present, a patient receiving prophylaxis for bacterial endocarditis should be given which of the following drugs?
   A. tetracycline
   B. mycostatin
   C. septra
   D. clindamycin

77. Diazepam (Valium™) is a commonly utilized anti-anxiety drug in dentistry. Caution should be used in extended prescription of the drug because
  A. drug tolerance may occur, evidenced by the need for increased dosage
  B. allergy develops rapidly and may require hospitalization
  C. the drug may produce primary herpetic gingivostomatitis
  D. it is a pure antihistamine and long-term therapy is not necessary

78. Oral cancer therapy by radiation may create a mucositis resulting in pain, ulceration, and difficulty in chewing. Which of the following therapies is BEST to control mucositis?
  A. fresh fruit juice three times daily
  B. petrolatum-based lip balms
  C. antihistamine solutions mixed with Kaopectate™
  D. continuance of smoking for patient comfort

79. When injecting a complete 1.8 ml carpule of 2% lidocaine, the patient receives how many milligrams of the anesthetic solution?
  A. 1.8 mg
  B. 15 mg
  C. 36 mg
  D. 72 mg

80. A dental prophylaxis patient admits to taking Coumadin™ for several months for a heart condition. Which of the following tests is MOST important to conduct prior to proceeding with any therapy for this patient?
  A. bleeding time
  B. vitamin C level
  C. heparin time
  D. prothrombin time

81. Renal dialysis produces concern as to when best to dentally treat this patient. A concern is the use of heparin in the dialysis process and its effect on oral bleeding. When is the BEST time to treat the dialysis patient?
  A. immediately prior to dialysis
  B. immediately after dialysis
  C. the day after dialysis
  D. do not treat these patients

82. Which of the following is NOT a pharmacologic effect of digitalis (a cardiac glycoside)?
  A. improves myocardial contractile force
  B. increases ventricular rate
  C. increases cardiac output
  D. decreases venous pressure
  E. decreases blood volume

83. Digitalis acts directly on the
  A. myocardium
  B. pericardium
  C. heart cell
  D. heart valves

84. Quinidine is used to treat which of the following conditions?
  A. cardiac arrhythmias
  B. cardiac insufficiency
  C. congestive heart failure
  D. hypertension
  E. hypotension

85. Which of the following drugs is used MOST commonly in the treatment of hypertension?
  A. neuronal blockers
  B. reserpine
  C. methyldopa
  D. thiazides

86. Which of the following is the MOST common of all cardiovascular diseases?

    A. coronary artery disease

    B. stroke

    C. angina

    D. hypertension

    E. cardiac arrythmia

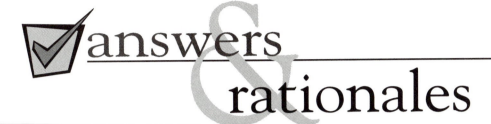

answers & rationales

1.

D. Amphetamines such as Benzedrine™ do not depress the central nervous system. They tend to produce increased alertness, wakefulness, and loss of sense of fatigue. Amphetamines have indirect adrenergic stimulant effects which cause increases in blood pressure and reflex cardiac slowing. They are potent central nervous system stimulants. (1:524)

2.

D. The inscription of the body of the prescription contains the names and quantities of the drugs prescribed. In addition to the active ingredients, the inscription also contains diluents, colors, flavors, or other nontherapeutically active components that are necessary for the formulation of the product. The pharmacist may legally add any component necessary for a pharmaceutically acceptable product. (1:64–67)

3.

A. The Justice Department is the federal agency that is responsible for enforcement of the Comprehensive Drug Abuse Prevention and Control Act of 1970. The Justice Department regulates all controlled substances including narcotic preparations. The nation's foods, drugs and medical devices, and cosmetics are protected by the federal Food, Drug, and Cosmetic Act, enforced by the Food and Drug Administration. (1:13, 70–71)

4.

A. Of the five schedules stated by the Controlled Substances Act of 1970, Schedule I substances have no accepted medical use in the United States. These Schedule I drugs may be used only for experimental research. Schedule I drugs include heroin, LSD, marijuana, and other hallucinogens. (1:71–72)

5.

D. Clark's rule is the formula used for computing children's dosages. It is as follows:

$$\frac{\text{child's weight (in lbs.)}}{150} \times \text{adult dose} = \text{child's dose}$$

Clark's rule is based on a scientific principle of dosage per body weight. (1:48)

6.

A. Anaphylaxis is an acute, life-threatening emergency that most frequently occurs after intravenous injection of a drug. Anaphylaxis is characterized by hypotension, bronchospasm, laryngeal edema, and cardiac arrhythmias. Fatal anaphylaxis is rare, but has occurred after a single oral dose of penicillin in highly sensitive individuals. (1:55–56)

7.

D. The abbreviation h.s. means at bedtime or hour of sleep. The abbreviation p.o. means by mouth. The abbreviation a.c. means as desired. The abbreviation b.i.d. means twice a day. (1:67)

8.

C. The abbreviation q.i.d. means 4 times a day. This can also be interpreted as "take every 6 hours." The abbreviation q3h means once every 3 hours. The abbreviation t.i.d. means 3 times a day. The abbreviation stat means immediately. (1:67)

9.

C. Healthcare workers or anyone who develops a positive tuberculin skin test may, after proper chest radiography and medical consultation, be placed on prophylactic long-term, generally one year, Isoniazid™ therapy. (1:186–188)

10.

B. Relative analgesia primarily employs the use of nitrous oxide–oxygen, but pain control must be given concomitantly with local anesthetic. Nitrous oxide offers comfort to the dental patient and an increased patient acceptance of dental procedures. Because of increased patient acceptance, the treatment administration is more relaxed. (1:267–268)

11.

C. Nitrous oxide is a nonirritating colorless gas. It has little or no odor. It is stored in a blue cylinder at 750 psi. (1:267)

12.

B. Because they do not involve the endocardium per se, cardiac pacemakers will not necessitate antibiotic prophylaxis. Cardiac pacemakers may be affected by electronic devices such as ultrasonic scaling devices, pulp testers, and electrosurgical equipment. Prosthetic joint replacements sometimes require antibiotic prophylaxis. (3:158)

13.

C. Phenytoin (Dilantin™) produces excessive gingival enlargement in some patients who are treated with this drug. It is a highly effective anticonvulsant drug. The severity of the gingival enlargement differs. It is not seen in every patient taking this drug. (1:315)

14.

A. A synonym for phenoxymethyl penicillin is penicillin V. The usual adult dose of penicillin V is 250 to 500 mg every 6 hours. Trade names for penicillin V include PenVeeK™ and Penicillin V K™. (2:484, 2576)

15.

D. Penicillin V is more resistant than penicillin G to acid inactivation in gastric secretions. Therefore, it has a measurably improved intestinal absorption because of its conversion into a soluble alkaline salt at the pH of the duodenal contents. Oral penicillin V gives higher and better-sustained levels of penicillin activity than does oral buffered penicillin G at various dosage levels. (1:165–166)

16.

A. Next to morphine, codeine is the most important alkaloid of opium. Codeine is only one-sixth as potent as morphine. It is less narcotic and less addictive and produces less constipation and less nausea. (1:131–134)

17.

D. Morphine is the standard to which all other strong analgesics are compared. Morphine promotes drowsiness, depresses reasoning, stimulates imagination, and produces euphoria. It depresses the respiratory and cough centers, contracts pupils, and elicits vomiting. (1:134, 138)

18.

C. Tetracycline is an antibiotic, and antibiotics are not controlled by the Drug Enforcement Administration. Methadone, meperidine, and alphaprodine require DEA numbers for prescription. The DEA is an arm of the Department of Justice. (1:67, 70)

19.

C. When a nitroglycerin tablet is placed beneath the tongue in a patient suffering pain from angina pectoris, it relieves the pain by reducing the workload of the heart and producing a dilation of the blood vessels. Angina pectoris is a syndrome of chest pain or discomfort that results from inadequate blood supply to a segment of the myocardium. (1:336)

20.

B. Long-term cortisone therapy produces an enhancement of gluconeogenesis and is contraindicated for patients who have diabetes mellitus. Corticosteroids decrease the resistance to infections because they cause a general depression of the inflammatory response. Most frequently, corticosteroids are used for their anti-inflammatory and anti-allergic actions. (1:409–411, 413–415)

21.

B. The trade names for mepivicaine hydrochloride are Carbocaine™ and Isocaine™. The trade name for procaine is Novacain™. The trade names for lidocaine are Xylocaine™ and Octocaine™. The trade names for prilocaine are Citanest™ and Citanest Forte™. (1:223–226)

22.

B. Acetaminophen does not produce gastric ulceration like aspirin does. Acetaminophen has approximately the same analgesic and antipyretic effects as aspirin. The anti-inflammatory properties of acetaminophen are not clinically significant. (1:123–125)

23.

B. The usual adult dose of aspirin is 650 mg every 4 hours. A mild toxic reaction to aspirin is termed salicylism. It is characterized by headache, nausea, tinnitus, vomiting, dizziness, and dimness of vision. (1:106–115)

24.

C. Nalorphine (Nalline™) is an antidote used for overdosage of narcotic agents. Levallorphan (Lorfan™) is another widely used narcotic antagonist, as is naloxone (Narcan™). All of these agents are capable of reversing respiratory depression induced by narcotics. (1:521)

25.

B. Drugs classified as sedatives and hypnotics have many of the same properties. However, a drug is not labeled hypnotic until its dosage produces sleep. Although agents may be promoted as either sedatives or hypnotics, the same drugs may be either, depending on the dose. (1:240, 252, 254–256)

26.

B. Thiopental sodium (Pentothal™) is an ultrashort-acting barbiturate. Intravenous doses have a rapid onset of about 30 to 40 seconds. If this drug is given in repeated doses, the drug will accumulate in body tissues and a prolonged recovery will result. (1:274)

27.

A. The alcohols ethanol and isopropanol are primarily bactericidal against vegetative forms of bacteria. Ethyl alcohol is most effective in concentrations of 50 to 70 percent. Isopropyl alcohol is more potent than ethyl alcohol and is used in concentrations of 30 to 90 percent. (10:65–66)

28.

C. Topical thrombin can be used for local bleeding. It acts to rapidly convert blood fibrinogen to fibrin. It cannot be used intravascularly. (9:1029)

29.

A. Triamcinolone acetonide (Kenalog™) has been used to treat some acute and chronic lesions of the oral mucosa, such as recurrent ulcerative stomatitis. As with all corticosteroids, triamcinolone acetonide is entirely suppressive, but not curative. It does not prevent recurrence of any oral lesions. (1:316, 412–413; 3:558–559)

30.

D. Two grams (2000 mg) of amoxicillin should be given 1 hour prior to the procedure for prophylaxis against bacterial endocarditis. (8:1794–1801)

31.

A. The acidic nature of inflamed tissues greatly decreases the action of an injected local anesthetic due to impairment of the release of local anesthetic base. Following an injection into inflamed areas, the drug is absorbed more rapidly because of the increased blood supply. This factor reduces the duration and effectiveness of the anesthetic and increases its toxicity. (1:218)

32.

B. The antibacterial spectrum of erythromycin closely resembles that of penicillin. It is a drug of choice for patients who are allergic to penicillin. If the patient is allergic to penicillin and erythromycin, clindamycin could be administered. (8:1794–1801)

33.

B. Talwin™ is marketed as the proprietary compound of the generic pentazocine. Talwin™ is a narcotic antagonist that is an effective analgesic when given orally. It is capable of producing hallucinations. (1:142, 520–521)

34.

A. Meperidine hydrochloride (Demerol™) is classified as a Schedule II drug by the Controlled Substances Act. Demerol™ is a narcotic-analgesic. It has one-tenth the analgesic activity of morphine. (1:141)

35.

C. Meperidine hydrochloride (Demerol™) has both morphine-like and atropine-like properties and can be used for patients showing intolerance to morphine. It is less likely to produce gastrointestinal disturbance than morphine. A tolerance may result from meperidine HCl therapy. (1:141, 504)

36.

D. The combination of diazepam (Valium™) and meperidine HCl (Demerol™) for preoperative sedation provides enhanced amnesia, relaxation, sedation, and analgesia. The purpose of preoperative sedation is to decrease salivation and mucoid secretions, raise pain thresholds, depress reflex irritability, and lessen metabolic activity. (1:249, 251)

37.

B. In general, barbiturates do not produce analgesia unless they are given in extremely high doses which are not generally acceptable. High concentrations of barbiturates can be lethal. Barbiturates in high concentrations depress liver and kidney functions, reduce gastrointestinal mobility, and lower body temperatures. (1:251–254)

38.

A. Promethazine (Phenergan™) is primarily antihistaminic, but it has side effects of local anesthesia and sedation. Its production of excessive sedation may be accompanied by dizziness, dryness of the mouth, uncoordination, blurred vision, and fatigue. (2:2578–2579)

39.

B. The drug of choice for treatment of symptoms of acute anaphylaxis is epinephrine. This drug is also administered for cardiac arrest. Epinephrine is not indicated for emergency treatment of shock. (1:482)

40.

A. Vasoconstrictors may be used to control diffuse bleeding following an oral surgical procedure (such as a gingivectomy). However, the action is transient and a longer-lasting method such as sutures or packs should then be used. Epinephrine therapy is only effective in controlling capillary oozing. (1:95–96)

41.

A. Methadone hydrochloride is a strong analgesic drug with little sedative action and is comparable in potency to morphine. Methadone can be substituted for morphine. It is used as an oral substitute for heroin in maintenance programs for drug abusers. (2:1222–1223)

42.

D. Phenobarbital is a useful sedative and hypnotic and may be used for continuous control of specific forms of epilepsy. Phenobarbital is a long-acting barbiturate. It is most effective in controlling seizures of grand mal epilepsy. (1:252-256, 367, 372)

43.

C. The addition of a vasoconstrictor to a local anesthetic delays systemic absorption and prolongs and increases the depth of anesthesia. It will render the area of injection less hemorrhagic. (1:226–228)

44.

C. Oxycodone is marketed as the multiple-entity preparation Percodan™. Oxycodone is more potent and more addictive than codeine. Oxycodone, in addition to being marketed as Percodan™, is also found in Percodan-Demi™, Percocet™, and Tylox™. (1:138–141)

45.

A. Large doses of aspirin increase the uric acid output and decrease the plasma urate concentration. Doses between 2 and 3 g per 24 hours usually do not alter the secretion of uric acid. Smaller doses of aspirin (1 to 2 g per 24 hours) may decrease the secretion of uric acid and elevate the plasma urate concentrations. (1:109)

46.

C. Tylenol™ (acetaminophen) may be substituted for aspirin when allergy is a problem. Acetaminophen has the same analgesic properties and antipyretic effects as aspirin. It does not, however, have the anti-inflammatory activity of aspirin. (1:123–125)

47.

A. Chlorothiazide, a diuretic used in the treatment of hypertension, may be one of the more common drugs encountered in hypertensive dental patients. Other commonly encountered diuretics include Hydro-Diuril™, Lasix™, and Aldactone™. (1:343–344)

48.

C. Local anesthetics produce loss of the following sensations and nerve pathways in this order: autonomics, cold, warmth, pain, touch, and pressure. (1:219–220)

49.

D. Amoxicillin is the most frequently prescribed antibiotic in physicians' offices. It is a semisynthetic, broad spectrum antibiotic. It is most effective with gram-positive and gram-negative organisms. (1:166–167)

50.

A. Ampicillin is a semisynthetic penicillin that is not resistant to penicillinase deactivation. Ampicillin has the ability to penetrate the cell walls so that they can exert their bactericidal effect. (1:166–167; 2:2569–2570)

51.

C. A serious adverse reaction to clindamycin therapy can be an enterocolitis. A more serious consequence of clindamycin therapy can be pseudomembranous colitis. Clindamycin is an antibiotic effective primarily against gram-positive organisms. (2:2399)

52.

D. Hypoglycemia may occur in diabetic patients who have taken their insulin but have not eaten. The dental team should recognize that sweating, weakness, hunger, tachycardia, and mental confusion are all signs of hypoglycemia. Overdosage of insulin or unaccustomed exercise or stress can also produce hypoglycemia in the diabetic patient. (3:341–359)

53.

D. Sjörgen's syndrome is a systemic disorder characterized by decreased salivary and lacrimal function that affects over one million Americans. A sequelae of the disease is increased caries activity, but is managed by daily application of topical fluoride in a custom tray. (6:74–84)

54.

B. Demerol™ is a narcotic analgesic and has no effect on the clotting mechanism. Aspirin, dicumarol, and warfarin are anticoagulants. Warfarin is marketed as Coumadin™. (1:141, 358–360)

55.

D. The cause of death in a barbiturate overdose is respiratory depression. Respiratory depression is easily produced with large doses of barbiturates; therefore, barbiturates are not used for anesthesia. (1:251–254)

56.

D. Corticosteroids are anti-inflammatory. They suppress the signs and symptoms of inflammation but not the underlying disease process. Corticosteroids, however, are not curative. (1:413)

57.

D. Acetaminophen is a nonnarcotic analgesic available without prescription. Codeine, meperidine, and oxycodone are all scheduled drugs that require a prescription. (1:123)

58.

D. Hypersensitivity (allergic) reactions are not uncommon with penicillin ingestion. They vary from skin eruptions to acute anaphylaxis. Allergic reactions occur in approximately 5 to 10 percent of patients treated with penicillin. (1:55–56, 164–165)

59.

A. The lethal dose of aspirin is 10 to 30 grams. High blood levels of salicylates produce poisoning. Young children are highly susceptible to salicylate poisoning. (1:113)

60.

D. The terms *antiseptic, germicide,* and *disinfectant* are often confused. Antiseptic compounds inhibit but do not necessarily destroy microorganisms. Germicides are capable of destroying microorganisms. Disinfectants are lethal for pathogenic microorganisms. (10:56)

61.

B. A virucide is an agent capable of killing viruses. A bactericide is an agent capable of destroying bacteria. A fungicide is an agent capable of killing fungi. (10:64–66)

62.

C. The only gaseous chemical agent that can be relied on for complete sterilization of instruments is ethylene oxide. The use of ethylene oxide requires special equipment, is time-consuming, and is expensive. Therefore, it is not practical for the average private dental office. (10:63–64)

63.

C. When administered during tooth formation, tetracyclines may be deposited in tooth substance, causing tooth discoloration which can be observed clinically. The discoloration varies in quality and intensity from light gray to yellowish to dark blue or brown. The discoloration may be generalized or affect varying regions of the crowns of the teeth. (1:172)

64.

A. Riboflavin deficiencies produce glossitis and cheilosis, not avitaminosis. Niacin deficiencies produce pellagra. Vitamin D deficiencies produce rickets. Vitamin C deficiencies produce scurvy. (1:277–301)

65.

C. The inclusion of epinephrine in an emergency kit is mandatory for the treatment of cardiac arrest and anaphylaxis. These are the only two emergency situations that would require its use in a dental office. Epinephrine is not indicated for treatment of shock. (1:96, 400)

66.

A. Within a few minutes of cardiac arrest, metabolic acidosis reaches a critical level. A safe rule of thumb is to administer 1 mEq/kg sodium bicarbonate intravenously, then one-half dose every 10 minutes. Not more than 3 or 4 ampules should be given before lab-monitoring of acid-base balance is available. (1:469)

67.

C. A patient in syncope should be placed in a supine position and allowed to inhale spirits of ammonia. Inhaled ammonia irritates the trigeminal nerve sensory endings, with a resulting reflex stimulation of medullary respiratory and vasomotor centers. The administration of oxygen will aid in combating tissue anoxia. (1:477, 483)

68.

B. Xerostomia, "dry mouth," can be caused by diseases affecting the salivary glands, radiation therapy, or drugs. Immediate symptoms can be relieved by the application of sodium carboxymethyl-cellulose. It is a nonirritating agent that moistens and lubricates the oral tissues and may be used for prolonged periods without adverse effects. Xero-lube™ is one trade name for this artificial saliva. (1:312–314)

69.

C. When a patient takes penicillin with salicylates, the resulting effect is the enhancement of the effect of the penicillin. Penicillin and tetracycline taken simultaneously inhibits the penicillin. Penicillin taken with oral anticoagulants can produce hemorrhage. (1:505–506)

70.

A. A recent report detailed a patient with excessive bleeding from a surgical site. The patient was a chronic drug abuser and "snorted" cocaine in the dental chair. (5:60–62)

71.

D. Procardia™ (nifedipine) is a calcium channel-blocking drug with vasodilator properties utilized in the management of hypertension. (1:335, 348)

72.

B. Allegra™ is a specific histamine antagonist that has major benefits in that it does not impair psychomotor function nor produce sedation. Recently, fexofenadine (Allegra™) replaced Seldane™ as a non-sedating antihistamine. (1:401)

73.

B. Patients who are diagnosed by their physicians as hypertensive are generally treated first in a nonpharmacologic manner or in combination with drugs to achieve and maintain a diastolic blood pressure below 90 mm/Hg. (3:164–166)

74.

A. Zidovudine™ (AZT) is frequently used in the systemic treatment of HIV disease. Acyclovir™ (Zovirax), an antiviral agent for herpetic lesions, Mycelex™ for fungal infection, and Dexamethasone™ (Decadron) for recurrent aphthous ulcerations are topically applied medications also utilized in treatment of oral lesions from HIV. (3:296–297)

75.

D. Persons who have had a single attack of rheumatic fever have residual heart damage in about 65% of the cases, whereas those patients having more than one attack of rheumatic fever result in almost 100% residual heart disease. If a patient with a history of rheumatic fever has to have emergency care, it is advised to provide antibiotic coverage if medical advice is not available. (3:117)

76.

D. The only drug with a similar bacterial spectrum to penicillin is clindamycin. The other drugs are more precise in their antibiotic spectrum and are not indicated for a patient allergic to penicillin in the case of bacterial endocarditis prophylaxis. (8:1794–1801)

77.

A. Diazepam (Valium™) is one of the most effective anti-anxiety drugs used today. Caution should be taken in giving long-term doses if the patient shows signs of drug tolerance by asking for additional strength of medication to achieve the same result. (3:498)

78.

C. The mucositis from radiation therapy can be severe and cause pain, sloughing of the tissue, and dysphagia. Fruit juices and petrolatum-based lip balms add to the irritant effect of the mucositis. Antihistamine solutions mixed with Kaopectate™ or like substances may provide a soothing effect for more comfortable chewing. (3:477)

79.

C. Multiplying the concentration of the administered solution by the volume equals the amount of milligrams injected. 20 mg/1 mL × 1.8 mL = 36 mg lidocaine. (1:234–235)

80.

D. Patients may be on anticoagulants for a variety of reasons. A dental prophylaxis should not be attempted until the patient has been cleared by the physician. The best test to gauge the level of anticoagulation is the prothombin time. Most physicians will suggest that the patient may be treated if the PT is 1 1/2 to 2½ times the normal control. (1:360; 3:433–434)

81.

C. The use of heparin in the dialysis patient is a must for successful therapy. Heparin has a half-life of four hours and its effects may be variable several hours after administration. The preferred time for dental care for the dialysis patient is the day after dialysis. (3:435; 9:521–523)

82.

B. Digitalis decreases ventricular rate. Digitalis is used to improve circulation in patients with congestive heart failure. Digitalis increases the force of myocardial contraction, increases cardiac output, and decreases heart size, venous pressure, and blood volume. Additionally, digitalis relieves edema due to a positive inotropic edema. (7:815)

83.

A. Digitalis acts directly on the myocardium and increases the force of myocardial contraction. Digitalis acts directly on the heart and modifies both its mechanical and electrical activity. (7:815)

84.

A. Quinidine is used to treat cardiac arrhythmias. Other drugs utilized to treat cardiac arrhythmias include procanimide, disopyramide, and moricizine. (7:847–850)

85.

D. Thiazides are the most frequently used antihypertensive agents in the United States. Thiazides are more effective than loop diuretics. (7:787–788)

86.

D. Hypertension is the most common cardiovascular disease in the United States. Hypertension is defined as an elevation of systolic and/or diastolic blood pressures above 140/90 mm Hg. (7:784)

16 Research and Statistics

DIRECTIONS Each of the questions below is followed by several suggested answers. Select the best answer in each case.

---

1. A study was conducted to determine which polishing agent is most effective in removing plaque. In this study, plaque is considered to be which kind of variable?

   A. dependent

   B. independent

   C. experimental

   D. extraneous

2. Five dental hygiene students who had extremely high plaque scores are assigned to complete a videotaped plaque control program. The rest of the students in the class were asked to review the chapter on prevention techniques. At the end of the month, the plaque scores of these five students are significantly improved in comparison to the rest of the class. Which of the following threats to internal validity MOST likely accounts for the improvement?
   A. history
   B. maturation
   C. instrumentation
   D. statistical regression
   E. mortality

3. In an alumni survey, respondents are asked to select the highest degree they have completed: 1) associate degree, 2) bachelors degree, 3) masters degree, or 4) doctorate. This variable, degree completed, utilizes which scale of measurement?
   A. nominal
   B. ordinal
   C. interval
   D. ratio

4. A study was conducted to determine if there is any relationship between decayed, missing, or filled (DMF) teeth and fluoride concentration in the water. Which statistical test would be MOST appropriate for the analysis of data?
   A. correlation coefficient
   B. chi-square
   C. student's t-test
   D. paired student's t-test
   E. analysis of variance

5. The following data represent the number of abstracts read by 11 dental hygiene students: 1, 1, 1, 1, 2, 2, 3, 4, 5, 8, 9. What is the mode?
   A. 1
   B. 2
   C. 3.36
   D. 8

6. The extent to which an instrument measures what one intends to measure is
   A. correlation
   B. probability
   C. reliability
   D. validity

7. The scores achieved by six students on an examination were: 93, 92, 91, 90, 89, 25. Which measure of central tendency would BEST be used to accurately describe the group's performance?
   A. mean
   B. median
   C. mode
   D. range

8. Which of the following correlation coefficients represents the weakest relationship?
   A. -.92
   B. -.10
   C. 0
   D. +.10
   E. +.92

9. At which level of significance can a researcher be the MOST confident that a real difference exists between two treatments?
   A. p = .06
   B. p = .05
   C. p = .01
   D. p = .001

10. In a positively skewed distribution,
   A. the mean will be greater than the median

B. the mean will be less than the median

C. the mean, median, and mode will have the same value

D. the curve will be symmetrical and uni-modal

11. The standard deviation is a measure of

    A. central tendency

    B. variability

    C. correlation

    D. regression

12. In collecting data, the advantage of using the interview technique over the questionnaire is that the interview technique

    A. is less time-consuming

    B. can reach a broader population

    C. is less expensive

    D. assures more adequate responses

13. Which type of sampling requires the researcher to select every *n*th subject from a list?

    A. random

    B. stratified

    C. systematic

    D. convenience

14. A research design in which the researcher studies the effects of more than one independent variable is called

    A. an experimental design

    B. a factorial design

    C. a quasi-experimental design

    D. a time series design

15. True experiments have which two characteristics?

    A. control group and random assignment

    B. pretest and posttest

    C. pilot study and control group

    D. random selection and random assignment

16. The student's t-test is an example of which type of statistics?

    A. descriptive

    B. inferential

    C. classical

    D. experimental

17. Which of the following is an adequate null hypothesis?

    A. Smoking is important in the development of cancer.

    B. There is a direct relationship between smoking and cancer.

    C. There is a negative relationship between smoking and cancer.

    D. There is no relationship between smoking and cancer.

18. The BEST way to control sequence-relevant extraneous variables is through the use of

    A. a control group

    B. random selection

    C. counterbalancing

    D. analysis of covariance

19. The BEST way to control history as a threat to internal validity is through the use of

    A. a control group

    B. random selection

    C. counterbalancing

    D. analysis of covariance

20. The degree to which the independent variable brings about change in the dependent variable is

    A. internal validity

    B. external validity

    C. reliability

    D. Hawthorne effect

21. While there is no single rule that governs sample size in research, what is the MINIMUM number that is generally recommended for sample size per group to meet the assumptions of certain statistical tests?
    A. 5
    B. 10
    C. 30
    D. 100

22. If two variables have a perfectly positive correlation, the correlation coefficient is
    A. 0
    B. 1
    C. 10
    D. 100
    E. -1

23. Which measure is MOST useful in describing the variability of a distribution?
    A. mean
    B. median
    C. range
    D. standard deviation

24. Which type of sampling BEST enables the researcher to study differences that might exist between different subgroups of a population?
    A. simple random
    B. stratified
    C. systematic
    D. convenience

25. A trial run of a study to determine feasibility and practicality is called a
    A. control study
    B. longitudinal study
    C. placebo
    D. pilot study

26. The number of new cases of a disease over a period of time is called
    A. incidence
    B. prevalence
    C. rate
    D. significance

27. In writing a review of the literature, what type of literature source will MOST likely provide the most current and accurate information?
    A. encyclopedia
    B. literature review
    C. research report
    D. textbook

28. Periodicals include all of the following EXCEPT
    A. journals
    B. magazines
    C. newspapers
    D. textbooks

29. What statistical test is used to determine if there are significant differences between two or more means?
    A. analysis of variance (ANOVA)
    B. chi-square
    C. Pearson r
    D. t-test

30. Simple dental indices measure whether or not a condition exists and do not describe severity. As an index becomes more complex, its use becomes less reliable.
    A. The first statement is true; second statement is false.
    B. The first statement is false; second statement is true.
    C. Both statements are true.
    D. Both statements are false.

31. The Patient Hygiene Performance Index requires that teeth numbered 3, 8, 14, 24, and 30 be scored. If one of the posterior teeth is missing or severely decayed, which tooth is then utilized?

    A. the corresponding tooth on the opposite side of the mouth

    B. the next tooth mesially

    C. the next tooth distally

    D. the corresponding tooth in the opposite jaw

    E. Teeth should not be substituted.

32. Most dental indices utilize which of the following?

    A. nominal/ordinal data

    B. interval/ratio data

33. In a clinical study, the term "washout" refers to which occurrence?

    A. After a given amount of time, groups switch products.

    B. Participant(s) withdraw.

    C. Alike groups are used to compare alike products at different points in time.

    D. A period of time is allowed for effects of agent/product/treatment to dissipate.

34. Questions of internal validity cannot be answered positively unless the research design provides adequate control of extraneous variables. Anything that contributes to the control of a design contributes to its internal validity.

    A. Both statements are true.

    B. Both statements are false.

    C. The first statement is true; second statement is false.

    D. The first statement is false; second statement is true.

Please refer to the excerpt on the following page from a survey of dental faculty to answer questions 35 through 37.

Excerpt from a Survey of Dental Faculty

A. Please indicate your current academic rank:
    ○ Professor   ○ Associate Professor
    ○ Assistant Professor   ○ Instructor

B. What is the year of your birth?

    _____

C. What is your citizenship status?
    ○ United States citizen, native
    ○ United States citizen, naturalized
    ○ Permanent resident of the United States (immigrant visa)
    ○ Temporary resident of the United States (nonimmigrant visa)

D. During the next three years, how likely is it that you will leave this job to:
    ○ Accept a full-time position   Highly Likely ____ ____ ____ Highly Unlikely
       at a different dental school.
    ○ Leave dental education to enter   Highly Likely ____ ____ ____ Highly Unlikely
       a private practice position.
    ○ Retire from the workforce.   Highly Likely ____ ____ ____ Highly Unlikely
    ○ Cut back to part-time teaching.   Highly Likely ____ ____ ____ Highly Unlikely
    ○ Move into an administrative   Highly Likely ____ ____ ____ Highly Unlikely
       position.

E. What is your approximate level of income?
    ○ $25,000–$50,000
    ○ $51,000–$75,000
    ○ $76,000–$100,000

---

35. Question A in the survey utilizes which of the following types of measurement for the answer?

    A. ratio
    B. nominal
    C. ordinal
    D. interval

36. Which question in the survey utilizes a Likert scale to collect data for the answer?

    A. question A
    B. question B
    C. question C
    D. question D
    E. question E

37. Question B in the survey will collect which of the following types of data in the answer?

    A. nominal
    B. ordinal
    C. ratio
    D. interval

38. The y-axis of a graph usually reflects

    A. the variable of interest
    B. scale used to measure the variable of interest
    C. frequency of scores along the scale
    D. cumulative frequency value

39. Which of the following represents the difference between a bar graph and a histogram?

    A. Bar graphs are 2-dimensional; histograms are 3-dimensional.

    B. Bar graphs are used to display nominal/ordinal data; histograms are used to display interval/ratio data.

    C. Bar graphs are used to display continuous data; histograms are used to display discrete data.

    D. Bar graphs are used to compare data pictorially by superimposing two or more distributions; histograms are used to compare data pictorially by superimposing three or more distributions.

40. Which of the following types of samples is LEAST representative?

    A. random

    B. convenience

    C. stratified

    D. systematic

41. Which of the following situations describes a double-blind study?

    A. Both the researcher and the examiners are unaware of the subjects' treatment assignments.

    B. Both the experimental and control group subjects are unaware of their treatment assignments.

    C. The researchers as well as the subjects are unaware of their treatment assignments.

    D. None of the above.

42. Which of the following is characteristic of stratified sampling?

    A. A cross section of subjects is chosen.

    B. There is a large number of subjects.

    C. Subjects are randomly chosen from a previously subdivided population.

    D. Subjects are randomly chosen from individuals with characteristics of interest that represent a subgroup from a defined population.

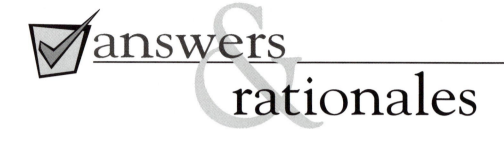

answers & rationales

1.

A. The dependent variable is the response to treatment that is measured in an experiment. In this example, the amount of plaque is measured in response to treatment. The independent variable is the treatment administered in an experiment or the variable that is manipulated by the investigator. In this example, the type of polishing agent used is the independent or experimental variable. Extraneous variables are other uncontrolled variables that are not intended but that influence the dependent variable and effect the results of the study. (1:4; 4:144–145; 151–153)

2.

D. Because of the extremely high scores, the improvement could most likely be accounted for by statistical regression. A variety of factors could account for the initial high scores including unpreparedness or measurement error. One month later, these extreme scores would be expected to regress toward the mean score, even without a plaque control program. Although history, maturation, and instrumentation could affect performance on the second plaque score, these factors would affect both groups. Unless students dropped out of the course, mortality would not be a problem. (1:55–57; 4:116–117)

3.

B. The type of degree from associate degree to doctorate is an example of a variable measured on the ordinal scale. The ordinal scale of measurement provides information about the rank order of objects or persons on some continuum. Although these types of degrees can be rank ordered from low (1) to high (4), there are not equal distances between each level or it

would be considered an interval scale of measurement. (2:120–125; 4:66–67, 211–212, 218)

4.

A. A correlation coefficient is a descriptive statistical measure used to determine the strength of the relationship between two sets of variables. The student's t-test and analysis of variance are parametric tests used to determine if there is a significant difference between two or more means. Chi-square is a nonparametric test used to determine if there are significant differences between groups on a variable which is nominally scaled. (1:116–130; 4:78–79, 106–107, 110)

5.

A. The mode is a measure of central tendency which tells you which response in a distribution occurred most frequently. (2:127; 4:36)

6.

D. Validity is the degree to which an instrument measures what it is designed to measure. Reliability is the consistency of measurement or the degree to which the instrument will produce the same results every time the same characteristic is measured. (2:256, 268; 4:11, 114)

7.

B. The median would best describe the performance of the group because this is a skewed distribution. The one extreme score of 25 would severely affect the mean, making it nonrepresentative of the group. The range is not a measure of central tendency. (2:131–132; 4:88)

314

8.

C. A correlation coefficient of 0 means that there is absolutely no relationship between two variables. The correlation coefficient is a number between -1.0 and +1.0. A correlation coefficient of -.92 represents a very strong inverse relationship between two variables. A correlation coefficient of +.92 represents a very strong direct relationship. (2:152–154; 4:106–107)

9.

D. A significance level of p = .001 indicates that the probability of a difference occurring by chance is approximately 1 in 1000. This is a very highly significant level of confidence. A significance level of p = .05 indicates that the probability of chance occurrence of the observed effect is 5 in 100. (2:186–188)

10.

A. A skewed distribution is one in which there are a few extreme scores, making the curve asymmetrical. A positively skewed distribution has a few extreme scores in the right or positive half of the curve. These extremely high scores pull the mean in their direction, always making the mean higher than the median in a positively skewed distribution. If the distribution is negatively skewed, the mean is pulled toward the direction of the skew, making the mean less than the median. In a normal curve, the mean, median, and mode will have approximately the same numerical value. (1:122; 4:93–97)

11.

B. The standard deviation is a statistic used to measure how the scores in a distribution are scattered around the mean. It is a measure of variability or dispersion. The higher the standard deviation, the greater the amount of variability or dispersion from the mean. (2:138–141; 4:77–78, 89)

12.

D. The interview technique allows the researcher to clarify any questions that are not clear and to discuss responses with participants to assure adequate depth. The disadvantage is that it is time-consuming and more expensive. With the questionnaire, a broader population can be reached simultaneously, requiring less of the researcher's time. (1:80–81)

13.

C. Systematic sampling requires that every nth subject is selected from a list. The entire population size is divided by the desired sample size to determine which nth subject is selected. A stratified sample is used to provide representation of subjects with different characteristics in the sample. A random sample requires the use of a table of random numbers or drawing numbers from a hat. (1:76)

14.

B. A factorial design allows the researcher to simultaneously study more than one independent variable in a single experiment. The advantage of using the factorial design is that it allows the researcher to identify any interaction that might occur when particular variables are combined. (1:70; 4:153–156)

15.

A. True experiments must include at least one control group in addition to the treatment groups. Also, subjects must be randomly assigned to one of these groups. (2:336; 4:134–136)

16.

B. The student's t-test is an example of inferential statistics. Inferential statistics involves the use of statistical tests to make decisions about the population based on data gathered from a sample. Descriptive statistics are used only to summarize and communicate data. (3:148; 4:78–79)

17.

D. A null hypothesis proposes that there is no difference between population groups or that there is no relationship between variables. If a difference is found statistically, then the null hypothesis is rejected. (1:37; 4:165–167)

18.

C. The effects of sequence-relevant variables are a problem when subjects are receiving more than one experimental treatment in a sequence. A design called counterbalancing is used so that half of the subjects receive treatment A, then treatment B. The other half of the subjects are exposed to treatment B, and then treatment A. A washout period is usually required between treatments to avoid a carryover effect from one treatment to the next. (1:63; 4:152–153)

19.

A. The use of a control group will not prevent events from occurring that could affect the dependent variable, but the effect of events would be present in both the control and the experimental groups. The differences found between the two groups could then be attributed to the independent variable. (1:55; 4:144–145, 158)

20.

A. Internal validity is the degree to which the change in the dependent variable is brought about by the independent variable and not by other, extraneous variables. External validity refers to the degree to which the experiment reflects the conditions in the real world. Reliability is consistency of measurement or the degree to which repeated measures with an instrument will produce consistent results. The Hawthorne effect is the inclination for subjects under experimentation to change behavior because of experimental conditions, causing a change in the dependent variable. (1:55–57; 4:144–145, 158)

21.

C. A minimum of 30 subjects must be selected for each sample group to enable the researcher to meet the assumptions of large sample statistics. Generally, the larger the sample size, the more representative it is of the population. (1:78; 4:122, 143, 176–178)

22.

B. Correlation coefficients express the degree and direction of a relationship between variables. The coefficients range from +1.00 through 0 to -1.00. A coefficient of +1.00 represents a perfect positive correlation; -1.00 represents a perfect inverse relationship; and a correlation of 0 indicates that no relationship exists between two variables. (2:147; 4:106–107, 110)

23.

D. The standard deviation describes how widely the scores are distributed about the mean. It takes into account the value of each score. The range describes

the variability of the distribution, but it only takes into account the highest and lowest scores. The mean and median are measures of central tendency, not variability. (2:136–138; 4:77–78, 89)

24.

B. In stratified sampling, the researcher identifies the subgroups of interest and randomly selects a specific number of subjects from each subgroup. (2:172–176; 4:182–184)

25.

D. A pilot study is a preliminary trial using a small sample. The purpose of a pilot study is to assess the feasibility of the data collection and analysis plan. Problems in the process can be corrected before the actual sample is tested. (1:5; 4:140)

26.

A. Incidence is the number of new cases of a disease in a specific population over a period of time. Prevalence is the total number of cases in a specific population. (1:11)

27.

C. Research reports are considered a source of primary literature. These are considered to be more accurate and unbiased sources because they are written by the direct observer of the information. Textbooks and literature reviews are considered secondary sources of literature which is information that has been summarized by another author. Encyclopedias are considered tertiary literature, the most diluted form of information. (1:16–17)

28.

D. Periodicals are sources of literature that are published on a regular basis, usually several times a year. Textbooks are not published on a regular basis and are not considered periodicals. Examples of periodicals are journals, magazines, and newspapers. (1:21)

29.

A. The analysis of variance (ANOVA) is a test that is used to determine differences between two or more means. The t-test is used only to test the differences between two means. The chi-square test is a nonparametric test used with categorical (nominal) data. Pearson r is a correlation coefficient. (2:199; 4:80–81, 90)

30.

C. Simple dental indices measure whether or not a condition exists and do not describe severity. As an index becomes more complex, its use becomes less reliable. However, simple dental indices cannot be measured quantifiably and therefore may not be as accurate for measuring dental disease conditions. (1:93)

31.

C. The teeth that are scored for the Patient Hygiene Performance Index are numbers 3, 8, 14, 24, and 30. If any of the posterior teeth that are to be scored are missing or severely decayed, the next tooth distally can be substituted. Not all dental indices allow for substitutions. (1:97)

32.

A. Most dental indices utilize nominal or ordinal data; however, quantitative comparisons made by researchers cannot always be based on one numerical value in relation to another. (1:93)

33.

D. In a cross-over study, one group will use Product A and the other group will use Product B for a specific period of time. After that time period, the two groups will switch products. If there is no washout period, it would be impossible for the researcher to determine which product was responsible for changes. A washout period is another method of controlling variables and protecting validity. (1:63)

34.

A. A study must be internally valid in order to contribute knowledge to the field. Therefore, any procedures that are utilized by the researcher to control extraneous variables will contribute to the validity of the design. (1:55)

35.

B. A nominal scale is used to organize data into mutually exclusive categories. Each category must be different and the criteria for inclusion into each category must be specified. (1:78)

36.

D. Likert scales can be considered ordinal or interval. Likert scales consist of a series of items worded favorably and unfavorably regarding the construct that is to be assessed. Likert-type scaling is frequently used by social science researchers. A disadvantage of Likert-type scaling is that the respondents may not have similar senses of the magnitude of each response. (4:200)

37.

C. A ratio scale is the highest level of measurement because it contains all of the characteristics of the nominal, ordinal, and interval scales. Common examples of variables measured with a ratio scale are height, age, and weight. (1:79)

38.

C. The x-axis usually reflects the scale employed to measure the variable of interest; the y-axis usually reflects the frequency of scores occurring along the scale of measurement. (1:108)

39.

B. A bar graph is used to pictorially represent nominal or ordinal data that are discrete in nature. A histogram is used to pictorially display interval or ratio scaled variables that are discrete in nature. (1:108)

40.

B. On occasion, access to the total population for study sampling is not feasible. Therefore, the researcher may utilize a readily available population for sampling, known as convenience sampling. However, even with convenience sampling, random assignment should be utilized. Convenience sampling may limit inference of results beyond the sample to the general population. (1:76)

41.

C. In a double-blind study, neither the researchers nor the subjects are aware of their treatment assignments. (1:57)

42.

D. Stratified sampling is the process of sampling subjects that have specific characteristics of interest from a defined population. (1:76)

17 Case Studies

CASE HISTORY I QUESTIONS

1. According to this patient's clinical examination findings, radiographic examination, and periodontal assessment, which periodontal classification is correct?
   A. Case Type I
   B. Case Type II
   C. Case Type III
   D. Case Type IV
   E. Case Type V

2. According to Angle's classification of malocclusion, what type of molar relationship exists in Class I, or neutroclusion?
   A. The buccal groove of the mandibular first permanent molar is mesial to the mesiobuccal cusp of the maxillary first permanent molar by at least the width of a premolar.
   B. The mesiobuccal cusp of the maxillary first permanent molar occludes with the buccal groove of the mandibular first permanent molar.
   C. The buccal groove of the mandibular first permanent molar is distal to the mesiobuccal cusp of the maxillary first permanent molar by at least the width of a premolar.

3. What could be the etiology of the recession (1 mm) found on teeth #6 and 11 (facial surfaces)?
   A. Periodontal infection (periodontitis)
   B. Instrumentation (initial therapy)
   C. Periodontal surgery
   D. Restorative procedures and oral surgery
   E. Orthodontic treatment
   F. Patient Self-Care (incorrect toothbrushing)

4. Susan M. has a DO amalgam on tooth #5. According to G.V. Black's classification of dental restorations, which classification is correct?
   A. Class I
   B. Class II
   C. Class III
   D. Class IV
   E. Class V
   F. Class VI

CASE HISTORY II QUESTIONS

1. The correct periodontal diagnosis for Jane S., based on her clinical examination, radiographic examination, and periodontal assessment is:
   A. Case Type III Periodontitis
   B. NUG (Necrotizing Ulcerative Gingivitis)
   C. NUP (Necrotizing Ulcerative Periodontitis)
   D. Case Type V Refractory Periodontitis

2. What caries classification (according to G.V. Black) is present on the mesial of tooth #6?
   A. Class I
   B. Class II
   C. Class III
   D. Class IV
   E. Class V
   F. Class VI

3. What oral hygiene change should be made immediately by Jane S. to alleviate her symptoms?
   A. She needs to begin flossing.
   B. She needs to rinse with Listerine.
   C. She needs to brush twice daily with a soft nylon brush.
   D. No changes need to be made.

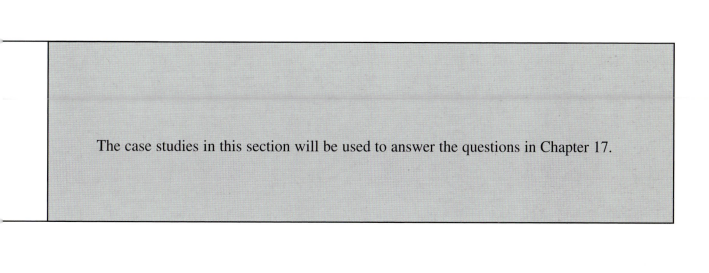

The case studies in this section will be used to answer the questions in Chapter 17.

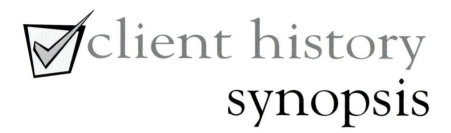

✓client history
synopsis

CASE HISTORY I

PATIENT HISTORY

Susan M. is 21 years old. Her overall health is good. She is aware of the importance of good oral care and brushes daily—after breakfast and after dinner. However, she claims that her work environment doesn't leave her time to brush or floss during the day. (She is a legal secretary.)

CLINICAL EXAMINATION

Susan has 28 natural teeth. She has Class I occlusion and her restorations are not defective. None of the interdental papillae have any visual signs of inflammation such as redness or swelling. Only one of her gingival margins indicates inflammation is present (slight swelling and redness). However, upon probing, an entirely different picture of her gingival health is obtained—gingivitis is confirmed with 19 bleeding sites.

RADIOGRAPHIC EXAMINATION

No loss of alveolar crestal bone. No supragingival or subgingival calculus present. No caries or defective restorations present.

PERIODONTAL ASSESSMENT

No pocket depths exceeding 3 mm.
1 mm recession on teeth # 6, 11 (facial surfaces)
Bleeding upon probing in 19 interdental sites

DIETARY HISTORY

Patient receives adequate intake of Recommended Daily Allowances of all food groups. Patient drinks 3 diet soft drinks per day. Patient denies use of chewing gum or candy.

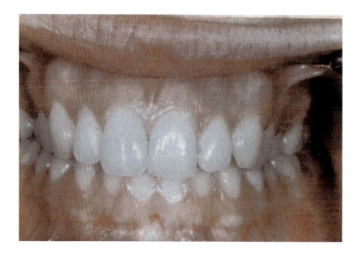

MEDICAL HISTORY

Patient Name	_Case History I_

EACH QUESTION MUST HAVE AN ANSWER. CIRCLE YES OR NO; WRITE IN ANSWERS WHERE APPROPRIATE.

A. GENERAL INFORMATION

* VITAL SIGNS

DATE	HT / WT	BP	HR
	5'3" / 130	128 / 86	72
	/	/	
	/	/	
	/	/	
	/	/	

* 1. Has there been any change in your general health within the past year . . . . YES **(NO)**
* 2. Have you had any serious illness or operation . . . . YES **(NO)**
  3. Have you been hospitalized within the past two (2) years? . . . . YES **(NO)**
  4. Any recent unexplained gain or loss of weight . . . . YES **(NO)**
* 5. If under the care of a physician, give

    Name: _____

    Address: _____

    Phone #: _____

B. CARDIOVASCULAR SYSTEM

DO YOU HAVE OR HAVE YOU HAD:
1. High Blood Pressure . . . . YES **(NO)**
2. Low Blood Pressure . . . . YES **(NO)**
* 3. Heart Attack . . . . YES **(NO)**
* 4. Heart Murmur (congenital heart disease) . . . . YES **(NO)**
* 5. Heart Surgery (bypass, valve) . . . . YES **(NO)**
  6. Shortness of breath . . . . YES **(NO)**
  7. Chest Pain Upon Exertion (angina) . . . . YES **(NO)**
  8. Swollen Ankles . . . . YES **(NO)**
* 9. Rheumatic Heart Disease or Fever . . . . YES **(NO)**
  10. A Stroke . . . . YES **(NO)**
  11. A Pacemaker . . . . YES **(NO)**
  12. Other . . . . YES **(NO)**

C. NERVOUS SYSTEM

DO YOU HAVE OR HAVE YOU HAD:
1. Nervous Breakdown, Psychotherapy . . . . YES **(NO)**
2. Epilepsy or Convulsions . . . . YES **(NO)**
3. Neuritis, Neuralgia, or Numbness . . . . YES **(NO)**
* 4. Fainting Spells or Seizures . . . . YES **(NO)**
  5. Other . . . . YES **(NO)**

D. RESPIRATORY SYSTEM

DO YOU HAVE OR HAVE YOU HAD:
1. Any Respiratory Disease . . . . YES **(NO)**
2. Tuberculosis . . . . YES **(NO)**
3. Sinus Trouble . . . . YES **(NO)**
4. Hay Fever . . . . YES **(NO)**
5. Pneumonia . . . . YES **(NO)**
6. Asthma or Emphysema . . . . YES **(NO)**
7. Chronic Cough, Sore Throat, or Coughing Up Blood . . . . YES **(NO)**
8. Did You Smoke . . . . YES **(NO)**
9. Do You Smoke . . . . YES **(NO)**
10. Other . . . . YES **(NO)**

E. GENITOURINARY SYSTEM

DO YOU HAVE OR HAVE YOU HAD:
1. Kidney Disease . . . . YES **(NO)**
2. Swollen Ankles . . . . YES **(NO)**
3. Difficulty in or Frequent Urination . . . . YES **(NO)**
4. Blood in Your Urine . . . . YES **(NO)**
5. Other . . . . YES **(NO)**

F. GASTROINTESTINAL SYSTEM

DO YOU HAVE OR HAVE YOU HAD:
1. Stomach or Intestinal Trouble . . . . YES **(NO)**
2. Indigestion, Diarrhea, Vomiting, or Constipation . . . . YES **(NO)**
3. Appetite Problem . . . . YES **(NO)**
* 4. Jaundice or Hepatitis . . . . YES **(NO)**
  5. Liver Disease . . . . YES **(NO)**
  6. Ulcers . . . . YES **(NO)**
  7. Other . . . . YES **(NO)**

G. ENDOCRINE SYSTEM

DO YOU HAVE OR HAVE YOU HAD:
* 1. Diabetes . . . . YES **(NO)**
     a. Do you have to urinate frequently . . . . YES **(NO)**
     b. Are you thirsty much of the time . . . . YES **(NO)**
     c. Is your mouth dry . . . . YES **(NO)**
  2. A Thyroid Problem . . . . YES **(NO)**
  3. Parathyroid Problem . . . . YES **(NO)**
  4. Hormone Therapy . . . . YES **(NO)**
  5. Other . . . . YES **(NO)**

H. BONES AND JOINTS

DO YOU HAVE OR HAVE YOU HAD:
1. Arthritis . . . . YES **(NO)**
2. Inflammatory Rheumatism . . . . YES **(NO)**
* 3. Joint Replacement . . . . YES **(NO)**
  4. Back or Neck Injury . . . . YES **(NO)**
  5. Other . . . . YES **(NO)**

I. BLOOD-LYMPHATICS

DO YOU HAVE OR HAVE YOU HAD:
* 1. Blood Disorder or Anemia . . . . YES **(NO)**
* 2. Abnormal Bleeding with Previous Extractions or Surgery . . . . YES **(NO)**
* 3. Transfusions . . . . YES **(NO)**
  4. Bruise Easily . . . . YES **(NO)**
  5. Swollen Lymph Nodes (glands) . . . . YES **(NO)**
  6. Other . . . . YES **(NO)**

J. INFECTIOUS DISEASE

DO YOU HAVE OR HAVE YOU HAD:
* 1. Hepatitis (type A, B, other) . . . . YES **(NO)**
* 2. AIDS, ARC, HIV, ANTI-HIV . . . . YES **(NO)**
* 3. Syphilis, Gonorrhea, Herpes . . . . YES **(NO)**
  4. Acute Pharyngitis (oral or strep) . . . . YES **(NO)**
  5. Childhood Diseases: Rubella, Rubeola, **(Chicken Pox)** Mumps . . . . **(YES)** NO
* 6. Are You or Have You Been an IV Drug User . . . . YES **(NO)**
  7. Other . . . . YES **(NO)**

K. **HEAD, EYES, EARS, NOSE, THROAT**

DO YOU HAVE OR HAVE YOU HAD:
* 1. Head or Jaw Injury .... YES *NO*
  2. Frequent Headaches .... YES *NO*
  3. Dizziness .... YES *NO*
  4. Vision Problems .... YES *NO*
  5. Hearing Problems .... YES *NO*
  6. Nose Bleeds .... YES *NO*
  7. Nasal Obstructions .... YES *NO*
  8. Chronic Sore Throat .... YES *NO*
  9. Halitosis .... YES *NO*
  10. Altered Taste Perceptions .... YES *NO*
  11. Dry Mouth .... YES *NO*
  12. Do You Wear Contact Lenses .... *YES* NO
  13. Other .... YES *NO*

L. **MEDICATIONS**

ARE YOU TAKING ANY OF THE FOLLOWING:
* 1. Antibiotics or Sulfa Drugs .... YES *NO*
* 2. Anticoagulants (blood thinners) .... YES *NO*
* 3. Medicine for High Blood Pressure .... YES *NO*
* 4. Cortisone (steroids) .... YES *NO*
* 5. Tranquilizers .... YES *NO*
* 6. Antihistamines .... YES *NO*
* 7. Aspirin (regular, ongoing basis) .... YES *NO*
* 8. Insulin, Orinase, or Similar Drug .... YES *NO*
* 9. Digitalis or Other Heart Drug .... YES *NO*
* 10. Nitroglycerin .... YES *NO*
* 11. Chemotherapy .... YES *NO*
* 12. Chemically Dependent (alcohol, drugs) ...... YES *NO*
* 13. Diet pills (Fen-phen, Dexfenfluramine) ..... YES *NO*
* 14. Other Medications .... YES *NO*

M. **ALLERGIES**

ARE YOU ALLERGIC TO OR HAD A REACTION TO:
* 1. Local Anesthetic (novocaine, etc.) .... YES *NO*
* 2. Penicillin, Sulfa Drugs or Other Antibiotics .... YES *NO*
* 3. Latex .... YES *NO*
* 4. Barbiturates, Sleeping Pills .... YES *NO*
* 5. Aspirin .... YES *NO*
* 6. Iodine .... YES *NO*
* 7. Codeine or Other Narcotics .... YES *NO*
* 8. Metals (rings, earrings, etc.) .... YES *NO*
* 9. Other Allergies .... YES *NO*

N. **RADIATION HISTORY**

1. Are you employed in any situation which exposes you to X-rays or other ionizing radiation? .... YES *NO*
* 2. Have you had radiation therapy .... YES *NO*

O. **DENTAL HISTORY**

* Are you having dental pain or discomfort at this time? .... YES *NO*
If you wear dentures, go to question #14.

DO YOU HAVE OR HAVE YOU HAD:
1. Frequent Toothaches .... YES *NO*
2. Periodontal (gum) Disease *gingivitis* ..... *YES* NO
3. Orthodontic Treatment .... YES *NO*
4. Difficulty in Opening or Closing Your Jaw .. YES *NO*
5. Grinding or Clenching Your Teeth .... YES *NO*
6. Chronic Facial Pain .... YES *NO*
7. Do You Brush Daily .... *YES* NO
8. Do You Floss Daily .... YES *NO*
9. Do You Want To Keep Your Teeth .... *YES* NO
10. Does Having Dental Treatment Make You Nervous .... YES *NO*
11. Have you had a bad experience in a dental office .... YES *NO*
12. Have Your Dental Experiences in General Been (circle) *GOOD* AVERAGE, POOR
13. Children
    Fluoride (Dietary Hx) .... *YES* NO
    Oral Habits .... YES *NO*
    Birth History Normal .... *YES* NO
14. Denture History
    a. Do You Think You Need Dentures .... YES *NO*
    b. How Long Have You Worn Dentures _____
    c. How Old Are Your Present Dentures_____

P. **WOMEN**

* Are You Pregnant .... YES *NO*

DO YOU HAVE OR HAVE YOU HAD:
1. Menstrual Problems .... YES *NO*
2. Breast Cancer/Tumor .... YES *NO*
* 3. Are You Taking Birth Control Pills .... YES *NO*
4. Have You Been Through Menopause .... YES *NO*
5. Other .... YES *NO*

Do you have any disease condition or problem not listed .... YES *NO*

_____
_____

To the best of my knowledge, all of the preceding answers are true and correct. If I ever have any change in my health, or if my medicines change, I will inform the faculty or student at the next appointment without fail.

* _____   * _____   * _____   * _____

Date   Student Signature   Faculty Signature   Signature of Patient, Parent, or Guardian.

MEDICAL HISTORY/PHYSICAL EVALUATION UPDATE

Date	Changes (See Comments)	Student Signature	Faculty Signature
_____	YES NO	_____	_____
_____	YES NO	_____	_____
_____	YES NO	_____	_____
_____	YES NO	_____	_____

ADULT EXISTING CONDITIONS

DATE _____

| Patient Name | *Case History I* |

Date	1	2	3	4	5	6	7	8	9	10	11	12	13	14	15	16
			.00.	.00.	.00.	no	depths	over	3 mm.			.00.	.00.			

F

L

Date	1	2	3	4	5	6	7	8	9	10	11	12	13	14	15	16
						no	depths	over	3 mm.							

1 mm. recession facials #6 + #11

Date	Tooth #	Cold[1]	Hot[1]	Perc[1]	Palp[1]	Ept No.	Pulp Diag.	Peri Diag.

[1]Use: + = norm.   0 = no res.   ++= abnorm. pos.

PULPAL DIAGNOSIS
N - Vital, normal
R - Reversible pulp infl.
I - Irreversible pulp infl.
NP - Necrotic pulp
O - Other

PERIAPICAL DIAGNOSIS
N - Normal
AP - Acute apical periodontitis
C - Chronic apical periodontitis
S - Chronic suppurative apical periodontitis
AA - Acute apical abscess
P - Periradicular osteosclerosis

PERIO DIAGNOSIS
Case Type [ ]   Prophy [ ]   Perio [ ]

Date	32	31	30	29	28	27	26	25	24	23	22	21	20	19	18	17
						no	depths	over	3 mm.							

L

F

Date	32	31	30	29	28	27	26	25	24	23	22	21	20	19	18	17
				0	no	depths	over 3mm.	00,	00,	00.				.00		

INITIAL TMD FINDINGS

Mandibular Range of Motion

☐Yes ☐No   Maximum vertical opening < 40mm
☐Yes ☐No   Lateral movements < 7mm
☐Yes ☐No   Differences between R and L
            lateral movement ≥ 2mm
☐Yes ☐No   Pain with any of the above
☐Yes ☐No   History of "Jaw Locking"
☐Yes ☐No   Past history of TMJ/TMD

Pain on Palpation

☐Yes ☐No   Lateral TMJ   R   L
☐Yes ☐No   Masseter   R   L
☐Yes ☐No   Temporalis   R   L
☐Yes ☐No   Coronoid process   R   L

Joint Sounds

☐Yes ☐No   Right TM Joint
☐Yes ☐No   Left TM Joint

Mandibular Deviation/Deflection

☐Yes ☐No   Opening > 2mm
☐Yes ☐No   Protrusion > 2mm

Panoramic evaluation suggests osseous changes
(erosion, flattening)
☐Yes ☐No   R   L

_____
_____
_____
_____

EXTRAORAL SOFT TISSUE FINDINGS:

_____
_____
_____

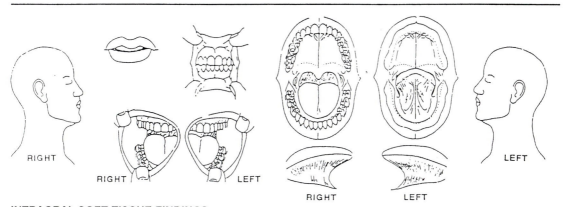

RIGHT   RIGHT   LEFT   RIGHT   LEFT   LEFT

INTRAORAL SOFT TISSUE FINDINGS:

_____
_____
_____

INITIAL OCCLUSAL FINDINGS

Angle's Molar Classification

☐Class I   R   L
☐Class II   R   L
☐Class III   R   L

☐Yes ☐No   Group function   R   L
☐Yes ☐No   Canine guidance   R   L

☐Yes ☐No   Reverse (R) articulation
☐Yes ☐No   Wear facets

ADDITIONAL OCCLUSAL FINDINGS

☐Yes ☐No   Horizontal overlap   ___mm
☐Yes ☐No   Vertical overlap   ___mm

☐Yes ☐No   CO to MIP discrepancies
    Ant._____mm   Vert._____mm
    Right_____mm   Left_____mm

Nonworking (N) Interferences
    ☐Yes ☐No   right side
    ☐Yes ☐No   left side

Protrusive (P) Interferences
    ☐Yes ☐No   right side
    ☐Yes ☐No   left side

PLEASE CIRCLE INITIAL (I) CONTACTS AND ANY INTERFERENCES (N,P) OR REVERSE (R) ARTICULATIONS.

1	2	3	4	5	6	7	8	9	10	11	12	13	14	15	16
32	31	30	29	28	27	26	25	24	23	22	21	20	19	18	17

4C

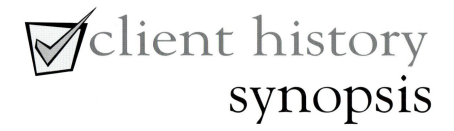

☑ client history synopsis

CASE HISTORY II

PATIENT HISTORY

Jane S. is a 17-year-old high school student. As a work-study student, she attends school half a day and works at a Dairy Queen the other half of the day. She rarely eats at home and is never in bed before 12:00 a.m. She is underweight and smokes 2 packs per day. She drinks beer occasionally. She states that her gums bleed and hurt to the extent that she has trouble eating. She tries to brush her teeth once a day using a hard bristle toothbrush. She has never used dental floss.

CLINICAL EXAMINATION

Jane had never had any previous dental treatment. Carious lesions were found on teeth #6, 11, 14, 19, 30, and 31. Scant amounts of supragingival calculus were noted; however, heavy subgingival calculus was found generalized throughout the mouth. The patient was found to have foul mouth odor. The gingiva was found to spontaneously hemorrhage.

RADIOGRAPHIC EXAMINATION

Carious lesions were found interproximally on teeth #5, 12, 13, 21, 28, and 29. Subgingival calculus was found generalized throughout the mouth. Moderate loss of alveolar bone was generalized throughout the mouth. No restorations were present.

PERIODONTAL ASSESSMENT

A generalized absence of interdental papillae was noted throughout the mouth. The gingiva was edematous, demonstrated a loss of stippling, and bled immediately upon probing. Generalized 4–5 mm pockets were found throughout the mouth.

DIETARY HISTORY

The patient has been referred to a nutritionist for dietary counseling by the school nurse. She states she only eats 1 meal per day, which often consists of just ice cream.

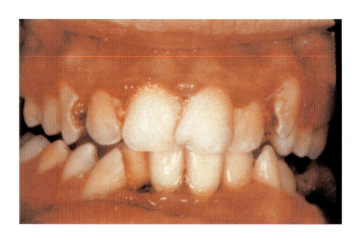

MEDICAL HISTORY

Patient Name 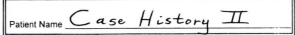 *Case History II*

EACH QUESTION MUST HAVE AN ANSWER. CIRCLE YES OR NO; WRITE IN ANSWERS WHERE APPROPRIATE.

A. GENERAL INFORMATION

* VITAL SIGNS

DATE	HT / WT	BP	HR
	5'4", 98	98 / 56	69
	/	/	
	/	/	
	/	/	
	/	/	

* 1. Has there been any change in your general health within the past year .... YES (NO)

* 2. Have you had any serious illness or operation .... YES (NO)

3. Have you been hospitalized within the past two (2) years? .... YES (NO)

4. Any recent unexplained gain or loss of weight .... (YES) NO

* 5. If under the care of a physician, give

Name: _____

Address: _____

Phone #: _____

B. CARDIOVASCULAR SYSTEM

DO YOU HAVE OR HAVE YOU HAD:

1. High Blood Pressure .... YES (NO)
2. Low Blood Pressure .... (YES) NO
* 3. Heart Attack .... YES (NO)
* 4. Heart Murmur (congenital heart disease) .... YES (NO)
* 5. Heart Surgery (bypass, valve) .... YES (NO)
6. Shortness of breath .... YES (NO)
7. Chest Pain Upon Exertion (angina) .... YES (NO)
8. Swollen Ankles .... YES (NO)
* 9. Rheumatic Heart Disease or Fever .... YES (NO)
10. A Stroke .... YES (NO)
11. A Pacemaker .... YES (NO)
12. Other .... YES (NO)

C. NERVOUS SYSTEM

DO YOU HAVE OR HAVE YOU HAD:

1. Nervous Breakdown, Psychotherapy .... YES (NO)
2. Epilepsy or Convulsions .... YES (NO)
3. Neuritis, Neuralgia, or Numbness .... YES (NO)
* 4. Fainting Spells or Seizures .... YES (NO)
5. Other .... YES (NO)

D. RESPIRATORY SYSTEM

DO YOU HAVE OR HAVE YOU HAD:

1. Any Respiratory Disease .... YES (NO)
2. Tuberculosis .... YES (NO)
3. Sinus Trouble .... YES (NO)
4. Hay Fever .... YES (NO)
5. Pneumonia .... YES (NO)
6. Asthma or Emphysema .... YES (NO)
7. Chronic Cough, Sore Throat, or Coughing Up Blood .... YES (NO)
8. Did You Smoke .... (YES) NO
9. Do You Smoke *2 packs / day* .... (YES) NO
10. Other .... YES (NO)

E. GENITOURINARY SYSTEM

DO YOU HAVE OR HAVE YOU HAD:

1. Kidney Disease .... YES (NO)
2. Swollen Ankles .... YES (NO)
3. Difficulty in or Frequent Urination .... YES (NO)
4. Blood in Your Urine .... YES (NO)
5. Other .... YES (NO)

F. GASTROINTESTINAL SYSTEM

DO YOU HAVE OR HAVE YOU HAD:

1. Stomach or Intestinal Trouble .... YES (NO)
2. Indigestion, Diarrhea, Vomiting, or Constipation .... YES (NO)
3. Appetite Problem .... (YES) NO
* 4. Jaundice or Hepatitis .... YES (NO)
5. Liver Disease .... YES (NO)
6. Ulcers .... YES (NO)
7. Other .... YES (NO)

G. ENDOCRINE SYSTEM

DO YOU HAVE OR HAVE YOU HAD:

* 1. Diabetes .... YES (NO)
    a. Do you have to urinate frequently .... YES (NO)
    b. Are you thirsty much of the time .... YES (NO)
    c. Is your mouth dry .... YES (NO)
2. A Thyroid Problem .... YES (NO)
3. Parathyroid Problem .... YES (NO)
4. Hormone Therapy .... YES (NO)
5. Other .... YES (NO)

H. BONES AND JOINTS

DO YOU HAVE OR HAVE YOU HAD:

1. Arthritis .... YES (NO)
2. Inflammatory Rheumatism .... YES (NO)
* 3. Joint Replacement .... YES (NO)
4. Back or Neck Injury .... YES (NO)
5. Other .... YES (NO)

I. BLOOD-LYMPHATICS

DO YOU HAVE OR HAVE YOU HAD:

* 1. Blood Disorder or Anemia .... YES (NO)
* 2. Abnormal Bleeding with Previous Extractions or Surgery .... YES (NO)
* 3. Transfusions .... YES (NO)
4. Bruise Easily .... YES (NO)
5. Swollen Lymph Nodes (glands) .... YES (NO)
6. Other .... YES (NO)

J. INFECTIOUS DISEASE

DO YOU HAVE OR HAVE YOU HAD:

* 1. Hepatitis (type A, B, other) .... YES (NO)
* 2. AIDS, ARC, HIV, ANTI-HIV .... YES (NO)
* 3. Syphilis, Gonorrhea, Herpes .... YES (NO)
4. Acute Pharyngitis (oral or strep) .... YES (NO)
5. Childhood Diseases: Rubella, Rubeola, (Chicken Pox) Mumps .... (YES) NO
* 6. Are You or Have You Been an IV Drug User .... YES (NO)
7. Other .... YES (NO)

3 A

K. HEAD, EYES, EARS, NOSE, THROAT

DO YOU HAVE OR HAVE YOU HAD:

* 1. Head or Jaw Injury .... YES (NO)
2. Frequent Headaches .... YES (NO)
3. Dizziness .... YES (NO)
4. Vision Problems .... YES (NO)
5. Hearing Problems .... YES (NO)
6. Nose Bleeds .... YES (NO)
7. Nasal Obstructions .... YES (NO)
8. Chronic Sore Throat .... YES (NO)
9. Halitosis .... (YES) NO
10. Altered Taste Perceptions .... (YES) NO
11. Dry Mouth .... YES (NO)
12. Do You Wear Contact Lenses .... YES (NO)
13. Other .... YES (NO)

L. MEDICATIONS

ARE YOU TAKING ANY OF THE FOLLOWING:

* 1. Antibiotics or Sulfa Drugs .... YES (NO)
* 2. Anticoagulants (blood thinners) .... YES (NO)
* 3. Medicine for High Blood Pressure ... YES (NO)
* 4. Cortisone (steroids) .... YES (NO)
* 5. Tranquilizers .... YES (NO)
* 6. Antihistamines .... YES (NO)
* 7. Aspirin (regular, ongoing basis) ... YES (NO)
* 8. Insulin, Orinase, or Similar Drug .. YES (NO)
* 9. Digitalis or Other Heart Drug ...... YES (NO)
* 10. Nitroglycerin .... YES (NO)
* 11. Chemotherapy .... YES (NO)
* 12. Chemically Dependent (alcohol, drugs) ... YES (NO)
* 13. Diet pills (Fen-phen, Dexfenfluramine) ... YES (NO)
* 14. Other Medications .... YES (NO)

M. ALLERGIES

ARE YOU ALLERGIC TO OR HAD A REACTION TO:

* 1. Local Anesthetic (novocaine, etc.) .... YES (NO)
* 2. Penicillin, Sulfa Drugs or Other Antibiotics ... YES (NO)
* 3. Latex .... YES (NO)
* 4. Barbiturates, Sleeping Pills .... YES (NO)
* 5. Aspirin .... YES (NO)
* 6. Iodine .... YES (NO)
* 7. Codeine or Other Narcotics .... YES (NO)
* 8. Metals (rings, earrings, etc.) .... YES (NO)
* 9. Other Allergies .... YES (NO)

N. RADIATION HISTORY

1. Are you employed in any situation which exposes you to X-rays or other ionizing radiation? ... YES (NO)
* 2. Have you had radiation therapy .... YES (NO)

O. DENTAL HISTORY

* Are you having dental pain or discomfort at this time? *my gums hurt* (YES) NO
If you wear dentures, go to question #14.

DO YOU HAVE OR HAVE YOU HAD:

1. Frequent Toothaches .... (YES) NO
2. Periodontal (gum) Disease .... (YES) NO
3. Orthodontic Treatment .... YES (NO)
4. Difficulty in Opening or Closing Your Jaw ... YES (NO)
5. Grinding or Clenching Your Teeth ... YES (NO)
6. Chronic Facial Pain .... YES (NO)
7. Do You Brush Daily *1 X* .... (YES) NO
8. Do You Floss Daily .... YES (NO)
9. Do You Want To Keep Your Teeth ... (YES) NO
10. Does Having Dental Treatment Make You Nervous ... (YES) NO
11. Have you had a bad experience in a dental office ... YES (NO)
12. Have Your Dental Experiences in General Been (circle) GOOD, AVERAGE, POOR *I have never been to the dentist.*
13. Children
Fluoride (Dietary Hx) .... YES (NO)
Oral Habits .... YES (NO)
Birth History Normal .... (YES) NO
14. Denture History
a. Do You Think You Need Dentures ... YES (NO)
b. How Long Have You Worn Dentures ____
c. How Old Are Your Present Dentures ____

P. WOMEN

* Are You Pregnant .... YES (NO)

DO YOU HAVE OR HAVE YOU HAD:

1. Menstrual Problems .... YES (NO)
2. Breast Cancer/Tumor .... YES (NO)
* 3. Are You Taking Birth Control Pills ... YES (NO)
4. Have You Been Through Menopause ... YES (NO)
5. Other .... YES (NO)

Do you have any disease condition or problem not listed ... YES (NO)

_____
_____
_____

To the best of my knowledge, all of the preceding answers are true and correct. If I ever have any change in my health, or if my medicines change, I will inform the faculty or student at the next appointment without fail.

* _____ * _____ * _____ * _____

Date | Student Signature | Faculty Signature | Signature of Patient, Parent, or Guardian.

MEDICAL HISTORY/PHYSICAL EVALUATION UPDATE

Date	Changes (See Comments)	Student Signature	Faculty Signature
_____	YES NO	_____	_____
_____	YES NO	_____	_____
_____	YES NO	_____	_____
_____	YES NO	_____	_____

ADULT EXISTING CONDITIONS

DATE _____

Patient Name Case History II

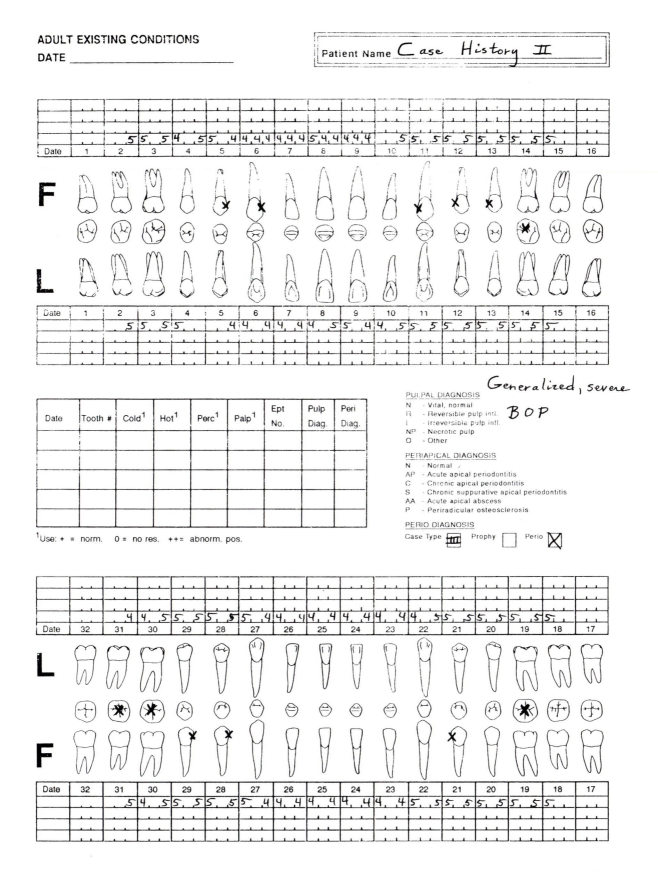

Date	1	2	3	4	5	6	7	8	9	10	11	12	13	14	15	16

F

L

Date	1	2	3	4	5	6	7	8	9	10	11	12	13	14	15	16

Date	Tooth #	Cold[1]	Hot[1]	Perc[1]	Palp[1]	Ept No.	Pulp Diag.	Peri Diag.

[1]Use: + = norm.   0 = no res.   ++= abnorm. pos.

Generalized, severe
BOP

PULPAL DIAGNOSIS
N - Vital, normal
R - Reversible pulp infl.
I - Irreversible pulp infl.
NP - Necrotic pulp
O - Other

PERIAPICAL DIAGNOSIS
N - Normal
AP - Acute apical periodontitis
C - Chronic apical periodontitis
S - Chronic suppurative apical periodontitis
AA - Acute apical abscess
P - Periradicular osteosclerosis

PERIO DIAGNOSIS
Case Type [▥]   Prophy [ ]   Perio [✗]

Date	32	31	30	29	28	27	26	25	24	23	22	21	20	19	18	17

L

F

Date	32	31	30	29	28	27	26	25	24	23	22	21	20	19	18	17

4C

INITIAL TMD FINDINGS

Mandibular Range of Motion
- ☐Yes ☐No Maximum vertical opening < 40mm
- ☐Yes ☐No Lateral movements < 7mm
- ☐Yes ☐No Differences between R and L
  lateral movement ≥ 2mm
- ☐Yes ☐No Pain with any of the above
- ☐Yes ☐No History of "Jaw Locking"
- ☐Yes ☐No Past history of TMJ/TMD

Pain on Palpation
- ☐Yes ☐No Lateral TMJ   R   L
- ☐Yes ☐No Masseter   R   L
- ☐Yes ☐No Temporalis   R   L
- ☐Yes ☐No Coronoid process   R   L

Joint Sounds
- ☐Yes ☐No Right TM Joint
- ☐Yes ☐No Left TM Joint

Mandibular Deviation/Deflection
- ☐Yes ☐No Opening > 2mm
- ☐Yes ☐No Protrusion > 2mm

Panoramic evaluation suggests osseous changes
(erosion, flattening)
- ☐Yes ☐No   R   L

_____
_____
_____
_____

EXTRAORAL SOFT TISSUE FINDINGS:

_____
_____
_____

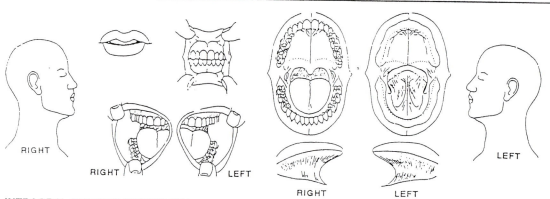

RIGHT   RIGHT   LEFT   RIGHT   LEFT   LEFT

INTRAORAL SOFT TISSUE FINDINGS:

_____
_____
_____

INITIAL OCCLUSAL FINDINGS

Angle's Molar Classification
- ☐Class I   R   L
- ☐Class II   R   L
- ☐Class III   R   L

- ☐Yes ☐No Group function   R   L
- ☐Yes ☐No Canine guidance   R   L

- ☐Yes ☐No Reverse (R) articulation
- ☐Yes ☐No Wear facets

ADDITIONAL OCCLUSAL FINDINGS

- ☐Yes ☐No Horizontal overlap   ___mm
- ☐Yes ☐No Vertical overlap   ___mm

- ☐Yes ☐No CO to MIP discrepancies
  Ant._____mm Vert._____mm
  Right_____mm Left_____mm

Nonworking (N) Interferences
- ☐Yes ☐No right side
- ☐Yes ☐No left side

Protrusive (P) Interferences
- ☐Yes ☐No right side
- ☐Yes ☐No left side

PLEASE CIRCLE INITIAL (I) CONTACTS AND ANY INTERFERENCES (N,P) OR REVERSE (R) ARTICULATIONS.

1	2	3	4	5	6	7	8	9	10	11	12	13	14	15	16
32	31	30	29	28	27	26	25	24	23	22	21	20	19	18	17

4C

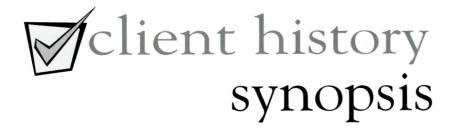

client history
synopsis

CASE HISTORY III

PATIENT HISTORY

Mrs. Jones is a 69-year-old widow whose only income is Social Security. She has had two previous heart attacks and is an insulin-dependent diabetic. She has no living family members and lives alone on a farm. The patient states she brushes her teeth whenever she gets around to it.

CLINICAL EXAMINATION

Mrs. Jones states that her last dental examination was 20 years ago. She states that she has had several fillings fall out over the years and that she has pulled three mandibular molars herself (after they became loose). She states that she wants her teeth fixed—even if they all have to be extracted and she has to have dentures.

RADIOGRAPHIC EXAMINATION

Extensive vertical bone loss was found on teeth #24 and 25 with periapical lesions on each tooth. The patient had severe generalized loss of alveolar crestal bone on all remaining teeth. Heavy subgingival calculus was generalized and supragingival calculus was found on the mandibular teeth.

PERIODONTAL ASSESSMENT

Ten millimeter pockets were located on the mesial and distal of teeth #24 and 25. Class III mobility was found on #24 and 25. Tooth #8 exhibited Class I mobility. Heavy plaque, calculus, and materia alba were generalized throughout the mouth. Gingiva was markedly inflamed in the mandibular right quadrant with generalized severe bleeding throughout the mouth.

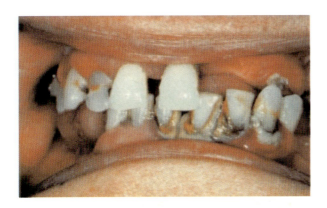

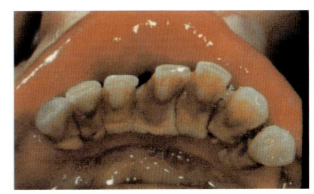

MEDICAL HISTORY

Patient Name __Case History III__

EACH QUESTION MUST HAVE AN ANSWER. CIRCLE YES OR NO; WRITE IN ANSWERS WHERE APPROPRIATE.

A. | GENERAL INFORMATION |

* VITAL SIGNS

DATE	HT / WT	BP	HR
	5'6" / 150	138 / 92	79
	/	/	
	/	/	
	/	/	
	/	/	

* 1. Has there been any change in your general health within the past year _Heart attack_ (YES) NO

* 2. Have you had any serious illness or operation _Diabetes, 2 heart attacks_ (YES) NO

3. Have you been hospitalized within the past two (2) years? _Heart attack_ (YES) NO

4. Any recent unexplained gain or loss of weight .... YES (NO)

* 5. If under the care of a physician, give

Name: __Dr. Jones__

Address: _____

Phone #: _____

B. | CARDIOVASCULAR SYSTEM |

DO YOU HAVE OR HAVE YOU HAD:
1. High Blood Pressure .... YES (NO)
2. Low Blood Pressure .... YES (NO)
* 3. Heart Attack _1984 , 1999_ .... (YES) NO
* 4. Heart Murmur (congenital heart disease) .... YES (NO)
* 5. Heart Surgery (bypass, valve) .... YES (NO)
6. Shortness of breath .... YES (NO)
7. Chest Pain Upon Exertion (angina) .... YES (NO)
8. Swollen Ankles .... (YES) NO
* 9. Rheumatic Heart Disease or Fever .... YES (NO)
10. A Stroke .... YES (NO)
11. A Pacemaker .... YES (NO)
12. Other .... YES (NO)

C. | NERVOUS SYSTEM |

DO YOU HAVE OR HAVE YOU HAD:
1. Nervous Breakdown, Psychotherapy .... YES (NO)
2. Epilepsy or Convulsions .... YES (NO)
3. Neuritis, Neuralgia, or Numbness .... YES (NO)
* 4. Fainting Spells or Seizures .... YES (NO)
5. Other .... YES (NO)

D. | RESPIRATORY SYSTEM |

DO YOU HAVE OR HAVE YOU HAD:
1. Any Respiratory Disease .... YES (NO)
2. Tuberculosis .... YES (NO)
3. Sinus Trouble .... YES (NO)
4. Hay Fever .... YES (NO)
5. Pneumonia .... YES (NO)
6. Asthma or Emphysema .... YES (NO)
7. Chronic Cough, Sore Throat, or Coughing Up Blood .... YES (NO)
8. Did You Smoke .... YES (NO)
9. Do You Smoke .... YES (NO)
10. Other .... YES (NO)

E. | GENITOURINARY SYSTEM |

DO YOU HAVE OR HAVE YOU HAD:
1. Kidney Disease .... YES (NO)
2. Swollen Ankles .... YES (NO)
3. Difficulty in or Frequent Urination .... YES (NO)
4. Blood in Your Urine .... YES (NO)
5. Other .... YES (NO)

F. | GASTROINTESTINAL SYSTEM |

DO YOU HAVE OR HAVE YOU HAD:
1. Stomach or Intestinal Trouble .... YES (NO)
2. Indigestion, Diarrhea, Vomiting, or Constipation .... YES (NO)
3. Appetite Problem .... YES (NO)
* 4. Jaundice or Hepatitis .... YES (NO)
5. Liver Disease .... YES (NO)
6. Ulcers .... YES (NO)
7. Other .... YES (NO)

G. | ENDOCRINE SYSTEM |

DO YOU HAVE OR HAVE YOU HAD:
* 1. Diabetes _Insulin - dependent_ .... (YES) NO
   a. Do you have to urinate frequently .... (YES) NO
   b. Are you thirsty much of the time .... (YES) NO
   c. Is your mouth dry .... (YES) NO
2. A Thyroid Problem .... YES (NO)
3. Parathyroid Problem .... YES (NO)
4. Hormone Therapy .... YES (NO)
5. Other .... YES (NO)

H. | BONES AND JOINTS |

DO YOU HAVE OR HAVE YOU HAD:
1. Arthritis .... YES (NO)
2. Inflammatory Rheumatism .... YES (NO)
* 3. Joint Replacement .... YES (NO)
4. Back or Neck Injury .... YES (NO)
5. Other .... YES (NO)

I. | BLOOD-LYMPHATICS |

DO YOU HAVE OR HAVE YOU HAD:
* 1. Blood Disorder or Anemia .... YES (NO)
* 2. Abnormal Bleeding with Previous Extractions or Surgery .... YES (NO)
* 3. Transfusions .... YES (NO)
* 4. Bruise Easily .... YES (NO)
5. Swollen Lymph Nodes (glands) .... YES (NO)
6. Other .... YES (NO)

J. | INFECTIOUS DISEASE |

DO YOU HAVE OR HAVE YOU HAD:
* 1. Hepatitis (type A, B, other) .... YES (NO)
* 2. AIDS, ARC, HIV, ANTI-HIV .... YES (NO)
* 3. Syphilis, Gonorrhea, Herpes .... YES (NO)
4. Acute Pharyngitis (oral or strep) .... YES (NO)
5. Childhood Diseases (Rubella) Rubeola, (Chicken Pox,) Mumps .... (YES) NO
* 6. Are You or Have You Been an IV Drug User .... YES (NO)
7. Other .... YES (NO)

K. **HEAD, EYES, EARS, NOSE, THROAT**

DO YOU HAVE OR HAVE YOU HAD:
* 1. Head or Jaw Injury . . . . YES (NO)
  2. Frequent Headaches . . . . YES (NO)
  3. Dizziness . . . . YES (NO)
  4. Vision Problems . . . . YES (NO)
  5. Hearing Problems . . . . YES (NO)
  6. Nose Bleeds . . . . YES (NO)
  7. Nasal Obstructions . . . . YES (NO)
  8. Chronic Sore Throat . . . . YES (NO)
  9. Halitosis . . . . (YES) NO
  10. Altered Taste Perceptions . . . . (YES) NO
  11. Dry Mouth . . . . (YES) NO
  12. Do You Wear Contact Lenses . . . . YES (NO)
  13. Other . . . . YES NO

L. **MEDICATIONS**

ARE YOU TAKING ANY OF THE FOLLOWING:
* 1. Antibiotics or Sulfa Drugs . . . . YES (NO)
* 2. Anticoagulants (blood thinners) *Coumadin* (YES) NO
* 3. Medicine for High Blood Pressure *H.C.T.* (YES) NO
* 4. Cortisone (steroids) . . . . YES (NO)
* 5. Tranquilizers . . . . YES (NO)
* 6. Antihistamines . . . . YES (NO)
* 7. Aspirin (regular, ongoing basis) *1/day* (YES) NO
* 8. (Insulin) Orinase, or Similar Drug . . . . . (YES) NO
* 9. Digitalis or Other Heart Drug . . . . YES (NO)
* 10. Nitroglycerin . . . . YES (NO)
* 11. Chemotherapy . . . . YES (NO)
* 12. Chemically Dependent (alcohol, drugs) . YES (NO)
* 13. Diet pills (Fen-phen, Dexfenfluramine) . YES (NO)
* 14. Other Medications . . . . YES (NO)

M. **ALLERGIES**

ARE YOU ALLERGIC TO OR HAD A REACTION TO:
* 1. Local Anesthetic (novocaine, etc.) . . . . YES (NO)
* 2. Penicillin, Sulfa Drugs or Other Antibiotics YES (NO)
* 3. Latex . . . . YES (NO)
* 4. Barbiturates, Sleeping Pills . . . . YES (NO)
* 5. Aspirin . . . . YES (NO)
* 6. Iodine . . . . YES (NO)
* 7. Codeine or Other Narcotics . . . . YES (NO)
* 8. Metals (rings, earrings, etc.) . . . . YES (NO)
* 9. Other Allergies . . . . YES (NO)

N. **RADIATION HISTORY**

* 1. Are you employed in any situation which exposes you to X-rays or other ionizing radiation? . . . . YES (NO)
* 2. Have you had radiation therapy . . . . . . YES (NO)

O. **DENTAL HISTORY**

* Are you having dental pain or discomfort at this time? . . . . (YES) NO
If you wear dentures, go to question #14.

DO YOU HAVE OR HAVE YOU HAD:
  1. Frequent Toothaches . . . . (YES) NO
  2. Periodontal (gum) Disease . . . . (YES) NO
  3. Orthodontic Treatment . . . . YES (NO)
  4. Difficulty in Opening or Closing Your Jaw . . . . YES (NO)
  5. Grinding or Clenching Your Teeth . . . . YES (NO)
  6. Chronic Facial Pain . . . . YES (NO)
  7. Do You Brush Daily . . . . YES (NO)
  8. Do You Floss Daily . . . . YES (NO)
  9. Do You Want To Keep Your Teeth *If I can.* (YES) NO
  10. Does Having Dental Treatment Make You Nervous . . . . YES (NO)
  11. Have you had a bad experience in a dental office . . . . (YES) NO
  12. Have Your Dental Experiences in General Been (circle) GOOD, (AVERAGE,) POOR
  13. Children
      Fluoride (Dietary Hx) . . . . YES (NO)
      Oral Habits . . . . YES (NO)
      Birth History Normal . . . . (YES) NO
  14. Denture History
      a. Do You Think You Need Dentures . . . (YES) NO
      b. How Long Have You Worn Dentures ___
      c. How Old Are Your Present Dentures ___

P. **WOMEN**

* Are You Pregnant . . . . YES (NO)

DO YOU HAVE OR HAVE YOU HAD:
  1. Menstrual Problems . . . . YES (NO)
  2. Breast Cancer/Tumor . . . . YES (NO)
* 3. Are You Taking Birth Control Pills . . . . . YES (NO)
  4. Have You Been Through Menopause . . . (YES) NO
  5. Other . . . . YES (NO)

Do you have any disease condition or problem not listed . . . . YES (NO)

_____
_____
_____

To the best of my knowledge, all of the preceding answers are true and correct. If I ever have any change in my health, or if my medicines change, I will inform the faculty or student at the next appointment without fail.

*_____   *_____   *_____   *_____

_____
Date   Student Signature   Faculty Signature   Signature of Patient, Parent, or Guardian.

MEDICAL HISTORY/PHYSICAL EVALUATION UPDATE

Date	Changes (See Comments)	Student Signature	Faculty Signature
_____	YES NO	_____	_____
_____	YES NO	_____	_____
_____	YES NO	_____	_____
_____	YES NO	_____	_____

3 A

ADULT EXISTING CONDITIONS

DATE _____

Patient Name	Case History III

Date	1	2	3	4	5	6	7	8	9	10	11	12	13	14	15	16
	6 7 6 5 5 5	3 4 4	4 4	4 4 44	6 6 5 6 6	5 5	7 7	6 5 4 5 5	6 6	7 7 6 5						

F

DR

I

Fx

L

Date	1	2	3	4	5	6	7	8	9	10	11	12	13	14	15	16
	6 7 6 6 5 3 3 4 4	4	4 4	44	6 6 4 6 6	5 5	7 7	6 5 4 5 5	6 6	7 7 5 5						

Date	Tooth #	Cold¹	Hot¹	Perc¹	Palp¹	Ept No.	Pulp Diag.	Peri Diag.

¹Use: + = norm.   0 = no res.   ++= abnorm. pos.

PULPAL DIAGNOSIS

N - Vital, normal
R - Reversible pulp infl.
I - Irreversible pulp infl.
NP - Necrotic pulp
O - Other

Severe generalized bone loss

PERIAPICAL DIAGNOSIS

N - Normal
AP - Acute apical periodontitis
C - Chronic apical periodontitis
S - Chronic suppurative apical periodontitis
AA - Acute apical abscess
P - Periradicular osteosclerosis

PERIO DIAGNOSIS

Case Type [IV]   Prophy [ ]   Perio [ ]

Date	32	31	30	29	28	27	26	25	24	23	22	21	20	19	18	17
		5 6 7		4 5 5	6 6		9 10	10 10	10 9	6 6	5 10 8	4				

L

F

A

III III

Date	32	31	30	29	28	27	26	25	24	23	22	21	20	19	18	17
		4 6 8		4 5 5	6 6		9 10	10 10	10 9	6 6	5 6 8	8 4				

INITIAL TMD FINDINGS

Mandibular Range of Motion
- ☐Yes ☐No Maximum vertical opening < 40mm
- ☐Yes ☐No Lateral movements < 7mm
- ☐Yes ☐No Differences between R and L
  lateral movement ≥ 2mm
- ☐Yes ☐No Pain with any of the above
- ☐Yes ☐No History of "Jaw Locking"
- ☐Yes ☐No Past history of TMJ/TMD

Pain on Palpation
- ☐Yes ☐No Lateral TMJ   R L
- ☐Yes ☐No Masseter   R L
- ☐Yes ☐No Temporalis   R L
- ☐Yes ☐No Coronoid process   R L

Joint Sounds
- ☐Yes ☐No Right TM Joint
- ☐Yes ☐No Left TM Joint

Mandibular Deviation/Deflection
- ☐Yes ☐No Opening > 2mm
- ☐Yes ☐No Protrusion > 2mm

Panoramic evaluation suggests osseous changes
(erosion, flattening)
- ☐Yes ☐No   R L

_____
_____
_____

EXTRAORAL SOFT TISSUE FINDINGS:

_____
_____
_____

RIGHT   RIGHT   LEFT   RIGHT   LEFT   LEFT

INTRAORAL SOFT TISSUE FINDINGS:

_____
_____
_____

INITIAL OCCLUSAL FINDINGS

Angle's Molar Classification
- ☐Class I   R L
- ☐Class II   R L
- ☐Class III   R L

- ☐Yes ☐No Group function   R L
- ☐Yes ☐No Canine guidance R L

- ☐Yes ☐No Reverse (R) articulation
- ☐Yes ☐No Wear facets

ADDITIONAL OCCLUSAL FINDINGS

- ☐Yes ☐No Horizontal overlap   ___mm
- ☐Yes ☐No Vertical overlap   ___mm

- ☐Yes ☐No CO to MIP discrepancies
  Ant._____mm   Vert._____mm
  Right_____mm Left_____mm

Nonworking (N) Interferences
- ☐Yes ☐No right side
- ☐Yes ☐No left side

Protrusive (P) Interferences
- ☐Yes ☐No right side
- ☐Yes ☐No left side

PLEASE CIRCLE INITIAL (I) CONTACTS AND ANY INTERFERENCES (N,P) OR REVERSE (R) ARTICULATIONS.

1	2	3	4	5	6	7	8	9	10	11	12	13	14	15	16
32	31	30	29	28	27	26	25	24	23	22	21	20	19	18	17

4C

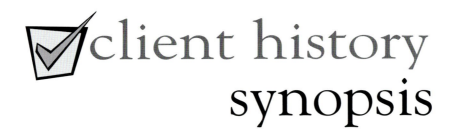

client history synopsis

CASE HISTORY IV

PATIENT HISTORY

Vonda Y. is 21 years old. Her overall health is good. She is aware of how important good oral hygiene is, but admits that she does not floss. She currently suffers from chronic toothaches and jaw pain resulting from a car accident in May 1998. She currently takes Estrastep for birth control.

CLINICAL EXAMINATION

Vonda has 28 natural teeth. She has Class II, Division 1 occlusion. She has numerous areas of class V caries. She has one occlusal carious lesion on tooth #19. Her tissues are much less inflamed at her maintenance visit. She has case type II periodontitis.

RADIOGRAPHIC EXAMINATION

There is generalized slight loss of alveolar bone. Moderate supragingival calculus reaccumulation has occurred on the mandibular anterior teeth. Rampant caries is noted radiographically, primarily of the class V type.

PERIODONTAL ASSESSMENT

Some 4 mm pockets remain. Generalized 1 mm recession was found in posterior areas. Slight bleeding upon probing was evident where pockets remain.

DIETARY HISTORY

Patient receives adequate intake of Recommended Daily Allowances of all food groups. She currently takes prenatal vitamins since the birth of her daughter. She admits a soda pop and sweet habit during her pregnancy.

MEDICAL HISTORY

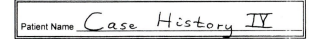

Patient Name _Case History IV_

EACH QUESTION MUST HAVE AN ANSWER. CIRCLE YES OR NO; WRITE IN ANSWERS WHERE APPROPRIATE.

A. | GENERAL INFORMATION |

* VITAL SIGNS

DATE	HT / WT	BP	HR
	5'5" / 130	28 / 86	67
	/	/	
	/	/	
	/	/	
	/	/	

* 1. Has there been any change in your general
health within the past year . . . . YES (NO)

* 2. Have you had any serious illness
or operation . . . . YES (NO)

3. Have you been hospitalized within the
past two (2) years? _child birth_ . . . . (YES) NO

4. Any recent unexplained gain or loss
of weight . . . . YES (NO)

* 5. If under the care of a physician, give

Name: _Dr. Jones, OB/GYN_

Address:_____

Phone #:_____

B. | CARDIOVASCULAR SYSTEM |

DO YOU HAVE OR HAVE YOU HAD:
1. High Blood Pressure . . . . YES (NO)
2. Low Blood Pressure . . . . YES (NO)
* 3. Heart Attack . . . . YES (NO)
* 4. Heart Murmur (congenital heart disease) . . . YES (NO)
* 5. Heart Surgery (bypass, valve) . . . . YES (NO)
6. Shortness of breath . . . . YES (NO)
7. Chest Pain Upon Exertion (angina) . . . . . . YES (NO)
8. Swollen Ankles . . . . YES (NO)
* 9. Rheumatic Heart Disease or Fever . . . . . . YES (NO)
10. A Stroke . . . . YES (NO)
11. A Pacemaker . . . . YES (NO)
12. Other . . . . YES (NO)

C. | NERVOUS SYSTEM |

DO YOU HAVE OR HAVE YOU HAD:
1. Nervous Breakdown, Psychotherapy . . . . . . YES (NO)
2. Epilepsy or Convulsions . . . . YES (NO)
3. Neuritis, Neuralgia, or Numbness . . . . YES (NO)
* 4. Fainting Spells or Seizures . . . . YES (NO)
5. Other . . . . YES (NO)

D. | RESPIRATORY SYSTEM |

DO YOU HAVE OR HAVE YOU HAD:
1. Any Respiratory Disease . . . . YES (NO)
2. Tuberculosis . . . . YES (NO)
3. Sinus Trouble . . . . YES (NO)
4. Hay Fever . . . . YES (NO)
5. Pneumonia . . . . YES (NO)
6. Asthma or Emphysema . . . . YES (NO)
7. Chronic Cough, Sore Throat,
or Coughing Up Blood . . . . YES (NO)
8. Did You Smoke . . . . (YES) NO
9. Do You Smoke _have smoked for 8 yrs._ (YES) NO
10. Other . . . . YES (NO)

E. | GENITOURINARY SYSTEM |

DO YOU HAVE OR HAVE YOU HAD:
1. Kidney Disease . . . . YES (NO)
2. Swollen Ankles . . . . YES (NO)
3. Difficulty in or Frequent Urination . . . . YES (NO)
4. Blood in Your Urine . . . . YES (NO)
5. Other . . . . (YES) NO

F. | GASTROINTESTINAL SYSTEM |

DO YOU HAVE OR HAVE YOU HAD:
1. Stomach or Intestinal Trouble . . . . YES (NO)
2. Indigestion, Diarrhea, Vomiting,
or Constipation . . . . YES (NO)
3. Appetite Problem . . . . YES (NO)
* 4. Jaundice or Hepatitis . . . . YES (NO)
5. Liver Disease . . . . YES (NO)
6. Ulcers . . . . YES (NO)
7. Other . . . . YES (NO)

G. | ENDOCRINE SYSTEM |

DO YOU HAVE OR HAVE YOU HAD:
* 1. Diabetes . . . . YES (NO)
a. Do you have to urinate frequently . . . . . . YES (NO)
b. Are you thirsty much of the time . . . . YES (NO)
c. Is your mouth dry . . . . YES (NO)
2. A Thyroid Problem . . . . YES (NO)
3. Parathyroid Problem . . . . YES (NO)
4. Hormone Therapy . . . . YES (NO)
5. Other . . . . YES (NO)

H. | BONES AND JOINTS |

DO YOU HAVE OR HAVE YOU HAD:
1. Arthritis . . . . YES (NO)
2. Inflammatory Rheumatism . . . . YES (NO)
* 3. Joint Replacement . . . . YES (NO)
4. Back or Neck Injury . . . . YES (NO)
5. Other . . . . YES (NO)

I. | BLOOD-LYMPHATICS |

DO YOU HAVE OR HAVE YOU HAD:
* 1. Blood Disorder or Anemia . . . . YES (NO)
* 2. Abnormal Bleeding with Previous
Extractions or Surgery . . . . YES (NO)
* 3. Transfusions . . . . YES (NO)
4. Bruise Easily . . . . YES (NO)
5. Swollen Lymph Nodes (glands) . . . . YES (NO)
6. Other . . . . YES (NO)

J. | INFECTIOUS DISEASE |

DO YOU HAVE OR HAVE YOU HAD:
* 1. Hepatitis (type A, B, other) . . . . YES (NO)
* 2. AIDS, ARC, HIV, ANTI-HIV . . . . YES (NO)
* 3. Syphilis, Gonorrhea, Herpes . . . . YES (NO)
4. Acute Pharyngitis (oral or strep) . . . . YES (NO)
5. Childhood Diseases: Rubella, Rubeola,
(Chicken Pox) Mumps . . . . (YES) NO
* 6. Are You or Have You Been an IV
Drug User . . . . YES (NO)
7. Other . . . . YES (NO)

I-20

K. **HEAD, EYES, EARS, NOSE, THROAT**

DO YOU HAVE OR HAVE YOU HAD:
* 1. Head or Jaw Injury *car accident 1998* *may* YES NO
2. Frequent Headaches .... YES (NO)
3. Dizziness .... YES (NO)
4. Vision Problems .... YES (NO)
5. Hearing Problems .... YES (NO)
6. Nose Bleeds .... YES (NO)
7. Nasal Obstructions .... YES (NO)
8. Chronic Sore Throat .... YES (NO)
9. Halitosis .... YES (NO)
10. Altered Taste Perceptions .... YES (NO)
11. Dry Mouth .... YES (NO)
12. Do You Wear Contact Lenses ..... YES (NO)
13. Other .... YES (NO)

L. **MEDICATIONS**

ARE YOU TAKING ANY OF THE FOLLOWING:
* 1. Antibiotics or Sulfa Drugs .... YES (NO)
* 2. Anticoagulants (blood thinners) .... YES (NO)
* 3. Medicine for High Blood Pressure ... YES (NO)
* 4. Cortisone (steroids) .... YES (NO)
* 5. Tranquilizers .... YES (NO)
* 6. Antihistamines .... YES (NO)
* 7. Aspirin (regular, ongoing basis) *1 each evening* (YES) NO
* 8. Insulin, Orinase, or Similar Drug .. YES (NO)
* 9. Digitalis or Other Heart Drug ...... YES (NO)
* 10. Nitroglycerin .... YES (NO)
* 11. Chemotherapy .... YES (NO)
* 12. Chemically Dependent (alcohol, drugs) .... YES (NO)
* 13. Diet pills (Fen-phen, Dexfenfluramine) ... YES (NO)
* 14. Other Medications *Estrastep, oral contraceptive* (YES) NO

M. **ALLERGIES**

ARE YOU ALLERGIC TO OR HAD A REACTION TO:
* 1. Local Anesthetic (novocaine, etc.) .... YES (NO)
* 2. Penicillin, Sulfa Drugs or Other Antibiotics ..... YES (NO)
* 3. Latex .... YES (NO)
* 4. Barbiturates, Sleeping Pills ..... YES (NO)
* 5. Aspirin .... YES (NO)
* 6. Iodine .... YES (NO)
* 7. Codeine or Other Narcotics ...... YES (NO)
* 8. Metals (rings, earrings, etc.) ... YES (NO)
* 9. Other Allergies .... YES (NO)

N. **RADIATION HISTORY**

1. Are you employed in any situation which exposes you to X-rays or other ionizing radiation? .... YES (NO)
* 2. Have you had radiation therapy .... YES (NO)

O. **DENTAL HISTORY**

* Are you having dental pain or discomfort at this time? *Jaw pain / occasional toothaches* (YES) NO
If you wear dentures, go to question #14.

DO YOU HAVE OR HAVE YOU HAD:
1. Frequent Toothaches *from car accident* (YES) NO
2. Periodontal (gum) Disease .... YES (NO)
3. Orthodontic Treatment .... YES (NO)
4. Difficulty in Opening or Closing Your Jaw *From car accident injury* (YES) NO
5. Grinding or Clenching Your Teeth ...... YES (NO)
6. Chronic Facial Pain .... (YES) NO
7. Do You Brush Daily .... (YES) NO
8. Do You Floss Daily .... (YES) NO
9. Do You Want To Keep Your Teeth .... (YES) NO
10. Does Having Dental Treatment Make You Nervous .... (YES) NO
11. Have you had a bad experience in a dental office .... YES (NO)
12. Have Your Dental Experiences in General Been (circle) GOOD, (AVERAGE) POOR
13. Children
Fluoride (Dietary Hx) .... (YES) NO
Oral Habits .... (YES) NO
Birth History Normal .... (YES) NO
14. Denture History
a. Do You Think You Need Dentures .... YES (NO)
b. How Long Have You Worn Dentures ____
c. How Old Are Your Present Dentures____

P. **WOMEN**

* Are You Pregnant .... (YES) NO

DO YOU HAVE OR HAVE YOU HAD:
1. Menstrual Problems .... YES (NO)
2. Breast Cancer/Tumor .... YES (NO)
* 3. Are You Taking Birth Control Pills ... YES (NO)
4. Have You Been Through Menopause ... YES (NO)
5. Other .... YES (NO)

Do you have any disease condition or problem not listed .... YES (NO)

_____
_____
_____

To the best of my knowledge, all of the preceding answers are true and correct. If I ever have any change in my health, or if my medicines change, I will inform the faculty or student at the next appointment without fail.

* _____   * _____   * _____   * _____

Date   Student Signature   Faculty Signature   Signature of Patient, Parent, or Guardian.

MEDICAL HISTORY/PHYSICAL EVALUATION UPDATE

Date	Changes (See Comments)	Student Signature	Faculty Signature
_____	YES NO	_____	_____
_____	YES NO	_____	_____
_____	YES NO	_____	_____
_____	YES NO	_____	_____

3 A

ADULT EXISTING CONDITIONS

DATE _____

Patient Name *Case History IV*

Upper chart

Date	1	2	3	4	5	6	7	8	9	10	11	12	13	14	15	16
3/30/00												(4)	(404)	(44)	(404)	
1/16/00		2,1,2	4,1,4	3,1,2	3,1,3	3,1,2	2,1,2	3,1,2	2,1,2	2,3,2	2,1,2	4,1,4	4,2,4	4,2,4	3,2,3	

F / L tooth diagrams (sealant, sealants marked)

Date	1	2	3	4	5	6	7	8	9	10	11	12	13	14	15	16
1/16/00		2,1,3	3,1,2	3,1,2	3,1,2	1,1,2	2,1,2	2,1,2	2,1,2	2,1,2	2,1,3	2,1,2	2,1,2	2,3,2	4,3,2,3	
3/30/00		(4)									(4)	(404)		(404)		

Date	Tooth #	Cold[1]	Hot[1]	Perc[1]	Palp[1]	Ept No.	Pulp Diag.	Peri Diag.

[1]Use: + = norm. 0 = no res. ++= abnorm. pos.

PULPAL DIAGNOSIS
N - Vital normal
R - Reversible pulpitis
I - Irreversible pulpitis
NP - Necrotic pulp
O - Other

PERIAPICAL DIAGNOSIS ...

PERIO DIAGNOSIS ...

Generalized sl.-mod. BOP

Lower chart

Date	32	31	30	29	28	27	26	25	24	23	22	21	20	19	18	17
3/30/00		(4)	(4)									(4)	(44)	(4)		
1/16/00	3,2,3	4,2,4	4,2,2	2,2,2	2,1,2	2,1,2	1,1,1	1,1,2	2,1,2	2,1,3	1,1,2	3,1,3	4,3,4	4,3,5	

L / F tooth diagrams (sealant marked)

Date	32	31	30	29	28	27	26	25	24	23	22	21	20	19	18	17
1/16/00	4,2,4	4,2,4	3,1,2	2,1,2	3,1,2	3,1,2	2,1,1	1,1,2	3,1,3	3,1,2	3,1,2	2,1,2	3,1,3	4,2,4	
3/30/00					*hone.*	*over.*	*3.mm.*								

40

INITIAL TMD FINDINGS

Mandibular Range of Motion

☐Yes ☐No Maximum vertical opening < 40mm
☐Yes ☐No Lateral movements < 7mm
☐Yes ☐No Differences between R and L
           lateral movement ≥ 2mm
☐Yes ☐No Pain with any of the above
☐Yes ☐No History of "Jaw Locking"
☐Yes ☐No Past history of TMJ/TMD

Pain on Palpation

☐Yes ☐No Lateral TMJ   R L
☐Yes ☐No Masseter   R L
☐Yes ☐No Temporalis   R L
☐Yes ☐No Coronoid process   R L

Joint Sounds

☐Yes ☐No Right TM Joint
☐Yes ☐No Left TM Joint

Mandibular Deviation/Deflection

☐Yes ☐No Opening > 2mm
☐Yes ☐No Protrusion > 2mm

Panoramic evaluation suggests osseous changes
(erosion, flattening)
☐Yes ☐No   R L

_____
_____
_____
_____

EXTRAORAL SOFT TISSUE FINDINGS:

_____
_____

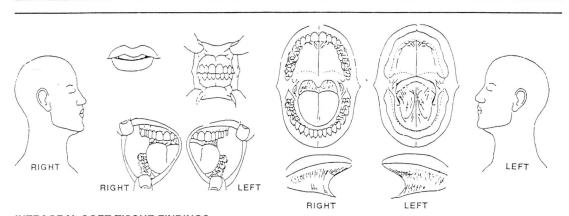

RIGHT   RIGHT   LEFT   RIGHT   LEFT   LEFT

INTRAORAL SOFT TISSUE FINDINGS:

_____
_____
_____

INITIAL OCCLUSAL FINDINGS

Angle's Molar Classification

☐Class I   R L
☐Class II   R L
☐Class III   R L

☐Yes ☐No Group function   R L
☐Yes ☐No Canine guidance R L

☐Yes ☐No Reverse (R) articulation
☐Yes ☐No Wear facets

ADDITIONAL OCCLUSAL FINDINGS

☐Yes ☐No Horizontal overlap   ___mm
☐Yes ☐No Vertical overlap   ___mm

☐Yes ☐No CO to MIP discrepancies
Ant._____mm Vert._____mm
Right_____mm Left_____mm

Nonworking (N) Interferences
☐Yes ☐No right side
☐Yes ☐No left side

Protrusive (P) Interferences
☐Yes ☐No right side
☐Yes ☐No left side

PLEASE CIRCLE INITIAL (I) CONTACTS AND ANY INTERFERENCES (N,P) OR REVERSE (R) ARTICULATIONS.

1	2	3	4	5	6	7	8	9	10	11	12	13	14	15	16
32	31	30	29	28	27	26	25	24	23	22	21	20	19	18	17

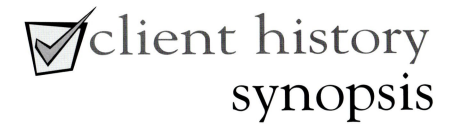

client history synopsis

CASE HISTORY V

PATIENT HISTORY

Ava N. is an 81-year-old female who resides in an assisted living center. She has a history of high blood pressure and currently takes Hyzaar to keep it well controlled. In April 1998, she had an angioplasty. She smoked from the age of 24 until the age of 58. Other surgeries include gallbladder removal, March 1999, a right knee replacement in August 1999, and a right hip replacement in February 1992. She takes Clindamycin for antibiotic prophylaxis. She is very diligent about homecare, especially since she has developed case type III Periodontitis.

CLINICAL EXAMINATION

Ava has 28 natural teeth. She has Class III occlusion and her restorations are not defective. Moderate gingival erythema and edema are generalized. Moderate bleeding on probing was also found to be generalized. Slight calculus reaccumulation has occurred in the mandibular anterior area.

RADIOGRAPHIC EXAMINATION

No caries or defective restorations are present. There is generalized moderate horizontal bone loss.

PERIODONTAL ASSESSMENT

A 7 mm pocket remains on the buccal aspect of tooth #2. There is generalized pocket depth decreases of 1–2 mm at the second (periodontal maintenance) visit. There is moderate, generalized bleeding upon probing.

MEDICAL HISTORY

Patient Name **Case History V**

EACH QUESTION MUST HAVE AN ANSWER. CIRCLE YES OR NO; WRITE IN ANSWERS WHERE APPROPRIATE.

A. **GENERAL INFORMATION** **81 years of age**

* VITAL SIGNS

DATE	HT / WT	BP	HR
	5'2" / 150	150 / 85	75
	/	/	
	/	/	
	/	/	
	/	/	

* 1. Has there been any change in your general health within the past year .... (YES) NO
* 2. Have you had any serious illness or operation .... (YES) NO
   3. Have you been hospitalized within the past two (2) years? .... (YES) NO
   4. Any recent unexplained gain or loss of weight .... YES (NO)
* 5. If under the care of a physician, give

   Name: **Dr. Smith**

   Address: _____

   Phone #: **(505) 555 - 0060**

B. **CARDIOVASCULAR SYSTEM**

DO YOU HAVE OR HAVE YOU HAD:
   1. High Blood Pressure .... (YES) NO
   2. Low Blood Pressure .... YES (NO)
* 3. Heart Attack .... YES (NO)
* 4. Heart Murmur (congenital heart disease) ... YES (NO)
* 5. Heart Surgery (bypass, valve) .... YES (NO)
   6. Shortness of breath .... YES (NO)
   7. Chest Pain Upon Exertion (angina) .... YES (NO)
   8. Swollen Ankles .... YES (NO)
* 9. Rheumatic Heart Disease or Fever .... YES (NO)
   10. A Stroke .... YES (NO)
   11. A Pacemaker .... YES (NO)
   12. Other **April 1998 Angioplasty** ...... (YES) NO

C. **NERVOUS SYSTEM**

DO YOU HAVE OR HAVE YOU HAD:
   1. Nervous Breakdown, Psychotherapy .... YES (NO)
   2. Epilepsy or Convulsions .... YES (NO)
   3. Neuritis, Neuralgia, or Numbness .... YES (NO)
* 4. Fainting Spells or Seizures .... YES (NO)
   5. Other .... YES (NO)

D. **RESPIRATORY SYSTEM**

DO YOU HAVE OR HAVE YOU HAD:
   1. Any Respiratory Disease .... YES (NO)
   2. Tuberculosis .... YES (NO)
   3. Sinus Trouble .... YES (NO)
   4. Hay Fever .... YES (NO)
   5. Pneumonia .... YES (NO)
   6. Asthma or Emphysema .... YES (NO)
   7. Chronic Cough, Sore Throat, or Coughing Up Blood .... YES (NO)
   8. Did You Smoke **quit 23 years ago** ... (YES) NO
   9. Do You Smoke .... YES (NO)
   10. Other .... YES (NO)

E. **GENITOURINARY SYSTEM**

DO YOU HAVE OR HAVE YOU HAD:
   1. Kidney Disease .... YES (NO)
   2. Swollen Ankles .... YES (NO)
   3. Difficulty in or Frequent Urination ...... YES (NO)
   4. Blood in Your Urine .... YES (NO)
   5. Other .... YES (NO)

F. **GASTROINTESTINAL SYSTEM**

DO YOU HAVE OR HAVE YOU HAD:
   1. Stomach or Intestinal Trouble .... YES (NO)
   2. Indigestion, Diarrhea, Vomiting, or Constipation .... YES (NO)
   3. Appetite Problem .... YES (NO)
* 4. Jaundice or Hepatitis .... YES (NO)
   5. Liver Disease .... YES (NO)
   6. Ulcers .... YES (NO)
   7. Other **gallbladder removed March 1999** (YES) NO

G. **ENDOCRINE SYSTEM**

DO YOU HAVE OR HAVE YOU HAD:
* 1. Diabetes .... YES (NO)
      a. Do you have to urinate frequently .... YES (NO)
      b. Are you thirsty much of the time .... YES (NO)
      c. Is your mouth dry .... YES (NO)
   2. A Thyroid Problem .... YES (NO)
   3. Parathyroid Problem .... YES (NO)
   4. Hormone Therapy .... YES (NO)
   5. Other .... YES (NO)

H. **BONES AND JOINTS**

DO YOU HAVE OR HAVE YOU HAD:
   1. Arthritis .... (YES) NO
   2. Inflammatory Rheumatism .... YES (NO)
* 3. Joint Replacement **® knee August 1999 ; ® Hip Feb. 1992** (YES) NO
   4. Back or Neck Injury .... YES (NO)
   5. Other .... YES (NO)

I. **BLOOD-LYMPHATICS**

DO YOU HAVE OR HAVE YOU HAD:
* 1. Blood Disorder or Anemia .... YES (NO)
* 2. Abnormal Bleeding with Previous Extractions or Surgery .... YES (NO)
   3. Transfusions .... YES (NO)
   4. Bruise Easily .... YES (NO)
   5. Swollen Lymph Nodes (glands) .... YES (NO)
   6. Other .... YES (NO)

J. **INFECTIOUS DISEASE**

DO YOU HAVE OR HAVE YOU HAD:
* 1. Hepatitis (type A, B, other) .... YES (NO)
* 2. AIDS, ARC, HIV, ANTI-HIV .... YES (NO)
* 3. Syphilis, Gonorrhea, Herpes .... YES (NO)
   4. Acute Pharyngitis (oral or strep) .... YES (NO)
   5. Childhood Diseases: Rubella, Rubeola, (Chicken Pox) Mumps .... (YES) NO
* 6. Are You or Have You Been an IV Drug User .... YES (NO)
   7. Other .... YES (NO)

3 A

K. HEAD, EYES, EARS, NOSE, THROAT

DO YOU HAVE OR HAVE YOU HAD:
* 1. Head or Jaw Injury .... YES (NO)
2. Frequent Headaches .... YES (NO)
3. Dizziness .... YES (NO)
4. Vision Problems .... YES (NO)
5. Hearing Problems .... YES (NO)
6. Nose Bleeds .... YES (NO)
7. Nasal Obstructions .... YES (NO)
8. Chronic Sore Throat .... YES (NO)
9. Halitosis .... YES (NO)
10. Altered Taste Perceptions .... YES (NO)
11. Dry Mouth .... YES (NO)
12. Do You Wear Contact Lenses .... YES (NO)
13. Other .... YES (NO)

L. MEDICATIONS

ARE YOU TAKING ANY OF THE FOLLOWING:
* 1. Antibiotics or Sulfa Drugs *Clindamycin (premed)* (YES) NO
* 2. Anticoagulants (blood thinners) .... YES (NO)
* 3. Medicine for High Blood Pressure *Hyzaar 1x/day* (YES) NO
* 4. Cortisone (steroids) .... YES (NO)
* 5. Tranquilizers .... YES (NO)
* 6. Antihistamines .... YES (NO)
* 7. Aspirin (regular, ongoing basis) ...... YES (NO)
* 8. Insulin, Orinase, or Similar Drug ..... YES (NO)
* 9. Digitalis or Other Heart Drug .... YES (NO)
* 10. Nitroglycerin .... YES (NO)
* 11. Chemotherapy .... YES (NO)
* 12. Chemically Dependent (alcohol, drugs) .... YES (NO)
* 13. Diet pills (Fen-phen, Dexfenfluramine) .... YES (NO)
* 14. Other Medications .... YES (NO)

M. ALLERGIES

ARE YOU ALLERGIC TO OR HAD A REACTION TO:
* 1. Local Anesthetic (novocaine, etc.) ..... YES (NO)
* 2. (Penicillin) Sulfa Drugs or Other Antibiotics .... (YES) NO
* 3. Latex .... YES (NO)
* 4. Barbiturates, Sleeping Pills .... YES (NO)
* 5. Aspirin .... YES (NO)
* 6. Iodine .... YES (NO)
* 7. Codeine or Other Narcotics .... YES (NO)
* 8. Metals (rings, earrings, etc.) .... YES (NO)
* 9. Other Allergies .... YES (NO)

N. RADIATION HISTORY

1. Are you employed in any situation which exposes you to X-rays or other ionizing radiation? .... YES (NO)
* 2. Have you had radiation therapy .... YES (NO)

O. DENTAL HISTORY

* Are you having dental pain or discomfort at this time? .... YES (NO)
If you wear dentures, go to question #14.

DO YOU HAVE OR HAVE YOU HAD:
1. Frequent Toothaches .... YES (NO)
2. Periodontal (gum) Disease .... (YES) NO
3. Orthodontic Treatment .... YES (NO)
4. Difficulty in Opening or Closing Your Jaw .... YES (NO)
5. Grinding or Clenching Your Teeth ..... YES (NO)
6. Chronic Facial Pain .... YES (NO)
7. Do You Brush Daily .... (YES) NO
8. Do You Floss Daily .... (YES) NO
9. Do You Want To Keep Your Teeth ...... (YES) NO
10. Does Having Dental Treatment Make You Nervous .... YES (NO)
11. Have you had a bad experience in a dental office .... YES (NO)
12. Have Your Dental Experiences in General Been (circle (GOOD,) AVERAGE, POOR
13. Children
Fluoride (Dietary Hx) .... YES (NO)
Oral Habits .... YES (NO)
Birth History Normal .... (YES) NO
14. Denture History
a. Do You Think You Need Dentures .... YES (NO)
b. How Long Have You Worn Dentures _____
c. How Old Are Your Present Dentures _____

P. WOMEN

* Are You Pregnant .... YES (NO)
DO YOU HAVE OR HAVE YOU HAD:
1. Menstrual Problems .... YES (NO)
2. Breast Cancer/Tumor .... YES (NO)
* 3. Are You Taking Birth Control Pills .... YES (NO)
4. Have You Been Through Menopause .... (YES) NO
5. Other .... YES (NO)

Do you have any disease condition or problem not listed .... YES (NO)

_____
_____
_____

To the best of my knowledge, all of the preceding answers are true and correct. If I ever have any change in my health, or if my medicines change, I will inform the faculty or student at the next appointment without fail.

*	*	*	*
Date	*Amy Smith* Student Signature	*Michelle L. Sensat* Faculty Signature	Signature of Patient, Parent, or Guardian.

MEDICAL HISTORY/PHYSICAL EVALUATION UPDATE

Date	Changes (See Comments)	Student Signature	Faculty Signature
_____	YES NO	_____	_____
_____	YES NO	_____	_____
_____	YES NO	_____	_____
_____	YES NO	_____	_____

ADULT EXISTING CONDITIONS

DATE _____

Patient Name *Case Study V*

Date	1	2	3	4	5	6	7	8	9	10	11	12	13	14	15	16
1/6/00		4 7 4 4	4											5 4		
10/30/99		5 9 5									4 4 4	4 4	5			

F

L

Date	1	2	3	4	5	6	7	8	9	10	11	12	13	14	15	16
10/30/99		5 5 5 5									4 4 5	5 4	6 7 7 5		
1/6/00		4 4 5 4										4 5 6 5 4			

Date	Tooth #	Cold [1]	Hot [1]	Perc [1]	Palp [1]	Ept No.	Pulp Diag.	Peri Diag.

[1] Use: + = norm. 0 = no res. ++ = abnorm. pos.

Moderate generalized BOP

PULPAL DIAGNOSIS
N - (normal)
C - reversible pulpitis
I - irreversible pulpitis
NP - necrotic pulp
O - Other

PERIAPICAL DIAGNOSIS
N - normal
AA - Acute apical periodontitis
C - Chronic apical periodontitis
S - Chronic suppurative apical periodontitis
AA - acute apical abscess
D - condensing osteosclerosis

PERIO DIAGNOSIS
Case Type ___III___ Prophy [ ] Perio [X]

Date	32	31	30	29	28	27	26	25	24	23	22	21	20	19	18	17
1/6/00		4 5 5 4												4 4 5		
10/30/99		5 6 6 5														

L

F

Date	32	31	30	29	28	27	26	25	24	23	22	21	20	19	18	17
10/30/99		4 4												4 4 4 4		
1/6/00					none	over	3	mm								

INITIAL TMD FINDINGS

Mandibular Range of Motion

- ☐Yes ☒No Maximum vertical opening < 40mm
- ☐Yes ☒No Lateral movements < 7mm
- ☐Yes ☒No Differences between R and L lateral movement ≥ 2mm
- ☒Yes ☐No Pain with any of the above
- ☐Yes ☒No History of "Jaw Locking"
- ☐Yes ☒No Past history of TMJ/TMD

Pain on Palpation

- ☐Yes ☒No Lateral TMJ
- ☒Yes ☐No Masseter
- ☐Yes ☒No Temporalis
- ☐Yes ☒No Coronoid process

Joint Sounds

- ☐Yes ☒No Right TM Joint
- ☐Yes ☒No Left TM Joint

Mandibular Deviation/Deflection

- ☐Yes ☐No Opening > 2mm
- ☐Yes ☐No Protrusion > 2mm

Panoramic evaluation suggests osseous changes (erosion, flattening)

- ☐Yes ☐No   R   L

_____
_____
_____
_____

EXTRAORAL SOFT TISSUE FINDINGS:

All WNL

_____
_____

RIGHT   RIGHT   LEFT   RIGHT   LEFT   LEFT

INTRAORAL SOFT TISSUE FINDINGS:

Buccal mucosa — bilateral cheek bites (petechiae); Tongue - slightly coated
Alveolar processes — #30 B - amalgam tattoo
Other - slight - moderate generalized attrition

INITIAL OCCLUSAL FINDINGS

Angle's Molar Classification

- ☒Class I   Ⓡ Ⓛ
- ☐Class II   R   L
- ☐Class III R   L

- ☐Yes ☐No Group function R   L
- ☐Yes ☐No Canine guidance R   L

- ☐Yes ☐No Reverse (R) articulation
- ☐Yes ☐No Wear facets

ADDITIONAL OCCLUSAL FINDINGS

- ☐Yes ☒No Horizontal overlap ___mm
- ☐Yes ☐No Vertical overlap ___mm

- ☐Yes ☐No CO to MIP discrepancies
  - Ant._____mm Vert._____mm
  - Right_____mm Left_____mm

Nonworking (N) Interferences

- ☐Yes ☐No right side
- ☐Yes ☐No left side

Protrusive (P) Interferences

- ☐Yes ☐No right side
- ☐Yes ☐No left side

PLEASE CIRCLE INITIAL (I) CONTACTS AND ANY INTERFERENCES (N,P) OR REVERSE (R) ARTICULATIONS.

1	2	3	4	5	6	7	8	9	10	11	12	13	14	15	16
32	31	30	29	28	27	26	25	24	23	22	21	20	19	18	17

4C

4. Which types of microorganisms are implicated in NUG/NUP periodontal disease?
   A. Cocci
   B. Cocci and rods
   C. Vibrios and spirochetes
   D. Fusiform bacilli and spirochetes
   E. Rods and filamentous forms

5. The clinical difference between NUG and NUP is:
   A. Clinical attachment loss
   B. Fetid odor
   C. Ulceration of interdental papillae
   D. Spontaneous hemorrhage

6. What risk factors are considered as predisposing factors in the development of NUP in this patient?
   A. Stress
   B. Neglected oral hygiene
   C. Inadequate diet
   D. Tobacco smoking
   E. All except A
   F. All of the above

7. What initial periodontal therapy is indicated for this patient?
   A. Scaling and root planing with hand instruments
   B. Scaling and root planing with ultrasonic instruments
   C. General debridement with hand instruments
   D. General debridement with hand and ultrasonic instruments as needed
   E. None of the above at the first appointment

8. What dietary modifications should be made to ensure proper nutrition for a person with NUG/NUP?
   A. Increase intake of breads/cereals
   B. Increase intake of foods from the meat group
   C. Increase intake of foods from the milk group
   D. Increase intake of foods from the fruit group.
   E. All except A
   F. All except C

9. According to the periodontal assessment, which oral hygiene aid is most appropriate for use as an adjunct to toothbrushing and flossing?
   A. Gauze strip
   B. Interdental (single-tuft) brush
   C. Pipe cleaner
   D. Toothpick in holder

10. What instrument is most appropriate for use in subgingival debridement of the mandibular anterior area?
    A. Goldman H6/H7 sickle scaler
    B. Columbia 13/14 universal curette
    C. Langer 1/2 curette
    D. Gracey 5/6 curette

CASE HISTORY III QUESTIONS

1. What is the appropriate course of periodontal therapy for this patient?
   A. General gross debridement
   B. Periodontal debridement by the quadrant
   C. Oral hygiene instruction only
   D. Periodontal debridement by the quadrant (under anesthesia)
   E. Hand instrumentation

2. According to this patient's clinical examination, radiographic examination, and periodontal assessment, what is the correct periodontal diagnosis?
   A. Case Type I—Gingivitis
   B. Case Type II—Early Periodontitis
   C. Case Type III—Moderate Periodontitis
   D. Case Type IV—Advanced Periodontitis
   E. Case Type V—Refractory Periodontitis

3. What type of malposition is depicted by tooth #26?
   A. Labioversion
   B. Linguoversion
   C. Buccoversion
   D. Torsiversion

4. The facial gingiva of tooth #22 can best be described as:
   A. Clefted
   B. Festooned
   C. Knife-edged
   D. Rounded

5. The stain apparent on the facials of the mandibular anterior teeth (anatomical crowns) is:
   A. Yellow stain
   B. Green stain
   C. Black line stain
   D. Orange stain

6. The best rinse for this patient's oral health needs is:
   A. Scope
   B. 0.12% Chlorhexidine gluconate rinse
   C. Listerine
   D. 0.05% NaF rinse
   E. Warm saline rinse

7. If Mrs. Jones had a heart attack one month before her scheduled periodontal debridements, what would be the appropriate course of action?
   A. Postpone appointments for 1 month and obtain physician consent before treatment
   B. Postpone appointments for 3 months or more and obtain physician consent before treatment
   C. Postpone appointments for 6 months and obtain physician consent before treatment
   D. Proceed with planned treatment

8. Which medication may cause xerostomia and exacerbate Mrs. Jones' oral health condition?
   A. Hydrochlorothiazide (HCT)
   B. Coumadin
   C. Aspirin
   D. Insulin

9. What types of microorganisms would most likely be found in the pockets around teeth #24 and 25?
   A. Gram-positive cocci
   B. Rods and filamentous forms
   C. Vibrios, spirochetes and other gram-negative organisms
   D. Gram-negative, motile spirochetes and rods

10. What is the name of the space between teeth #8 and 9?
    A. Embrasure
    B. Marginal discrepancy
    C. Diastema
    D. Contact

11. To perform a Simplified Oral Hygiene Index (OHI-S), which tooth surfaces are assessed?
    A. #3 L, #8 F, #14 L, #19 B, #24 F, #30 B
    B. #3 B, #8 F, #14 B, #19 L, #24 F, #30 L
    C. #3 B, #8 L, #14 B, #19 L, #24 L, #30 L
    D. #3 L, #8 L, #14 B, #19 L, #24 L, #30 B

12. If a molar tooth used in the OHI-S index is missing, which tooth would you use to replace it?
    A. The second molar
    B. The third molar
    C. The second premolar
    D. The first premolar
    E. Either A or B

13. When using the Patient Hygiene Performance (PHP) index, into how many subdivisions do you divide each tooth examined?
    A. 2
    B. 3
    C. 4
    D. 5
    E. 6

14. If this women were to go into cardiac arrest, what would be the rate of compression necessary during CPR?
    A. 80 to 100 times per minute
    B. 60 to 80 times per minute
    C. 50 to 60 times per minute
    D. 40 to 50 times per minute
    E. 30 to 40 times per minute

15. In what position would you place your patient in the event of syncope?
    A. Supine
    B. Semi-upright
    C. Trendelenburg
    D. Maxillary positioning (chin-up)
    E. Mandibular positioning (chin-down)

16. If this patient were to experience keto-acidosis (diabetic coma), what would be the appropriate course of action?
    A. Terminate oral procedure
    B. Activate 911
    C. Keep patient warm
    D. Administer oxygen by nasal cannula
    E. All of the above

17. Which local anesthetic would be most appropriate for this patient based on her medical history?
    A. 2% Lidocaine with 1:100,000 epinephrine
    B. 4%Prilocaine
    C. 2%Lidocaine
    D. 3% Mepivacaine

CASE HISTORY IV QUESTIONS

1. What is most likely the etiology of Vonda's rampant decay?
    A. Pregnancy gingivitis
    B. 1 mm generalized recession
    C. High sucrose intake and frequency
    D. Lack of regular flossing

2. What is the relationship between the maxilla and mandible in a Class II Division 1 occlusion?
    A. The mesiobuccal cusp of the maxillary first permanent molar occludes with the buccal groove of the mandibular first permanent molar.
    B. The buccal groove of the mandibular first permanent molar is distal to the mesiobuccal cusp of the maxillary first permanent molar by at least the width of a premolar and all maxillary incisors are protruded.
    C. The buccal groove of the mandibular first permanent molar is distal to the mesiobuccal cusp of the maxillary first permanent molar by at least the width of a premolar and one or more maxillary incisors are retruded.
    D. The buccal groove of the mandibular first permanent molar is mesial to the mesiobuccal cusp of the maxillary first permanent molar by at least the width of a premolar.

3. What type of fluoride supplementation would be most appropriate for use at home?
    A. 0.05% NaF rinse used once daily
    B. 0.4% SnF_2 brush-on gel used once daily
    C. 1.1% neutral NaF brush-on gel used once daily
    D. 1.23% APF gel used once daily

4. What dietary recommendation would most benefit this patient?
    A. Increase intake of vitamins A, C, and D
    B. Increase calcium intake
    C. Omit sucrose solids and liquids from diet
    D. No recommendation is necessary

5. Which restorative material would be most beneficial in restoring Vonda's Class V carious lesions?
    A. Amalgam
    B. Composite
    C. Gold
    D. Glass-ionomer

CASE HISTORY V QUESTIONS

1. For someone not allergic to penicillin, the appropriate prophylactic regimen would be:
    A. Cefazolin, 1.0 g, IM or IV within 30 minutes before procedure
    B. Azithromycin, 500 mg, 1 hour before procedure
    C. Clindamycin, 600 mg, 1 hour before procedure
    D. Amoxicillin, 2.0 g orally, 1 hour before procedure

2. Hyzaar is implicated in causing xerostomia because it is of the drug class of:
    A. Anticholinergics
    B. Antidepressants
    C. Diuretics
    D. Antihistamines
    E. Antihypertensives

3. Which instrument is most appropriate for use in the 7 mm pocket of tooth #2?
    A. S204SD sickle scaler
    B. Gracey 5/6 curette
    C. Columbia 13/14 curette
    D. Gracey 11/12 After-five curette

4. Due to this patient's caries history, what fluoride regimen should be recommended?
    A. APF 0.5% gel
    B. NaF1.1%gel
    C. SnF_2 0.4% gel
    D. NaF 0.05% gel

5. Which polishing agent should be used to polish this patient's gold restorations?

   A. Pumice

   B. Calcium carbonate

   C. Emery

   D. Iron oxide (Rouge)

6. The restoration on tooth #21 would be classified as a class _____ restoration according to G.V. Black's classification system.

   A. I

   B. II

   C. III

   D. IV

   E. V

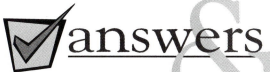
answers & rationales

CASE HISTORY I ANSWERS

1.

A. American Academy of Periodontology's Case Type I refers to inflammation of the gingiva, characterized clinically by changes in color, gingival form, position, surface appearance, and presence of bleeding and/or exudate. Bone loss has not occurred. (1:225, 2:128–129)

2.

B. In a normal occlusal relationship, the mesiobuccal cusp of the maxillary first permanent molar occludes with the buccal groove of the mandibular first permanent molar. (1:258–259)

3.

F. This patient has no history of periodontitis or dental surgery of any kind. She does not report orthodontic treatment history or exhibit history of restorative work in anterior areas. The most likely explanation is inadequate/incorrect self-care. Overvigorous or incorrect toothbrushing traumatizes the gingival tissues and can lead to recession. (1:595–596)

4.

B. Class II is defined as a restoration (or caries) involving the proximal surfaces of premolars and molars. Included in this class are MO, DO, and MOD restorations. (1:283, 241)

CASE HISTORY II ANSWERS

1.

C. By definition, necrotizing ulcerative periodontitis is a destructive infection of the periodontal tissues with ulceration of the interdental papillae, cratering of interdental bone and soft tissue, clinical attachment loss, pain, spontaneous gingival bleeding, poor appetite, fetid mouth odor, and a pseudomembrane formation over the necrotic areas. NUG does not, by definition, include loss of clinical attachment. Case Type III is a chronic periodontal infection and Case Type V does not fit the case history description. (1:225, 576–578)

2.

C. Class III carious lesions are defined as cavities in proximal surfaces of incisors and canines that do not involve the incisal angle. (1:241)

3.

C. Flossing is not indicated until acute symptoms subside. Listerine rinse contains high amounts of alcohol. Weak saline rinses or warm water rinses are indicated. Occasionally, hydrogen peroxide (3%) with equal parts water for rinsing is preferred. A soft bristle brush should be used several times a day. (1:581)

4.

D. Fusiform bacilli and medium-sized spirochetes are the predominate bacterial species implicated in NUG/NUP infections. (1:579)

5.

A. All clinical manifestations of NUG and NUP are the same except that NUP includes clinical attachment loss and cratering of interdental bone. (1:577)

6.

E. All except stress are predisposing factors for this patient; however, all of these risk factors may predispose the development of NUG/NUP in a susceptible individual. (1:578)

7.

D. It is most appropriate to perform general debridement with a combination of manual and ultrasonic instruments and to manage the pain associated with NUP with topical anesthetic or block anesthesia as appropriate. (1:580)

8.

E. Recommended dietary increases for those with NUG/NUP include the following: milk, meat, and fruit groups. (1:581)

9.

B. A small, cylindrical single-tufted interdental brush softened in warm H_2O is appropriate for the individual with wide embrasures due to loss of attachment and cratered interdental papillae. (1:377)

10.

D. A Gracey 5/6, by design, is used to gain access to subgingival areas due to its rounded toe and back. The 5/6 is used on anterior sextants and premolar teeth. (3:295)

CASE HISTORY III ANSWERS

1.

D. For diabetic patients, the clinician should limit the number of teeth treated at each visit. Allow short appointments for stress management. Debridement by the quadrant under anesthesia is appropriate for pain control, thorough deposit removal, and hemostasis. (1:890)

2.

D. The American Academy of Periodontology's Case Type IV, by definition, is further progression of periodontitis with major loss of alveolar bone support usually accompanied by increased tooth mobility. There is furcation involvement in multirooted teeth. (1:225)

3.

A. Tooth #26 is in a position labial to normal position. Linguoversion refers to a tooth lingual to normal position, buccoversion is buccal to normal position, and torsiversion is when a tooth is turned or rotated about its axis. (1:257–258)

4.

B. McCall's festoons are described as an enlargement of the marginal gingiva with the formation of a lifesaver-like gingival prominence. A Stillman's cleft is a v-shaped or slitlike indentation in the gingiva. Knife-edged tissue is healthy. Rounded tissue may be found in healthy or slightly inflamed tissues. (1:196)

5.

D. Orange stain more frequently occurs on anterior teeth, cervical third, on facial and lingual surfaces. It is rare and is caused by chromogenic bacteria. (1:287–288)

6.

B. Chlorhexidine gluconate has been shown to be the most effective antiplaque and antigingivitis chemotherapeutic agent available. Scope and Listerine are antimicrobial rinses, with Listerine having a therapeutic effect on gingivitis only. Sodium fluoride prevents dental caries. Warm saline rinses only serve to soothe tissues after instrumentation and promote tissue healing. (1:385–386)

7.

B. Elective dental and dental hygiene appointments may need to be postponed 3 months or more until the patient's physician has given consent for treatment. (1:858)

8.

A. Hydrochlorothiazide (HCT), a diuretic, is implicated in causing xerostomia. None of this patient's other medications specifically cause xerostomia. (1:691)

9.

D. In a diseased pocket, the microflora consists primarily of gram-negative, motile spirochetes and rods. (1:268)

10.

C. A diastema is a space or abnormal opening between two adjacent teeth in the same dental arch. (1:226)

11.

B. The six surfaces used to assess oral cleanliness by the Simplified Oral Hygiene Index (OHI-S) are: #3 B, #8 F, #14 B, #19 L, #24 F, and #30 L. (1:303)

12.

E. If a molar tooth used in the OHI-S index is missing, you could use either the second molar or third molar directly behind the missing first molar. The only stipulation is that it be fully erupted. (1:303)

13.

D. Each tooth is divided into 5 subdivisions: mesial third, middle third, and distal third, whereby the middle third is further subdivided into cervical, middle, and occlusal/incisal thirds. (1:303)

14.

A. The rate of compression for one-man, adult CPR is 80 to 100 times per minute. (1:904)

15.

C. Trendelenburg position (supine with the heart higher than the head on a surface inclined downward about 45°) is preferred for those patients experiencing syncope. (1:893, 911)

16.

E. All steps listed would be appropriate for the emergency management of ketoacidosis. (1:913)

17.

D. Due to her cardiac condition, epinephrine is contraindicated. The others listed are not long-acting enough for periodontal debridement. (1:501)

CASE HISTORY IV ANSWERS

1.

C. Smooth-surface decay most likely arises from a sticky, high-sucrose diet. Retention of these foods is for relatively long periods of time, whereby acid-forming bacteria break down the sugar to an acid, producing demineralization and subsequent caries. (1:273)

2.

B. The answer is appropriate because there is no mention of retruded anterior teeth and the mandible is in a retruded relationship with the maxilla. (1:258–259)

3.

C. Neutral sodium fluoride at high concentrations used once daily is preferred over NaF rinse and SnF_2 gel, particularly in one with rampant decay. 1.23% APF gel is used in-office only. (1:473)

4.

C. Omitting cariogenic foodstuffs from the diet at this time would benefit this patient. She currently receives supplementation from prenatal vitamins. (1:273)

5.

D. Glass ionomer restorations would be most beneficial because they adhere to dentin and enamel, release fluoride, reduce microleakage, and prevent secondary dental caries. Amalgam and gold would not be esthetic in anterior areas. Composite materials do not provide fluoride release to the surrounding enamel. (1:457)

CASE HISTORY V ANSWERS

1.

D. The appropriate antibiotic prophylactic regimen for patients who are not allergic to penicillin is Amoxicillin, 2.0 g orally, 1 hour before the procedure. (1:102)

2.

E. Hyzaar belongs to the drug class of antihypertensives. (1:345)

3.

D. After-five shanks are elongated to reach the depths of deep periodontal pockets. The Gracey 11/12 is appropriate for use on this tooth surface. All other instruments listed would not be appropriate for this tooth surface and pocket depth. (1:515)

4.

B. Due to this patient's dry mouth (xerostomia), a nonacidic fluoride supplement should be recommended. A 1.1% concentration is recommended for maximum uptake and optimum fluoride exposure. (1:469–471)

5.

D. Iron oxide is a fine red powder sometimes impregnated on paper discs and used to polish gold and precious metal alloys. (1:609)

6.

E. Cavities in the cervical 1/3 of facial or lingual surfaces (not pit or fissure) are class V caries. Class I cavities involve pits or fissures of teeth. Class II cavities involve proximal surfaces of premolars and molars. Class III cavities involve proximal surfaces of incisors and canines that do not involve the incisal angle. Class IV cavities involve proximal surfaces of incisors or canines that involve the incisal angle. (1:241)

References

Below is a numbered list of reference works. At the end of each explained answer in the chapters, there is a number combination in parentheses that refers to this list. The first number indicates a work on the list; the second number or set of numbers indicates the page or pages on which the relevant information may be found.

Chapter 1

1. Jacob SW, Francone CA: *Elements of Anatomy and Physiology,* 2nd ed. Philadelphia: Saunders, 1989

2. Moore KL: *Before We Are Born: Basic Embryology and Birth Defects,* 2nd ed. Philadelphia: Saunders, 1983

3. Jacob SW, Francone CA, Lossow WJ: *Structure and Function in Man,* 5th ed. Philadelphia: Saunders, 1982

4. Hiatt JL, Gartner LP: *Textbook of Head and Neck Anatomy,* 2nd ed. Baltimore: Williams & Wilkins, 1987

5. Moore KL, Dalley AF: *Clinically Oriented Anatomy,* 4th ed. Philadelphia: Lippincott Williams & Wilkins, 1999

Chapter 2

1. Jacob SW, Francone CA: *Elements of Anatomy and Physiology,* 2nd ed. Philadelphia: Saunders, 1989

2. Moore KL, Dalley AF: *Clinically Oriented Anatomy,* 4th ed. Philadelphia: Lippincott Williams & Wilkins, 1999

3. Brand RW, Isselhard DE: *Anatomy of Orofacial Structures,* 4th ed. St. Louis: C.V. Mosby, 1990

4. Hiatt JL, Gartner LP: *Textbook of Head and Neck Anatomy,* 2nd ed. Baltimore: Williams & Wilkins, 1987

5. Short MJ: *Head, Neck and Dental Anatomy.* Albany, NY: Delmar Publishers, 1994

Chapter 3

1. Phillips RW, Moore BK: *Elements of Dental Materials for Dental Hygienists and Dental Assistants,* 5th ed. Philadelphia: Saunders, 1994

2. Craig RG, Powers JM, Wataha JC: *Dental Materials Properties and Manipulation,* 7th ed. St. Louis: Mosby, 2000

3. Craig RG: *Restorative Dental Materials,* 9th ed. St. Louis: Mosby, 1993

4. Wilkins, EM: *Clinical Practice of the Dental Hygienist,* 8th ed. Philadelphia: Lippincott Williams & Wilkins, 1999

Chapter 4

1. Perry DA, Beemsterboer P, Carranza FA: *Techniques and Theory of Periodontal Instrumentation.* Philadelphia: Saunders, 1990

2. Grant DA, Stern IB, Everett FG: *Orban's Periodontics: A Concept in Theory and Practice,* 5th ed. St. Louis: C.V. Mosby, 1979

3. Carranza FA: *Glickman's Clinical Periodontology,* 6th ed. Philadelphia: Saunders, 1984

4. Regezi JA, Sciubba J: *Oral Pathology: Clinical-Pathologic Correlations,* 2nd ed. Philadelphia: Saunders, 1993

5. Wilkins EM: *Clinical Practice of the Dental Hygienist,* 8th ed. Philadelphia: Lippincott Williams & Wilkins, 1999

6. Pattison AM, Pattison GL: *Periodontal Instrumentation,* 2nd ed. Norwalk: Appleton & Lange, 1992

7. Cottone JA, Terezhalmy GT, Molinari JA: *Practical Infection Control in Dentistry.* Philadelphia: Lea & Febiger, 1991

8. Malamed SF: *Medical Emergencies in the Dental Office,* 4th ed. St. Louis: C.V. Mosby, 1993

9. Homiak AW, Cook PA, DeBoer J: Effect of hygiene instrumentation on titanium abutments: A scanning electron microscopy study. *J of Pros Dent* 67:364–368, 1992

10. Brough Muzzin KM, Johnson R, Carr P, Daffron P: The dental hygienist's role in the maintenance of osseointegrated dental implants. *J Dent Hyg* 62:448–453, 1988

11. Stefani LA: The care and maintenance of the dental implant patient. *J Dent Hyg* 62:447–466, 1988

12. Balshi TJ: Hygiene maintenance procedures for patients treated with the tissue integrated prosthesis (osseointegration). *Quintessance Int* 17:95–102, 1986

13. Dmytryk JJ, Fox SC, Moriarty JD: The effects of scaling titanium implant surfaces with metal and plastic instruments on cell attachment. *J Periodontol* 61:491–495, 1990

14. Wardlaw GM, Insel PM: *Perspectives in Nutrition,* 2nd ed. St. Louis: C.V. Mosby, 1993

15. Melfi RC: *Permar's Oral Embryology and Microscopic Anatomy,* 9th ed. Philadelphia: Lea & Febiger, 1994

16. Bhaskar SN: *Orban's Oral Histology and Embryology,* 10th ed. St. Louis: C.V. Mosby, 1986

17. Woodall IR, Dafoe BR, Young NS, Weed-Fonner L, Yankell SL: *Comprehensive Dental Hygiene Care,* 4th ed. St. Louis: C.V. Mosby, 1993

18. Hoag PM, Pawlak, EA: *Essentials of Periodontics,* 4th ed. St. Louis: C.V. Mosby, 1990

19. Dejani et al. Prevention of bacterial endocarditis. *J Am Med Assoc* 277(22):1794–1801, 1997

20. Weinberg MA, Westphal C, Palat M, Froum SJ: *Comprehensive Periodontics for the Dental Hygienist,* Upper Saddle River, New Jersey: Prentice Hall, 2001.

Chapter 5

1. Perry DA, Beemsterboer P, Carranza FA: *Techniques and Theory of Periodontal Instrumentation.* Philadelphia: Saunders, 1990

2. Grant DA, Stern IB, Everett FG: *Orban's Periodontics: A Concept in Theory and Practice,* 5th ed. St. Louis: C.V. Mosby, 1979

3. Carranza FA: *Glickman's Clinical Periodontology,* 6th ed. Philadelphia: Saunders, 1984

4. Regezi JA, Sciubba J: *Oral Pathology: Clinical-Pathologic Correlations,* 2nd ed. Philadelphia: Saunders, 1993

5. Wilkins EM: *Clinical Practice of the Dental Hygienist,* 8th ed. Philadelphia: Lippincott Williams & Wilkins, 1999

6. Pattison AM, Pattison GL: *Periodontal Instrumentation,* 2nd ed. Norwalk: Appleton & Lange, 1992

7. Lozada JL, James RA, Boskovic M, Cordova C, Emanuelli S: Surgical repair of peri-implant defects. *J Oral Implantology* 16:22–26, 1990

8. Bauman GR, Mills M, Rapley JW, Hallmon WW: Plaque-induced inflammation around implants. *Int J Oral Maxilofac Implant* 7:330–334, 1992

9. Woodall IR, Dafoe BR, Young NS, Weed-Fonner L, Yankell SL: *Comprehensive Dental Hygiene Care,* 4th ed. St. Louis: C.V. Mosby, 1993

10. Fedi PF: *The Periodontic Syllabus,* 2nd ed. Philadelphia: Lea & Febiger, 1989

11. Hoag PM, Pawlak EA: *Essentials of Periodontics,* 4th ed. St. Louis: C.V. Mosby, 1990

12. Weinberg MA, Westphal C, Palat M, Froum SJ: *Comprehensive Periodontics for the Dental Hygienist,* Upper Saddle River, New Jersey: Prentice Hall, 2001.

Chapter 6

1. Burt BA, Eklund SA: *Dentistry, Dental Practice, and the Community,* 5th ed. Philadelphia: W.B. Saunders Company, 1999

2. Dunning JM: *Principles of Dental Public Health,* 4th ed. Cambridge, MA: Harvard University Press, 1986

3. Marshall E: The fluoride debate one more time. *Science* 247:276–277, 1990

4. Cole SJ, Huether KJ, Proctor L: Access: Dental Health Professionals and the Deaf Community. Materials developed by the University of Minnesota, School of Dentistry and the Gallaudet College, Washington, DC

5. Jong AW (ed): *Community Dental Health,* 3rd ed. St. Louis: C.V. Mosby, 1993

6. Haring JI, Lind LJ: *Radiographic Interpretation for the Dental Hygienist.* Philadelphia: Saunders, 1993

7. U.S. Department of Health and Human Services, Public Health Service, National Institutes of Health: How to help your patients stop using tobacco: A National Cancer Institute manual for the oral health team. NIH Publication 91-3191, December 1990

8. Wilkins, EM: *Clinical Practice of the Dental Hygienist,* 8th ed. Philadelphia: Lippincott Williams & Wilkins, 1999

9. Nathe CN: *Dental Public Health Contemporary Practice for the Dental Hygienist.* Upper Saddle River, New Jersey: Prentice Hall, 2001

Chapter 7

1. Ash MM: *Wheeler's Dental Anatomy, Physiology and Occlusion,* 7th ed. Philadelphia: Saunders, 1993

2. Brand RW, Isselhard DE: *Anatomy of Orofacial Structures,* 6th ed. St. Louis: Mosby, Inc., 1998

3. Woelfel JB: *Dental Anatomy: Its Relevance to Dentistry,* 4th ed. Philadelphia: Lea & Febiger, 1990

Chapter 8

1. Goaz PW, White SC: *Oral Radiology, Principles and Interpretation.* 2nd ed. St. Louis: C.V. Mosby, 1987

2. Manson-Hing LR: *Fundamentals of Dental Radiography,* 3rd ed. Philadelphia: Lea & Febiger, 1990

3. Kasle MJ: *An Atlas of Dental Radiographic Anatomy,* 4th ed. Philadelphia: Saunders, 1994

4. Haring JI, Lind LJ: *Radiographic Interpretation for the Dental Hygienist.* Philadelphia: W.B. Saunders Company, 1993

5. Johnson ON, McNally MA, Essay CE: *Essentials of Dental Radiography for Dental Assistants and Hygienists,* 6th ed. Upper Saddle River, New Jersey: Prentice Hall 1999.

6. Wilkins EM: *Clinical Practice of the Dental Hygienist,* 8th ed. Philadelphia: Lippincott Williams & Wilkins, 1999

Chapter 9

1. Ten Cate AR: *Oral Histology: Development, Structure and Function,* 5th ed. St. Louis: Mosby-Yearbook, Inc., 1998

2. Riviere HL: *Lab Manual of Normal Oral Histology.* Chicago: Quintessence, 2000

3. Stevens A, Lowe J: *Human Histology,* 2nd ed. St. Louis: Mosby, 1997

4. Moore KL, Persuad TSN: *The Developing Human, Clinically Oriented Embryology,* 6th ed. Philadelphia: W.B. Saunders, 1998

5. Bath-Balogh M, Febrenbach MJ: *Illustrated Dental Embryology, Histology, and Anatomy.* Philadelphia: W.B. Saunders, 1997

6. Melfi RC, Alley KE: *Permar's Oral Embryology and Microscopic Anatomy,* 10th ed. Philadelphia: Lippincott Williams & Wilkins, 2000

7. Moore KL, Persaud TSN: *Before We Are Born: Essentials of Embryology and Birth Defects.* Philadelphia: W.B. Saunders, 1998

Chapter 10

1. Roitt I: *Essentials of Immunology,* 7th ed. Oxford: Blackwell Scientific Publications, 1991

2. Murray PR, Kobayashi GS, Phaller MA, Rosenthall KS: *Medical Microbiology,* 2nd ed. St. Louis: C.V. Mosby, 1994

3. Balows A, Hausler WJ, Herman KL, Isenberg HD, Shadomy HJ: *Manual of Clinical Microbiology,* 5th ed. Washington, DC: American Society for Microbiology, 1991

4. Sherris JC, Champoux JJ, Corey L, Neidhardt FC, Plorde JJ, Ray GC, Ryan KJ: *Medical Microbiology: An Introduction to Infectious Diseases,* 2nd ed. New York: Elsevier, 1990

5. Slots J, Taubman MA: *Contemporary Oral Microbiology and Immunology.* St. Louis: Mosby-Yearbook, Inc., 1992

6. Howard BJ, Keiser JF, Smith TF, Weissfield AS, Tilton RC: *Clinical and Pathogenic Microbiology,* 2nd ed. St. Louis: C.V. Mosby, 1994

7. Stites P, Stobo JD, Wells JV: *Basic and Clinical Immunology*, 6th ed. Norwalk, CT: Appleton & Lange, 1987

8. Gilardi GL: *Microbiological Terminology Update II, Clinically Significant Gram-Negative Rods and Cocci*. Nutley, NJ: Hoffman-LaRoche, Inc., 1988

9. MMWR, June 1992, Vol. 41, No. RR-11

10. Anderson WAD, Scotti TM: *Synopsis of Pathology*, 10th ed. St. Louis: C.V. Mosby, 1980

11. Cawson RA, McCracken AW, Marcus PB, Zaatari GS: *Pathology: The Mechanisms of Disease*, 2nd ed. St. Louis: C.V. Mosby, 1989

12. Ash MM: *Kerr and Ash's Oral Pathology: An Introduction to General and Oral Pathology for Hygienists*, 5th ed. Philadelphia: Lea & Febiger, 1986

Chapter 11

1. Shafer WG, Hine MK, Levy BML: *A Textbook of Oral Pathology*, 4th ed. Philadelphia: Saunders, 1983

2. Willet NP, White RR, Rosen S (eds): *Essential Dental Microbiology*. Norwalk, CT: Appleton & Lange, 1991

3. Anderson WAD, Scotti TM: *Synopsis of Pathology*, 9th ed. St. Louis: C.V. Mosby, 1976

4. Slots J, Taubman MA: *Contemporary Oral Microbiology and Immunology*. St. Louis: Mosby-Yearbook, Inc., 1992

5. Madigan MT, Martinko JM, Parker J: *Biology of Microorganisms*, 9th ed. Upper Saddle River, NJ: Prentice Hall International, Inc., 2000

6. Bhaskar SN: *Synopsis of Oral Pathology*, 7th ed. St. Louis: C.V. Mosby, 1986

7. Regezi JA, Sciubba J: *Oral Pathology: Clinical-Pathologic Correlations*, 2nd ed. Philadelphia: Saunders, 1993

8. Schuster GS (ed): *Oral Microbiology and Infectious Disease*, 3rd ed. Philadelphia: Decker, 1990

9. Holroyd SV, Wynn RL, Requa-Clark B: *Clinical Pharmacology in Dental Practice*, 4th ed. St. Louis: C.V. Mosby, 1988

10. Grant DA, Stern IB, Listgarten MA: *Periodontics in the Tradition of Gottlieb and Orban*, 6th ed. St. Louis: C.V. Mosby, 1988

Chapter 12

1. Nizel AE, Papas AS: *Nutrition in Clinical Dentistry*, 3rd ed. Philadelphia: Saunders, 1989

2. Wardlaw GM, Insel PM: *Perspectives in Nutrition*, 2nd ed. St. Louis: Mosby-Yearbook, Inc., 1993

3. Davis JR, Stegeman CA. *The Dental Hygienist's Guide to Nutritional Care*. Philadelphia: W. B. Saunders Company, 1998

Chapter 13

1. Anderson WAD, Scotti TM: *Synopsis of Pathology*, 10th ed. St. Louis: C.V. Mosby, 1980

2. Shafer WG, Hine MK, Levy BM: *A Textbook of Oral Pathology*, 4th ed. Philadelphia: Saunders, 1983

3. Kent TH, Hart MN, Shires TK: *Introduction to Human Disease*. Norwalk, Connecticut: Appleton & Lange, 1993

4. Cawson RA, McCracken AW, Marcus PB, Zaatari GS. *Pathology: The Mechanisms of Disease*, 2nd ed. St. Louis: C.V. Mosby, 1989

5. Ash MM: *Kerr and Ash's Oral Pathology: An Introduction to General and Oral Pathology for Hygienists*, 5th ed. Philadelphia: Lea & Febiger, 1986

6. Moore KL, Dalley AF. *Clinically Oriented Anatomy*, 4th ed. Philadelphia: Lippincott Williams & Wilkins, 1999

Chapter 14

1. Neville BW, Damm DD, Allen CM, Bouquot JE: *Oral & Maxillofacial Pathology*. Philadelphia: W.B. Saunders Company, 1995

2. Langlais RP, Miller CS: *Color Atlas of Common Oral Diseases*. Philadelphia: Lea & Febiger, 1993

3. Ash MM, Ward ML: *Kerr and Ash's Oral Pathology: An Introduction to General and Oral Pathology for Hygienists*. Philadelphia: Lea & Febiger, 1986

4. Kent TH, Hart MN: *Introduction to Human Disease*, 3rd ed. Norwalk, CT: Appleton & Lange, 1993

5. Eversole, LR: *Clinical Outline of Oral Pathology: Diagnosis and Treatment*, 2nd ed. Philadelphia: Lea & Febiger, 1984

6. Regezi JA, Sciubba JS: *Oral Pathology: Clinical-Pathologic Correlations*, 2nd ed. Philadelphia: Saunders, 1993

7. Ibsen OAC, Phelan JA: *Oral Pathology for the Dental Hygienist*. Philadelphia: Saunders, 1992

Chapter 15

1. Requa-Clark B: *Applied Pharmacology for the Dental Hygienist,* 4th ed. St. Louis: Mosby, Inc., 2000

2. *Physician's Desk Reference*, 48th ed. Montvale, New Jersey: Medical Economics, Inc., 1994

3. Little JW, Falace DA: *Dental Management of the Medically Compromised Patient*, 4th ed. St. Louis: C.V. Mosby, 1993

4. Kutscher AH, Goldberg MR, Hyman GA, et al: *Pharmacology for the Dental Hygienist*, 2nd ed. Philadelphia: Lea & Febiger, 1982

5. Johnson C, Brown R: How cocaine abuse affects post-extraction bleeding. *Journal of the American Dental Association* 124(12): 60–62, 1993

6. Atkinson JC, Fox PC: Sjörgen's syndrome: Oral and dental considerations. *Journal of the American Dental Association* 124:74–84, 1993

7. Gilman AG, Rall TW, Nies AS, Taylor P: *Goodman and Gilman's The Pharmacological Basis of Therapeutics*, 8th ed. New York: Pergamon Press, 1990

8. Dejani et al. Prevention of bacterial endocarditis. *Journal of the American Medical Association* 227(22):1794–1801, 1997

9. Wynn RL, Meiller TF, Crossley HL: *Drug Information Handbook for Dentistry*, 6th ed. Hudson: Lexi-Comp, Inc., 2000

10. Wilkins, EM: *Clinical Practice of the Dental Hygienist*, 8th ed. Philadelphia: Lippincott Williams & Wilkins, 1999

Chapter 16

1. Darby ML, Bowen DM: *Research Methods for Oral Health Professionals: An Introduction*. Pocatello, ID: The J.T. McCann Company, 1990

2. Ary D, Jacobs LC, Razavieh A: *Introduction to Research in Education*, 4th ed. Fort Worth, TX: Holt, Rinehart and Winston, 1990

3. Oyster CK, Hanten WP, Llorens LA: *Introduction to Research: A Guide for the Health Science Professional*. Philadelphia: Lippincott, 1987

4. Brunette DM: *Critical Thinking, Understanding and Evaluating Dental Research*. Chicago: Quintessence Publishing Co., 1996

5. DePoy, Elizabeth and Gitlin, LN: *Introduction to Research*. St. Louis: Mosby, 1994

Case Studies

1. Wilkins EM: *Clinical Practice of the Dental Hygienist*, 8th ed. Philadelphia: Lippincott Williams & Wilkins, 1999.

2. Haring JI, Lind LJ: *Radiographic Interpretation for the Dental Hygienist*. Philadelphia:W.B. Saunders Company, 1993

3. Nield-Gehrig JS, Houseman GA: *Fundamentals of Periodontal Instrumentation*, 3rd ed. Baltimore: Williams & Wilkins, 1996

Index